LECTURE NOTES

GASTROENTERO

LECTURE NOTES ON
GASTROENTEROLOGY

Elwyn Elias
BSc, MB, FRCP
Consultant Physician
Queen Elizabeth Hospital
Birmingham

Senior Clinical Lecturer
University of Birmingham

Clifford Hawkins
MD, FRCP
Honorary Consultant Physician
Queen Elizabeth Hospital
Birmingham

BLACKWELL SCIENTIFIC PUBLICATIONS

OXFORD LONDON EDINBURGH

BOSTON PALO ALTO MELBOURNE

© 1985 by
Blackwell Scientific Publications
Editorial offices:
Osney Mead, Oxford, OX2 oEL
8 John Street, London, WC1N 2ES
23 Ainslie Place, Edinburgh, EH3 6AJ
52 Beacon Street, Boston
  Massachusetts 02108, USA
744 Cowper Street, Palo Alto
  California 94301, USA
107 Barry Street, Carlton
  Victoria 3053, Australia

First published 1985

Set, printed and bound at
The Alden Press, Oxford

DISTRIBUTORS

USA
  Blackwell Mosby Book Distributors
  11830 Westline Industrial Drive
  St Louis, Missouri 63141

Canada
  Blackwell Mosby Book Distributors
  120 Melford Drive, Scarborough
  Ontario M1B 2X4

Australia
  Blackwell Scientific Book Distributors
  31 Advantage Road, Highett
  Victoria 3190

British Library
Cataloguing in Publication Data

Elias, Elwyn
  Lecture notes on gastroenterology.
  1. Gastrointestinal system — Diseases
  I. Title   II. Hawkins, Clifford
  616.3′3   RC801

  ISBN 0-632-00846-6

Contents

Preface, vii

Part I · The Clinical Approach

1 Symptoms, 3

2 Signs of Disease, 23

Part II · Investigations

3 The Value of Blood Tests, 41

4 Blood Chemistry, 50

5 The Upper Alimentary Tract, 61

6 The Liver, Biliary System and Pancreas, 71

7 The Small Intestine, Colon and Rectum, 92

Part III · Essential Background Information

8 General Problems, 117 GIT BLEEDING, JAUNDICE ACUTE ABDOMEN CHRONIC ABD. PAIN.

9 Disorders of the Oesophagus, 141

10 Peptic Ulcer, 158

11 Dyspepsia, Gastritis and Tumours of the Stomach, 183

12 Disorders of the Gallbladder, Biliary Tree and Pancreas, 194

13 Acute and Chronic Hepatitis, 212

14 Cirrhosis and Other Disorders of the Liver, 233

15 Malabsorption, 259

16 Occasional and Rare Disorders of the Small Intestine, 272

17 Inflammatory Bowel Disease, 285

18 Motility Disorders of the Colon and Rectum, 317

Preface

We have emphasized the clinical approach to the subject, as it is easily overlooked in this age of technology. We have also tried to avoid neglecting common symptoms like chronic abdominal pain which can be a bane to the general practitioner as well as accounting for many patients attending hospital clinics. The abdomen is a sounding board of the emotions, so psychological factors when relevant have been stressed.

Lists, cherished by some though disliked by others, are provided—not as catalogues but with causes given in their approximate order of occurrence: common, occasional and rare. These are personal and based on our combined experience and closely related, we hope, to clinical practice. Understandably, some readers may not always agree with their allotment and the lists, of course, relate to the situation in the UK.

Gastroenterology is advancing at a rapid pace so that new conditions are continually being discovered and old labels discarded. Many new techniques are coming onto the scene and some, though still at the stage of research, are likely to be of clinical use; this section has been made comprehensive but we hope that we have encouraged a discriminating approach. Details of new therapeutic methods now available to the gastroenterologist have also been included.

We would like to thank Mr T.F. Dee of the Clinical Photography Department, Queen Elizabeth Hospital, Birmingham, who has kindly made prints of the radiographs. We also especially thank Mrs Dawn Campbell who has patiently and painstakingly typed and retyped the various versions of the manuscript.

Elwyn Elias
Clifford Hawkins

PART 1
THE CLINICAL APPROACH

More mistakes are made from want of a proper
history than for any other reason.

Anon

Chapter 1
Symptoms

Diagnosis in most patients depends upon obtaining a good history. Unfortunately, this can easily be overlooked in a busy clinic: a form is written for a barium meal or endoscopy instead of listening to a description of the symptoms—just as the general practitioner may write a prescription for someone with dyspepsia to keep the queue of patients moving.

A detailed analysis of gastrointestinal symptoms (Table 1.1) takes time. The presence of other complaints is often important: for example, irritability, fatigue without obvious cause, loss of interest, insomnia, and sexual dysfunction point towards psychosomatic disease. Do not overlook the previous and family history: peptic ulcer is occasionally familial and cancer in the family may cause cancerophobia. Finally, discover the patient's own diagnosis and fears—which occasionally may be correct—and always take into account any social factor. The holistic (from the Greek ὅλος = whole) approach, where the doctor treats the patient as well as the disease, is especially important in gastroenterology.

However, patients do not always say what they mean and their own diagnoses may mislead. 'Biliousness' is unrelated to liver or biliary systems. The complaint of 'heartburn' has often nothing to do with this symptom; true heartburn is transient whereas burning feelings lasting for hours are often psychosomatic. 'Wind' covers various sensations from belching to feelings of fullness. So never accept the patient's word at face value; by 'stomach' is often meant abdomen and 'vomiting' may signify acid regurgitation.

Symptoms vary in their discriminating value: epigastric pain which wakes the patient at night and is relieved by alkali or milk is almost specific for peptic ulcer. Incidental findings are common: many with nervous dyspepsia have a symptomless hiatus hernia or gallstones.

Definition and meaning of symptoms

Appetite
This is a pleasant sensation related to previous experience of the smell and taste of food whereas hunger is disagreeable and associated with hunger pangs. Changes in appetite (Table 1.2) can be due to organic disease or psychological factors. Anorexia is a late sign and so of little value in diagnosing carcinoma of the stomach; pathological increase (bulimia) is a psychiatric disorder. Appetite in the healthy is unrelated to the needs of the body and depends upon social and environmental factors.

Table 1.1. Detailed analysis of symptoms.

Duration
Continuous or intermittent
Severity
Site and radiation
Relationships to time (day or night), to food, bowel action,
    menstrual cycle or stress
Aggravating or relieving factors (e.g. alkali)
Any change of appetite, bowel action, or weight

Taste
The taste of food is appreciated more by the sense of smell than by taste organs on the tongue; hence appreciation of taste may disappear when one has a cold. Many patients complain of unusual tastes, and no explanation—foul teeth or obvious disease in throat or nose—is found. These, especially when described as metallic or constantly bitter, are usually due to neurosis and other nervous symptoms are often present. Various drugs alter taste and penicillamine has a specific affect upon the taste mechanism, sparing the sense of smell; this is usually temporary and treatment can be continued. Bizarre tastes may arise during normal pregnancy, some may yearn for watercress while others even enjoy munching coal—preferring the black shiny type as it tastes more crisp and nutty.

Bad breath (halitosis)
Bad breath (halitosis) is occasionally caused by sepsis around teeth or in the nose, pharynx or lungs. Other odours may be excreted from the bloodstream into the breath from the lungs; these are produced during metabolism of food and are not due to disease. Halitosis after eating onions continues long after their digestion and

Table 1.2. Changes in appetite.

Increase	Decrease
Fresh air and exercise	Systemic disease
Aperitives like sherry	Fevers, hepatitis, alcoholism,
Sight and smell of food	hypercalcaemia, carcinoma etc.
Emotional	Depression
Drugs (e.g. insulin)	Anorexia nervosa
Thyrotoxicosis	
Bulimia	

absorption and is due to smell being discharged in the breath; garlic rubbed into soles of feet can be detected in breath. A persistent complaint of bad breath not apparent to others is a symptom of psychoneurosis.

Dry mouth (xerostomia)
Flow of saliva depends upon intact parotid and submaxillary glands, the usual stimulus to secretion being sight, smell or thought of food. Produced at the rate of about 1 litre daily, its function is mechanical—aiding mastication and swallowing, facilitating speech, helping to dilute irritants and to cool hot food; its weak digestive action due to the enzyme ptyalin is unimportant. Causes of diminished secretion are listed in Table 1.3. To confirm the diagnosis, the flow of saliva from the orifice of the

Table 1.3. Causes of dry mouth (xerostomia).

Dehydration
Diabetes mellitus, Addison's disease or diarrhoea
Fevers
Drugs
Anticholinergics, antidepressants and many others
Sjögren's syndrome
Disease of salivary glands (e.g. Mikulicz syndrome)

parotid ducts can be inspected after stimulation by sight or smell of a lemon or by massage of the parotid gland.

In Sjögren's syndrome, dry eyes occur with dry mouth. This is a chronic inflammatory and autoimmune disease of the salivary and lacrymal glands often associated with rheumatoid arthritis, and sometimes with autoantibody positive liver disease. The presence of dry eyes (sicca syndrome) is suggested by a positive Schirmer test—less than 5 mm of wetting by tears per 5 min on a piece of filter paper.

Increased salivation (ptyalism)
Increased salivation is caused by irritation in the mouth from stomatitis, teething in babies, or new dentures. Ptyalism may precede vomiting, occur in pregnancy or be psychogenic. It can be a troublesome symptom of post-encephalitic Parkinsonism because of a lesion of mid-brain or pons which cuts off the hypothalamus from the salivary nuclei. This must be distinguished from ptyalism due to inability to swallow a normal flow of saliva as in pharyngeal obstruction, or the drooling of saliva in imbeciles.

Waterbrash
Waterbrash is a curious form of ptyalism: the mouth suddenly and unexpectedly

fills with clear tasteless salivary fluid; it comes in paroxysms and may occur with peptic ulcer.

Heartburn

Heartburn (pyrosis) is an intense substernal burning sensation lasting a few minutes relieved immediately by alkali, particularly sodium bicarbonate. Heartburn, especially postural when patient bends down or sleeps at night, is often due to oesophagitis from hiatus hernia; the oesophagitis is caused by reflux of hydrochloric acid, against which oesophageal mucosa has no protection. Heartburn afflicts half pregnant women and disappears after delivery, being due to acid reflux because of raised abdominal pressure and reduced sphincter tone, or temporary hiatus hernia. Chemical oesophagitis due to alcohol is common. Certain foods like chocolate reduce the lower oesophageal sphincter pressure and can cause heartburn from reflux. Reflux of bile as well as acid can cause oesophagitis both in hiatus hernia and after partial gastrectomy.

Heartburn can occur when the oesophagus is normal. It is then due to disturbance of motility, for distension of a balloon placed in the lower oesophagus in normal subjects can produce a burning sensation associated with pain which radiates upwards in wave-like fashion as high as the throat; sometimes it is dull and gripping as in angina. Heartburn in patients with duodenal ulcer is probably due to a similar mechanism when there is no evidence of reflux or oesophagitis.

Difficulty in swallowing (dysphagia)

Dysphagia is a precise symptom that must never be ignored. The diagnostic net must be cast widely (Table 1.4) but three likely causes (Fig. 1.1.) are hiatus hernia, carcinoma and achalasia—the most important to exclude being carcinoma. Accurate diagnosis is possible in most cases if the taking of a careful history is combined with careful X-ray and/or endoscopy. It is often helpful to see the patient eat or drink. In achalasia, trick movements such as attempts to breathe out forcibly through a closed glottis may help to force food through the cardia. High oesophageal obstruction may cause the patient to eat with rabbit-like movements of the jaw for fear of letting food leave the mouth. One patient complained of a lump in the throat when drinking beer quickly, and he needed little encouragement to demonstrate this; later a barium swallow showed a pharyngeal pouch.

Hysterical dysphagia (globus hystericus) consists of a feeling of a lump in the throat rather than food sticking. This should not be diagnosed without excluding other possibilities. For example, a middle-aged woman with nervous symptoms complained to her general practitioner of dysphagia. He diagnosed globus hystericus and told her that it was 'the change', as she was at the menopause. He was in a way correct for she had swallowed some coins—the change which she had received when shopping. Removal of a foreign body is an urgent matter for it may lead to ulceration and cause fatal mediastinitis.

Table 1.4. Causes of dysphagia.

Common
- Hiatus hernia (spasm or stricture from oesophagitis)
- Carcinoma of oesophagus
- Achalasia

Occasional
- Neoplasms of tongue or nasopharynx
- Retropharyngeal abscess
- Foreign body
- Scleroderma
- Motility disturbance (more in elderly)
- Tumours in neck or mediastinum
- Palatal and pharyngeal paralysis from bulbar palsy or myasthenia gravis

Rare
- Strictures (from inflammation, damage from tablets, or fibrosis from prolonged intubation, or webs associated with iron deficiency—the Plummer–Vinson syndrome)
- Pharyngeal pouch
- Aneurysms or large goitres
- Dysphagia lusoria (from compression by the arteria lusoria, a congenital variation of right subclavian artery)

Food and digestion

Erroneous physiological ideas about the digestion of food are common. These notions have been encouraged by drug advertisements. For example, many dyspeptics complain of 'acidity' but this is an assumption on their part, for hyperchlorhydia never causes symptoms and their HCl output may in fact be normal or low.

Many without organic disease find that certain foods disagree with them and these are called indigestible, an idea disproved by gastric aspiration which shows that digestion proceeds normally. Similarly discomfort after 'acid' food or drink is not due to the pH, for substances like orange juice are more alkali than patients' gastric juice. Studies of intestinal motility fail to show any cause for discomfort after these foods or drinks, and food to which the patient is 'allergic' can seldom be detected if given without that person's knowledge through a tube. Many foods are called indigestible according to folklore rather than fact, so that any discomfort in a dyspeptic is likely to have been preceded by eating such a food during the previous few days; that food is then wrongly blamed for symptoms. Allergy to food usually lies in the psyche rather than in the gastric mucosa and these patients are often suffering from nervous dyspepsia. Eating fats upsets some patients whatever the cause of their dyspepsia. It is no more common in gallbladder disease and most patients with gallstones enjoy fat until their doctor implants belief that fat will cause

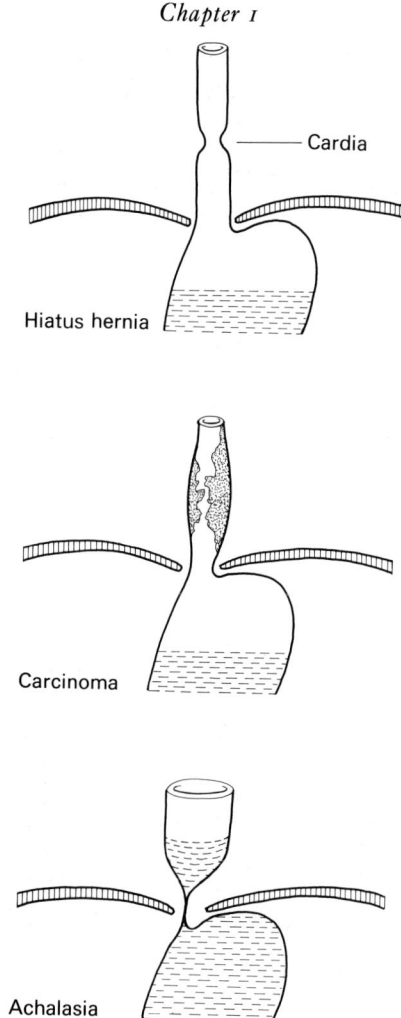

Fig. 1.1. Common causes of dysphagia.

discomfort. Duodenal ulcer patients sometimes first notice that fats, like bacon and eggs, cause pain and stop eating them. The explanation of this is not known, for fat neither stimulates gastric motility nor acidity—indeed the opposite usually occurs. Fat, chocolate and some other substances reduce tone of lower oesophageal sphincter and may cause heartburn due to reflux.

Food allergy
Gastrointestinal allergy to food is unusual. Sometimes cow's milk causes enteritis in children. Skin tests are as useless for detecting alimentary allergy, as is searching for

eosinophils in the stools. Elimination diets are of doubtful value unless relapse is shown to occur when the suspected substance is reintroduced (preferably without the patient's knowledge), for any improvement may be due to suggestion.

Certain diseases are caused by specific food intolerances as, for example, gluten in adult coeliac disease and sugars in the disaccharidase deficiencies. Yet the nature of the offending food has rarely been identified either by the patient or physician on the basis of cause and effect.

'Wind'

Wind or flatulence is a common complaint. Many think the 'wind' which they belch is due to fermentation in the stomach or improper digestion of food; but it is mostly swallowed air (aerophagy). The patient mistakenly diagnoses discomfort as due to wind and tries to disperse it by eructation. This results in the swallowing of air, for a gulp usually precedes belching. This air either merely distends the oesophagus or, with repeated efforts, is forced into the stomach (Fig. 1.2).

Accumulation of large volumes of air in the stomach may push up the diaphragm and cause dyspnoea in those with poor respiratory reserve; in others, the

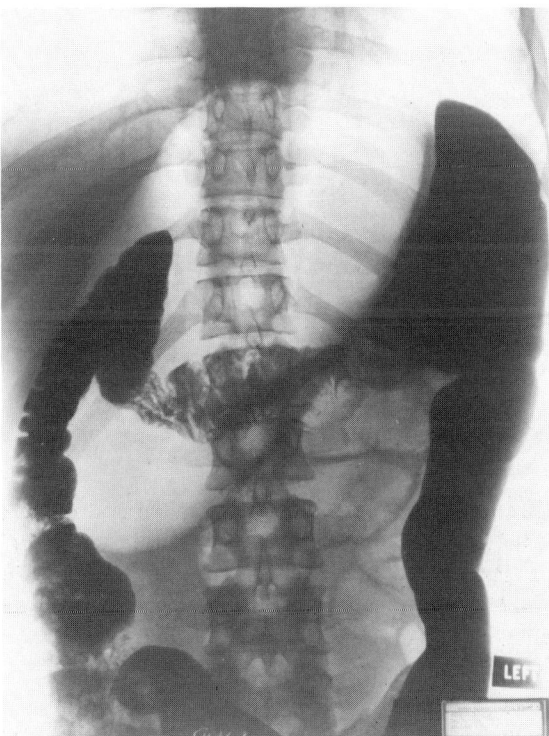

Fig. 1.2. Gross distension of stomach with air from aerophagy.

abdomen may be distended but suddenly subsides after a noisy belch. Mostly the feeling of being filled with gas is imaginary and can be proved so by X-ray. Those whose abdomens are distended with gas through faulty absorption, as in mal-absorption, seldom complain of it. Sometimes the air passes through the intestinal tract, causing borborygmi on its way and is discharged as flatus. The eructed 'wind' of gastric flatulence is odourless except when mixed with the aroma of recent food; this flavoured belch may be mistakenly regarded as another sign of indigestion.

When eructation is foul, the patient is probably suffering from pyloric obstruction with fermentation from bacteria or, if faecal, a gastro-colic fistula. This belch can be inflammable if it occurs at the moment when a cigarette is being lit, for hydrogen or methane is produced—a rare but alarming hazard.

Aerophagy is usually nervous and repeated swallowing movements may be seen during the consultation. Occasionally this is due to excess saliva from irritating lesions in the mouth. Discomfort in the chest from oesophagitis or angina, or in the abdomen from peptic ulcer or gallstones may initiate efforts in 'bringing up wind', and so cause aerophagy. Air swallowing is common after abdominal operations where there may be several causes: soreness of mouth or throat from tubes used by the anaesthetist, the fluid diet of frequent small drinks, and atonic distension of stomach and intestine from ileus.

It is often cured by explaining the mechanism to the patient. Belching must stop, and if this habit has become fixed, a cork or empty pipe placed between the teeth will help as swallowing is impossible with the mouth slightly open, though any air regurgitates naturally; this can be done after meals when aerophagy is more likely. An alkali or carminative can be prescribed for the feeling of gastric discomfort. Rarely, severe epigastric pain may occur from loculation of air and this is relieved by passing a stomach tube; it is more likely with a minor degree of volvulus of the stomach occasionally seen by barium meal as an incidental finding, or in para-oesophageal hiatus hernia where the thoracic portion of the stomach may undergo acute distension.

Some who complain of wind really mean farting, a less socially acceptable habit than the belch. However, it is normal to pass 500 ml in 24 h and most can be reassured; certain vegetables such as brussel sprouts may increase the flatus as the cellulose content protects them from normal digestion and provides material for fermentation by colonic bacteria. This can be a symptom of irritable colon perhaps because of diminished capacity of the colon due to spasm. The passing of flatus after intestinal surgery is a vital sign of improving intestinal function.

Nausea and vomiting

Nausea alone without evidence of organic disease is usually psychogenic—and vomiting is usually preceded by nausea except when psychogenic or due to a cerebral tumour. Many conditions cause vomiting (Table 1.5); ones that are easily missed are migraine, drugs (e.g. digoxin) and early pregnancy. Bronchitics may vomit at the end of a bout of coughing to clear their chests in the morning. When

Table 1.5. Causes of vomiting.

Migraine
Drugs (e.g. digoxin)
Pregnancy
Food poisoning
Hysteria
Alcoholism
Chronic bronchitis
Systemic diseases
    Fevers (especially pertussis), uraemia, Addison's disease
Abdominal conditions
    Peptic ulcer, carcinoma of stomach, appendicitis, peritonitis and intestinal obstruction
Cerebral diseases
    Abscess, tumour, meningitis, encephalitis

---

diarrhoea occurs as well, the cause is usually food poisoning. Hysteria may explain some outbreaks in schools as well as in the adult who remains remarkably well nourished in spite of it.

Vomit should be kept for inspection. The morning 'vomit' of alcoholics consists of mucus collected overnight in the oesophagus due to a chemical oesophagitis. It will be alkaline and contain particles of undigested food if due to oesophageal obstruction like achalasia. The colour of blood in the vomit depends up the rapidity of bleeding; if quick, it is bright red but if slow or retained in stomach for some time, haemoglobin is converted into haematin and the vomit resembles coffee-grounds. Vomit containing dark green bile may mimic that containing blood though the green colour of bile becomes obvious on dilution with water. Large quantities of vomit suggests pyloric stenosis; the specific symptom of this is the presence of food remnants like tomato skins in vomit after being eaten hours or even days before; and bile which cannot be regurgitated from the duodenum is usually though not always absent. When obstruction is below the ampulla of Vater, vomit is bile-stained and sometimes faecal.

Dyspepsia

Dyspepsia has been defined as pain or other symptoms (excluding dysphagia) in the upper abdomen or lower chest associated with eating. However, recent studies show that more than half the patients with peptic ulcer notice no relation to meals—there is just *belly ache*, localized to the epigastrium and occurring in attacks with pain-free intervals in between. Another misconception has been that ulcer pain is aggravated by food and occurs at a certain time after eating. This is not so, for it is relief of pain by eating or drinking which is typical, especially for duodenal ulcer; patients tell of immediate relief by neutralizing the acid with milk or antacids. Pain or discomfort after eating is not a good discriminating symptom as many with nervous dyspepsia have it.

Investigations are negative in nearly half the dyspeptics seen in the outpatient clinic; most of these will be cured by a sympathetic doctor who reassures and corrects faulty physiological ideas. Otherwise peptic ulcer is most likely, but there are many other causes (Table 1.6).

Table 1.6. Causes of dyspepsia.

Common
    Peptic ulcer
    Nervous
    Drugs (aspirin, phenylbutazone, corticosteroids and many others)
Occasional
    Carcinoma of stomach
    Gallbladder and pancreatic disease (intermittent epigastric pain)
    Disorders of the small intestine (pain is produced when food residue reaches narrowed ileum)
    Systemic diseases: uraemia, diabetes mellitus, and others

Abdominal pain
A thorough and detailed analysis of the pain prompts diagnosis in most patients and saves unnecessary investigations and operations.

Site of pain. Pain from a peptic ulcer is in the upper abdomen, and pain below the umbilicus virtually excludes it. Gallbladder disease causes pain in the epigastrium and right hypochondrium; pain only on the left excludes it. Colonic pain is referred mainly to the lower abdomen, especially left iliac fossa as in irritable colon.

Quality of pain. Typical colic with cycles occurring in crescendo-diminuendo fashion (Fig. 1.3) results only from intestinal obstruction and labour. The pain from gallbladder or renal stones impacted in the ducts is continuous with exacerbations—rarely intermittent.

Pain from peptic ulcer is less severe but steady over a period of an hour or so; some with ulcers use the word gnawing in contrast to those without organic disease who often use the terms hot, burning or bloated and their pain is commonly continuous. Organic pain is intermittent and fluctuates, and diagnosis depends upon its relation to food or defaecation, effect of alkalis, together with associated symptoms like vomiting, jaundice or diarrhoea.

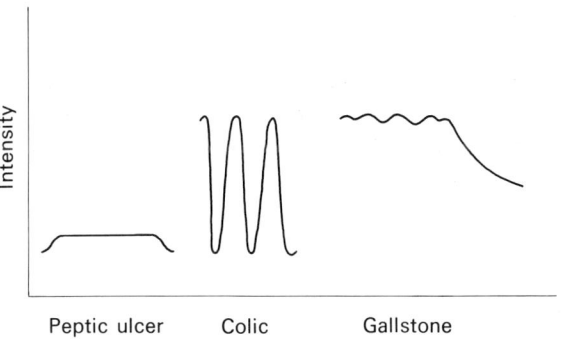

Fig. 1.3. Patterns of pain.

Mechanism of pain. Observations upon patients undergoing laparotomy under local anaesthesia show that no pain arises from manipulation of the stomach, but pain can easily be produced by squeezing inflamed tissues of a gastric ulcer or by stimulating it with chemical agents. This proves the presence of pain fibres. Hydrochloric acid is the most important stimulus of ulcer pain, and explains why relief of pain can be got by a meal, by alkali, by aspirating gastric contents, and by vomiting—the common factor being removal of hydrogen ions from the stomach. Some features of ulcer pain, however, remains unexplained: its absence in some in spite of high acidity and the rapid relief from rest in bed (although little if any alteration takes place in gastric acidity). The insensitivity of the pain-producing mechanism that precedes clinical healing is curious but the answer is probably that inflammation and tissue damage alters the visceral pain threshold as it does the somatic pain in the skin (e.g. a burn), so that a stimulus which produces no sensation in normal tissue may evoke pain when applied to damaged tissue; this causes a normal insensitive bowel to become sensitive to acids in the presence of an ulcer and its accompanying inflammation—then peristalsis, touch or pressure may evoke pain.

Visceral pain, such as from distension or engorgement of the bowel, is only vaguely localized and often associated with nausea or vomiting. Somatic pain due to inflammation of the parietal peritoneum is different, being a steady severe pain localized accurately over the site of the inflammation. Pressure there causes tenderness and reflex spasm in the overlying muscles (guarding or rigidity), and the patient lies still because pain is aggravated by movement. Acute and 'chronic' appendicitis illustrate three different forms of pain.

Acute appendicitis
There is usually a gradual onset of colicky central peri-umbilical pain which lasts a few hours, associated with nausea and vomiting; this is the visceral phase when the appendix has become obstructed and acts as a closed loop so that bacteria proliferate in the lumen and invade the appendix wall. The pain next shifts to the right iliac

fossa (Fig. 1.4), or rather to the site of the inflamed appendix; this is the parietal phase due to involvement of the sensitive peritoneum by the inflammation. The pain may be aggravated by movement and the patient prefers to lie still with the knees flexed. If the appendix hangs into the pelvis, the pain may be suprapubic and enteritis may be suggested because of vomiting and diarrhoea, and tenderness or an abscess may be felt on rectal examination. When retrocaecal, symptoms may become localized in the right loin.

Most patients with acute appendicitis present at the second phase with marked localized pain and tenderness in the right iliac fossa. Diagnosis is often easy but can be very difficult and it has achieved a sinister reputation—mimicking other abdominal conditions. There is usually fever, tachycardia and constipation and the blood may show a polymorphonuclear leucocytosis. Early diagnosis is essential as appendicectomy is then easier; later, with perforation and abscess formation, the condition becomes serious and this accounts for the annual death rate. Conservative treatment is only considered when the opportunity for removing the appendix has passed; then interval appendicectomy is carried out when the attack has settled down.

'Chronic appendicitis'

It is a clinical axiom that pain that starts in the right iliac fossa is unlikely to be due to appendicitis though there are exceptions to this as to every other rule. The site has become a notorious area for unnecessary surgery; and the frequent opportunity for removal and study of the appendix provides no evidence that a condition of 'chronic appendicitis' even exists.

However, this diagnosis is often given to a condition seen in young women

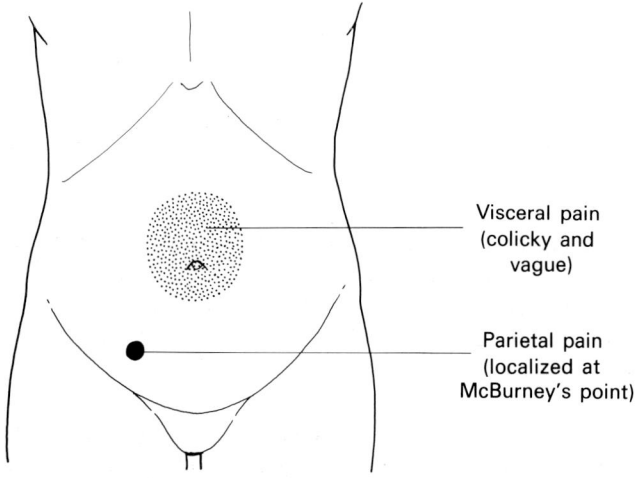

Visceral pain
(colicky and
vague)

Parietal pain
(localized at
McBurney's point)

Fig. 1.4. Stages of pain in acute appendicitis.

between 20 and 30 years. The description of the pain is a *continuous aching or nagging, with occasional sharp stabs*; it is unaffected by eating, defaecation, micturition, menses, or movement, but is worse when the patient is worried or fatigued. Many cases are psychogenic, and it is interesting that the description of their pain is identical to that of cardiac neurosis, where there is a continuous ache in the left breast and precordium with occasional stabs of pain. Organic disease seldom produces continuous pain. Many will have an underlying fear of appendicitis or other disease, and this fear may have been perpetuated by the doctor's lurid suggestion of a 'grumbling appendix'. Frequently the appendix is removed and although it may be described as abnormally long or kinked, or the pathologist may find minor inflammatory changes, the appendix is really within normal limits. However, the pain may disappear after operation, probably from suggestion; though if it continues, a diagnosis of 'adhesions' is often made. Adhesions, however, cause no symptoms except by mechanical obstruction and are common in the healthy. Inflammatory bowel disease is excluded by the absence of fever and a normal ESR and other blood tests.

Diagnosis of its psychogenic origin is supported by the presence of other anxiety symptoms, though this pain alone may occur in women with no obvious neurotic traits. If a confident and definite approach is taken at the onset, many will be cured by reassurance. Sometimes it is associated with the irritable bowel syndrome and this may be the explanation of some cases.

Constipation

Frequency of defaecation in healthy people varies so greatly, from twice daily to twice or three times weekly, that definition of constipation is difficult. The consistency of the stools is often diagnostic, for these are usually hard and dark from excessive dehydration during their prolonged stay in the colon. Causes of constipation are:

Physiological. Constipation is expected when the intake of food and fluid is diminished, as in febrile illness or after operation. A week or longer may pass without any desire to defaecate, and the only precaution necessary is to examine the rectum to exclude an unsuspected faecal accumulation.

Organic. Constipation may be an ominous symptom, the herald of a carcinoma or other lesion causing subacute intestinal obstruction. Hypothyroidism or hypercalcaemia may cause it, or sometimes it is part of a depressive illness. Hirschsprung's disease (p. 328), due to an aganglionic segment of rectum and sigmoid colon, usually occurs in children.

Drugs. Many drugs may cause constipation and even intestinal obstruction: opiates like morphine or codeine and other analgesics, anti-histaminics, anticholinergics like atropine and propantheline, or orphenadine hydrochloride (Disipal) prescribed for Parkinsonianism, tricyclic antidepressants, and drugs used for hypertension. Constipation may occur in drug addicts.

Anal lesions. Especially fissures.

Irritable colon. This spastic constipation is due to abnormal motility in the large bowel.

Faulty bowel habits. Constipation is due to loss of the conditioned reflex upon which defaecation normally depends. The sensation from the loaded rectum, the usual call to stool, is ignored so that it becomes chronically distended with faeces and no longer gives the signal for the mass peristalsis reflex to begin. It often originates from the early morning rush to catch the train to work, or a chilly lavatory. It may be precipitated by weakness of the muscles of defaecation in the elderly or debilitated, and may begin after an illness or operation when the stimulus of the distended rectum passes unnoticed by the patient and is untreated by the nursing staff. An extreme form is megacolon—often due to psychological factors in children.

Patients are occasionally seen who have been brought up to believe that the traditional daily motion is essential for the maintenance of proper health, a belief that was fostered by advertisers of proprietory purgatives, and they think that missing a bowel movement is of serious consequence. Those of nervous disposition may attribute their symptoms of being run down, or headache to constipation. But simple constipation without cathartic addiction is symptomless except for feelings of distension in the lower abdomen and rectum. Straining at stool from constipation may be dangerous in the patient with cardiac failure or cause pulmonary emboli from thrombophlebitis in the leg and pelvic vein. Otherwise, perfect health is usual and has been maintained in people who have had no bowel action for periods of up to 2 or 3 months. The idea that absorption of toxins gives symptoms of vague ill health is obsolete, though this possibly occurs when the bowel mucosa is damaged by repeated insults from purgatives. One of the great advances in gastroenterology has been the debunking of the importance of the bowel and its symptoms in the patient's mind.

Diagnosis. A careful history establishes the diagnosis of true constipation, as distinct from normal variations of bowel action, erroneously self-diagnosed as constipation by the patient. A colon loaded with faeces may be palpable, and a mobile hard mass of stool may simulate a neoplasm, but disappears after defaecation. Rectal examination is essential; the rectum is normally empty, and when it is full of faeces it should be felt later when empty to exclude a carcinoma of the rectum or sigmoid colon, and sigmoidoscopy carried out if necessary. A barium enema is often indicated, especially when constipation develops suddenly in a middle-aged person, to exclude a growth or diverticulitis, and it may be necessary in children and younger people to exclude megacolon.

Treatment. A definite diagnosis of the type of constipation must first be made, and investigations undertaken when necessary to exclude serious disease. No treatment is needed for physiological constipation as the bowel usually regains its normal functions spontaneously. It may be necessary to start this in the bed-bound patient by a suppository, and there is little to choose between glycerine or bisacodyl (Dulcolax), or by a single dose of a laxative such as magnesium sulphate in the morning.

The first approach to curing faulty bowel habits (diagnosed by a loaded rectum) is to explain the normal physiology so that misconceptions and fear concerning the bowel can be corrected. The habit of going to the lavatory at the same time each day should be restarted even though there is initial failure. The lavatory should be warm and the seat preferably low to allow more efficient function of the muscles of defaecation.

Dietetic advice must be given. The fibre content is increased so that stools become larger and softer and provide a better stimulus to the colon and rectum. Bran is the important source of cereal fibre which is lacking in the average diet in the Western world and provides a cheap and natural way of adding roughage to the diet. Obtainable from health stores or pet shops, it can be taken with milk (adding raisins or nuts if wished), water or fruit juice, or it can be mixed with cereals, porridge or soups. Bran goes well with muesli, mixed half of each, a plateful being taken each morning. In making bread, 25% of bran by weight can be added to the whole meal flour. The patient starts by taking 1 or 2 teaspoonsful a day and increases the daily dose of bran to about 2 tablespoonsful daily or until the motions have become bulkier and softer, and can be passed easily without straining. Other advice should be that portions of vegetables should be doubled or trebled and fruit like apples should not be peeled but eaten whole including the core. To relieve feelings of hunger between meals, fruit or raw vegetables such as celery and carrots, radishes or cucumber, should be nibbled instead of chocolate. Fruit like apple is helpful when eaten before retiring at night. Preparations used as purgatives are as follows:

1 Substances which provide bulk. These contain materials which swell in the bowel by absorbing water and promote peristalsis like a high residue diet. Examples are substances made from Sterculia gum (Normocol), from Psyllium seeds which contain much mucilage (Isogel), and preparations containing the synthetic hydrophilic substance, methylcellulose (Celevac).

2 Faecal softeners. Liquid paraffin lubricates and softens faeces, being useful when faeces must be kept soft after haemorrhoidectomy or when straining at stool must be avoided as in patients with hernia or heart disease. It is tasteless but many dislike its consistency, an objection that can be overcome using fruit juice or by using emulsified preparations such as liquid paraffin emulsion BP. Although liquid paraffin has been used for many years without trouble, other than lipoid pneumonia, there are theoretical risks as minute quantities are absorbed and remain in lymph nodes, with a hypothetical possibility of neoplasia, and it may interfere with absorption of fat-soluble vitamins, perhaps important in children.

3   Osmotic laxatives. Magnesium sulphate or other salts act by their osmotic effect in holding fluid in the bowel. Lactulose, a disaccharide, causes stools with a low pH and discourages ammonia-producing organisms and is useful in hepatic encephalopathy. Mannitol, a sugar, is used for preparing patients for colonoscopy.

4   Stimulant laxatives: In this group are bisacodyl, cascara and senna. These should only be taken occasionally, perhaps at the start of a regime for relieving constipation. They may, with discretion, be given in single doses to initiate defaecation in the bedridden patient but generally the habitual addict to them should be weaned from their use. This may be done gradually and glycerine suppositories or simple enemas can be used to stimulate the rectum and to start the normal conditioned reflex of defaecation. The cholinesterase inhibitor neostigmine can be used to stimulate the contractions of the colon.

Treatment for constipation is virtually without danger, providing there is no underlying lesion such as an early intestinal obstruction. Rarely, liquid paraffin may gain access to the lungs in debilitated or elderly people and cause lipoid pneumonia. The bulk-forming cathartics are free from side-effects, but oesophageal obstruction has been reported when the powder has been swallowed dry instead of with plenty of water and intestinal obstruction has occurred. Large amounts of tap water in enemata has caused water intoxication, especially in megacolon, in surgical patients receiving parenteral therapy, or in those with poor renal function. The regular use of purgatives causes semi-liquid stools, may occasionally cause potassium deficiency, usually after self-medication. Weakness and apathy due to lack of potassium is an ironical contrast to the belief that regular medication of the bowel gives vigour, well-being and strength.

Diarrhoea

Diarrhoea can be defined as too rapid an evacuation of too fluid stools. However, the excess of faecal water is more important than the frequency, and diarrhoea is present when the stool exceeds 200–300 ml liquid daily. It is not only a humiliating complaint but may lead to dehydration and electrolyte disturbances, such as potassium deficiency. The patient's history, together with naked-eye examination of the stools leads to the probable diagnosis in many patients. Disorders of the small intestine tend to cause voluminous stools, often pale and fatty, whereas those due to colonic disorders may be small and contain fresh blood, pus and mucus. Rectal examination must never be omitted and sigmoidoscopy is necessary to exclude cancer of the rectum and ulcerative colitis.

Pathophysiology. Anyone with acute diarrhoea will imagine that this is due to the overactive gut, but it is more often due to failure of fluid absorption with reduced peristalsis. The volume secreted into the small intestine each 24 h is tremendous. The various secretions entering the alimentary tract are shown in Fig. 1.5 and about 2 or 3 litres of fluid are added by food and drink. About 0.5 litre passes from the small intestine into the colon but the final produce (faeces) normally weighs only about 100–150 g daily and contains 100 ml of water. In disease of the small intestine, the volume of the 'faeces' may reach 5 litres or more a day. Fortunately, the reserve capacity of the normal colon is great: volunteers drank up to 20 litres water without diarrhoea and perfusion studies with a tube in the caecum showed that the colon can absorb 3 litres fluid daily, six times the normal 500 ml from ileostomy. So the colon, together with an efficient anal sphincter—the sentinel of

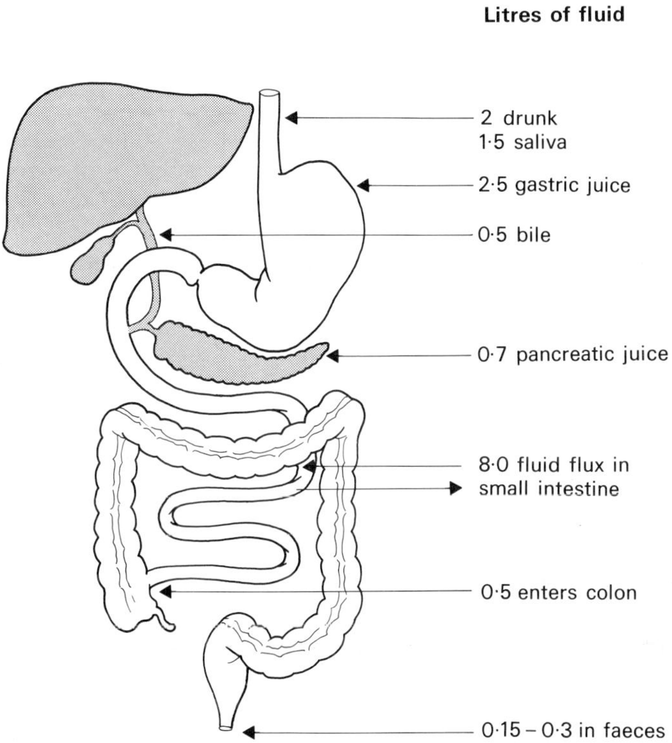

Litres of fluid

2 drunk
1·5 saliva

2·5 gastric juice

0·5 bile

0·7 pancreatic juice

8·0 fluid flux in small intestine

0·5 enters colon

0·15 – 0·3 in faeces

Fig. 1.5. The gastrointestinal tract handles 10 litres fluid daily.

social security—allows social life which would be impossible if, as in lower species, waste material was discharged at random.

Mechanisms of diarrhoea are as follows:

Failures in the fluid flux. The mechanism is usually mixed, being a failure of active ion absorption as well as stimulation of intestinal ion secretion. The rare congenital chloridorrhoea is the only example of the former occurring alone. Cholera is a striking example of a secretory diarrhoea where fluid pours from the small intestine though jejunal biopsy shows that the mucosa is normal; glucose potentiates the ionic pump helping to drive sodium together with water back into the circulation and is used in treatment. Other forms of acute infective diarrhoea probably have the same mechanism. This type of diarrhoea is recognized as it persists in spite of fasting.

Osmotic diarrhoea. Saline purgatives such as magnesium sulphate cause diarrhoea by the osmotic effect in holding a volume of water in the bowel. Products of food digestion which remains unabsorbed in malabsorption syndromes have a similar effect. Disaccharidase deficiency causes unabsorbed sugar to remain in the bowel; for example; in lactase deficiency, lactose remains in the gut and acts as an osmotic purgative. The diarrhoea stops when the patients fasts, or when the offending substance is no longer eaten.

Defective intestinal mobility. Motility studies on the colon have proved that this is the cause of diarrhoea in the irritable bowel syndrome. Other examples are the diarrhoea due to diabetic neuropathy from damage to autonomic nerves, postvagotomy diarrhoea, and diarrhoea resulting from thyrotoxicosis. Reduced peristalsis as in scleroderma may also allow bacterial overgrowth, causing the stagnant bowel syndrome.

Acute diarrhoea

Acute attacks of diarrhoea are usually due to food poisoning by salmonella or other (Table 7.2) organisms or bacterial dysentery (Table 1.7). The former is diagnosed clinically because of its explosive onset, several people being affected simultaneously and the outbreak subsiding in a few days; in contrast, dysentery has a longer incubation period and epidemics last a few weeks. When food poisoning is caused by salmonella the incubation period is 12–24 h with headache, malaise, nausea, vomiting and diarrhoea and the organism can be isolated on stool culture. However, sometimes it is due to the toxin of an organism and the organisms are killed by cooking; then the onset of diarrhoea and vomiting is 2–6 h after eating the food and organisms cannot be found in the faeces but may be detected in samples of the contaminated food before cooking. Traveller's diarrhoea (p. 359) may be due to

Table 1.7. Causes of acute diarrhoea.

Food contaminated with organisms or toxins produced by organisms
    Viruses causing 'gastroenteritis'
    Enterotoxin producers e.g. staphylococcus pyogenes, campylobacter, salmonella,
        clostridia, botulism etc.
    Traveller's diarrhoea
Drugs
Food allergy, e.g. to shellfish etc.

---

different food or drink, but more likely to organisms; pathogenic organisms are often not isolated and it may be due to unusual strains of coliform organisms—or pathogenic *E. coli*—and occasionally *Giardia lamblia*.

If no pathogen is found, a viral origin is assumed as in epidemic diarrhoea. Now that people fly across the world so swiftly, tropical diseases such as cholera may appear in temperate climates.

Chronic diarrhoea

Causes of diarrhoea which has been present for 6 weeks or longer are given in Table 1.8.

Some patients who complain of diarrhoea are really constipated; this 'spurious diarrhoea' is diagnosed by rectal examination as the rectum is full of impacted faeces and a faecal discharge leaks out—retention with overflow. Irritation in the rectum, as by a neoplasm, may provoke an urgent desire to open the bowels though no stool is passed—just blood and mucus. This ineffectual straining at stool is called tenesmus.

Treatment of diarrhoea

It is an important aphorism that treatment should not be started until the cause is found, but this is often not practicable. In acute diarrhoea drugs can be used to slow transit in the gut though this is not always appropriate as often the watery diarrhoea is due to a failure of water exchange in the small intestine without increased peristalsis. However, drugs commonly used are codeine phosphate (10–60 mg every 4 h—the maximum being 200 mg daily), diphenoxylate (Lomotil 10 mg then 5 mg every 6 h), and loperamide (4 mg at start then 2 mg after each loose stool up to 16 mg daily). In chronic diarrhoea, investigation is especially necessary to exclude serious disease. Codeine phosphate or loperamide can be used to control diarrhoea due to organic disease in addition to treatment aimed at the underlying process.

Table 1.8. Causes of chronic diarrhoea.

Motility disturbances, nervous diarrhoea and irritable colon

Organic disease of alimentary tract: neoplasms, inflammatory bowel disease, and diverticulitis

Drugs: antibiotics which change the flora or have a direct toxic effect on the mucosa (including pseudomembranous colitis), hypotensive agents, hypoglycaemic agents (e.g. metformin), analgesics and many other drugs

Infection and infestation: amoebiasis, *Giardia lamblia* and hookworm disease

Malabsorption

Systemic disease: thyrotoxicosis, uraemia, amyloidosis, and scleroderma

Self-induced by purgatives

Rare endocrine disorders, e.g. carcinoid syndrome

Chapter 2
Signs of Disease

Physical examination

Every patient must be examined and there are three objectives:

1 To detect disease.
2 To reassure.
3 To develop rapport with the patient.

Students and even some doctors assume that the only reason is to find some abnormality. Yet the real purpose of requesting a consultation—often not expressed—may be the erroneous fear that a chronic duodenal ulcer has become malignant, so all that is needed is a hand laid on the abdomen with a word of reassurance—and this may boost the morale of any patient. Extracting data about emotional problems is often easier with someone lying relaxed on the couch; for example a routine question 'Are you happily married?' may be answered with an unthinking 'Yes' when taking the history, though later the opposite may be found.

Diseases of the mouth

Inspection of the mouth and pharynx may reveal signs of systemic as well as local disease, and must be carried out thoroughly and with a good light.

The tongue

Coating, due to epithelial thickening together with débris from bacteria, yeast and food particles, is common in the healthy, particularly smokers, and is seldom a sign of disease. It is unconnected with constipation or any abdominal disorder and results from mouth breathing or eating food which needs no chewing. It is expected in any respiratory tract infection or fever. Coating is more marked at the back of the tongue where mobility is restricted and filliform papillae desquamate less readily and appear denser. The importance of movement of the tongue in preventing coating may be seen when one side is paralysed, for coating is thicker on the paralysed side.

Black hairy tongue (*lingua nigra*) is due to papillae over the posterior part being greatly elongated and appearing black or brown because of keratin. The cause is unknown. It is symptomless and difficult to eradicate, and reassurance is usually all that is needed. Antibiotics sometimes cure it because of their desquamating effect on the tongue. Geographical tongue is seen in many normal people; there are slightly raised irregular grey rings surrounded by reddish areas known as erythema migrans. There is a localized area of atrophy or desquamation of the filiform papillae demarcated by a clear greyish border. It comes and goes and may make the tongue painful, though more often it is symptomless. It is of no clinical significance and no treatment is effective except anaesthetic lozenges for relieving pain. The benign nature of geographical tongue contrasts with leucoplakia which is a whitish thickening of the mucosa of the tongue or cheek and is probably premalignant.

Neurosis. The tongue, too easily inspected by its owner, is an organ from which neurotic symptoms commonly arise; cancerophobia is readily induced by worry concerning the shape and size of the papillae, and pricking and burning sensation are complaints. Introspective people may study their tongue in the mirror each morning, using this as a barometer to foretell their feelings for the day; the greater the coating, the worse they feel. Cure is effected by simple explanation of normal oral physiology and by persuading them not to look at their tongue.

The smooth tongue (glossitis). The reason that the tongue is so often a sensitive index of nutritional deficiencies is probably because the rate of replacement of its cells is greater than in other parts of the body. The smooth tongue is a useful guide to deficiencies of iron and of vitamin B groups as may occur in malabsorption syndrome, though some cases of glossitis, especially in elderly people, are impossible to explain.

Visible changes may be preceded by burning sensations. Redness with soreness and increased salivation follow atrophic changes in the papillae, with later shedding of the epithelium and shallow ulceration. This process may be slowly progressive, or occurs with episodes of painful inflammation, involving the tip, sides or entire tongue. Finally there is complete atrophy of the filiform and fungiform papillae leaving a smooth tongue with a shiny glazed appearance. This last stage is common to all deficiencies; variations in the preceding pattern are probably due to differences in the severity and rapidity of the process. The 'glossitis' of iron deficiency is not so severe as in vitamin B_{12} deficiency; and oedema of the tongue as seen by indentation of the edges (also occasionally in normals) seems more likely in deficiencies of the B complex; then the colour is scarlet or when darker, beefy red; the purplish colour giving the magenta tongue of riboflavin deficiency may be due to stasis of blood in superficial capillaries. Glossitis is associated with angular stomatitis, and with cheilosis where there is slight oedema, soreness, and crusting of the exposed mucosa of the lips at the angles of the mouth.

Large tongue. This may be due to amyloid disease, acromegaly, or hypothyroidism, especially when congenital.

Ulcers in the mouth
Traumatic ulcers may be due to badly fitting dentures, biting the cheek or other injuries; they heal quickly when the cause is removed. If single ulcers persist for longer than 2 weeks the possibility of carcinoma should be considered. Both

malignant and syphilitic ulcers are painless, whereas the tuberculous one is painful and is due to tubercle bacilli present in the sputum of patients with open pulmonary tuberculosis.

There are many causes of recurrent oral ulceration and these are listed in Table 2.1. The commonest cause is aphthous stomatitis.

Table 2.1. Causes of mouth ulcers.

Common
    Aphthous (minor and major)
    Drugs (e.g. gold)
Occasional
    Traumatic (e.g. dentures, cheek biting)
    Coeliac disease
    Behçet's syndrome
    Reiter's disease
    Herpes zoster
Rare
    Crohn's disease
    Pemphigus
    Lichen planus
    Hand, foot and mouth disease (from coxsackie virus in children)
    Deliberate disability (self-inflicted)
    Herpes simplex
    Foot and mouth disease (from cattle)
    Erythema multiforme

Aphthous stomatitis. Clarity of nomenclature is usually inversely related to knowledge about the cause of a condition, and the twelve or more synonyms of this common lesion, so accessible to study, emphasize our ignorance. The ulcers occur in all age groups, though particularly afflict women of middle age. They begin as vesicles, are small (2 or 3 mm in diameter) superficial and very painful, particularly on eating and drinking. Crops come and go for no apparent reason, except that some may follow emotional stress. They heal spontaneously with intervals of freedom lasting many months, although the condition may persist for years.

No cause has been found and only palliative treatment is possible. The patient has to be reassured and protected from unnecessary measures such as dental extractions. Anaesthetic lozenges containing benzocaine, or a 2% lignocaine mouth wash can be used before eating. Topical steroids help if applied during the prodromal period of ulceration: the most useful preparations are 0.1% triamcinolone, 2.5 mg tablets of hydrocortisone sodium succinate, and 0.1 mg tablets of betamethasone 17-valerate. Systemic corticosteroids may have to be used in the rare severe case (major aphthous ulcers) and small doses of prednisolone may suffice. Some women with recurrent premenstrual ulceration may gain relief in pregnancy and improve with hormonal treatment. Oestrogens and the contraceptive pill occasionally are beneficial.

Examination of the abdomen

A complete examination of the alimentary system involves not only inspection of the tongue, mouth, teeth and throat, but also looking at the entire patient especially for the following: loss of weight (striae atrophicae may give the clue), clubbing, jaundice, anaemia and, for example, spider naevi.

Examining the abdomen depends especially upon feel and this can lead the tyro to detect non-disease and to worry the patient unnecessarily: imaginary lumps are found or structures palpable in a normal abdomen (Fig. 2.1) are misinterpreted as evidence of disease.

Technique

Relaxation of abdominal muscles is a *sine qua non* and the following may help:

1   The patient must lie flat with one pillow unless breathless or kyphotic as in the elderly; the arms are by the side and the body is covered except for the abdomen.
2   The examiner's hand should be warm; immersion in hot water is better than warming it at a fire, or a small hot-water bottle can be kept in the pocket.
3   The patient can be asked to breathe through the open mouth and the knees flexed by a pillow placed under them.

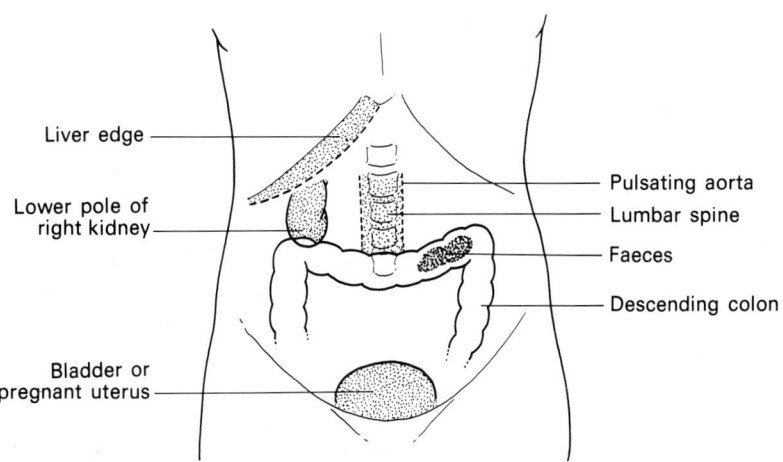

Fig. 2.1. Structures palpable in a normal abdomen.

Inspection. Look carefully and one of the following may be seen:

1   Distension, the causes being: fat (umbilicus is deep), fluid (umbilicus is shallow or everted), flatus (tympanic note as in obstruction), faeces (hard masses which alter after defaecation), fetus.

2   Scars of previous operations.

3   Striae atrophicae which may mean loss of weight or former pregnancy.

4   Abnormal pulsation: this is more likely to indicate nervousness than aortic reflux or aneurysm (walls of aneurysms are often covered with thrombus so they do not pulsate).

5   Visible peristalsis: typical of obstruction but can be normal in very thin people; gastric waves from left to right are diagnostic of pyloric obstruction—usually benign as carcinomas seldom allow time for hypertrophy of the gastric muscle to develop.

6   Skin lesions: pigmentation, or the vesicles of herpes zoster which can present as an acute abdomen before the rash occurs, or sepsis.

7   Outline of a lump or large organ which may move on respiration.

8   Distended venous collaterals (Fig. 2.2); the direction of blood flow should be checked by the classical experiment which enabled William Harvey to discover the circulation of the blood—by occluding the vein with finger pressure and emptying the vein above and below. In veins *below* the umbilicus, blood flowing upwards indicates obstruction to the inferior vena cava, blood flowing downwards suggests portal hypertension. In portal hypertension the flow is centrifugal from the umbilicus so in both conditions blood will probably flow upwards in veins above the umbilicus. A caput medusae is rare, being a large collection of veins emerging at the umbilicus in portal hypertension. The snake-like appearance gave rise to the term medusae: in mythology Medusa's golden hair had captivated Neptune and her hair was turned into snakes by Minerva.

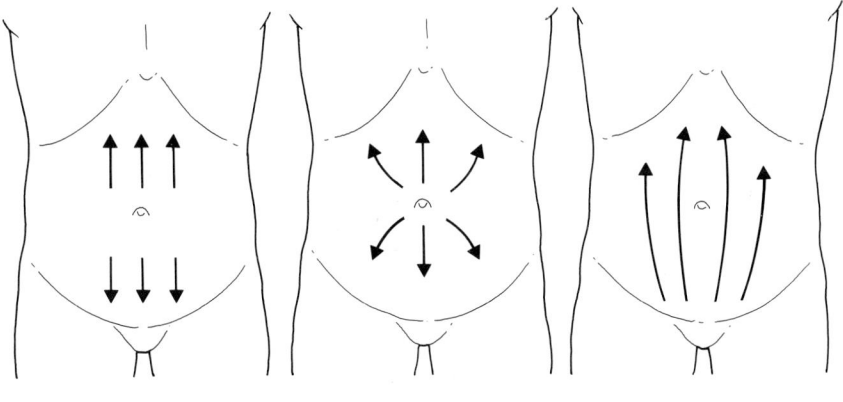

| Normal | Portal hypertension | Inferior vena cava obstruction |

Fig. 2.2. Venous patterns on the abdomen.

Palpation. Ask the patient to point to the site where the pain is felt and start at a distance from this. The abdomen is caressed and not prodded and the face watched to spot any wincing.

Palpation should first be light to gain the patient's confidence, and later deep and bimanual. Tenderness is commonly of no significance and is often widespread and exaggerated in the nervous patient, disappearing when the attention is directed elsewhere. True tenderness is constant and usually localized. Rebound tenderness may indicate peritoneal involvement, but also occurs in the healthy apprehensive patient.

Guarding may also be due to apprehension and an attempt should be made to abolish it by diverting the attention and by making sure that the patient is relaxed. Rigidity, which is constant and associated with tenderness, indicates peritoneal involvement as in appendicitis. Hernial orifices and lymph nodes should be felt and a rectal examination usually done.

Any lump must be carefully studied as to its size, consistency, mobility, movement with respiration and the nature of its surface. Then the following questions should be considered:

1   Could it be anything felt in a normal abdomen (Fig. 2.1) or enlargement of a viscera?

2   List the structures present in the vicinity.

3   Consider which of the following is likely:

    (a) Congenital (rare), for example Riedel's lobe of the liver (Fig. 2.3).

    (b) Inflammatory: any inflammation especially if treated by an antibiotic or Crohn's disease can be hard and mimic neoplasm.

    (c) Cystic: for example an ovarian cyst or cysts in the kidneys or pancreas.

    (d) Neoplastic.

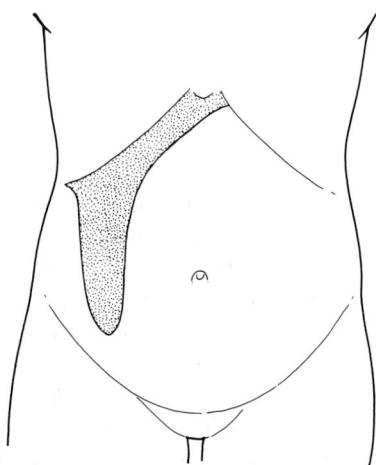

Fig. 2.3. Riedel's lobe of the liver (a normal variation).

Rectal examination

Abdominal examination is seldom complete unless a rectal examination is done, especially when symptoms point towards the colon or rectum. Lives would be saved if cancer of the rectum were detected early by feeling it in patients with a change of bowel action or rectal bleeding.

Explain and reassure the patient as there may be a desire to defaecate. First look carefully: redundant skin tags are common in the perianal area and small and slightly bluish external haemorrhoids are often visible; asking the patient to bear down may reveal an anal fissure. Go gently through the anal sphincter and let it relax. In the male, the firm, flat and rubbery prostate gland can be felt anteriorly just above the sphincter; and in the female, slightly higher anteriorly, the smooth firm cervix can be felt. The finger is then introduced as far as possible and moved in a full circle to examine the whole circumference and the patient is asked to bear down so that the tip of the finger can explore the upper reaches of the rectum. Posteriorly in either sex, the tip of the coccyx can be felt. The material on the gloved finger is studied; steatorrhoea may be diagnosed by pallor, ulceration when the occult blood test is positive, parasites may be seen by microscopy and the rest can be sent for culture to detect pathogenic organisms. Abnormalities found at rectal examination may be as follows:

1 Tumours (polyps or carcinomas).
2 Strictures or ulcers (as in Crohn's disease).
3 Pelvic abscess or diseases of the female adnexa.
4 Foreign bodies.

An anal fissure makes examination very painful and local anaesthetic may help. Proctoscopy is necessary to see internal haemorrhoids and to exclude ulcerative colitis by finding a normal rectum mucosa. Rectal examination can be a misnomer when an obese patient has enormous buttocks and the examiner a short finger; cancer cannot be excluded without sigmoidoscopy.

Special problems

Enlarged liver

Hepatomegaly is detected by resting the hand gently on the abdomen during inspiration. Starting in the right iliac fossa it is moved upwards during expiration and re-positioned for the next inspiration until either the liver edge or costal margin is felt. Light percussion confirms the lower edge and determines the level of the upper edge, so distinguishing between an enlarged liver and a normal sized liver palpable because of a wide costal margin or because it is low-lying due to emphysema. A systemic disease such as congestive cardiac failure (an enlarged liver may persist after other signs of failure have gone) must be excluded and the causes of hepatomegaly are shown in Table 2.2. If cirrhosis is thought likely, other signs of liver disease should be sought (Fig. 2.4), especially spider naevi (Fig. 8.2).

Table 2.2. Causes of hepatomegaly (those marked with an asterisk usually have splenomegaly as well).

Common
  Cirrhosis*
  Alcoholic fatty liver
  Malignant disease (usually metastatic carcinoma)
  Congestive cardiac failure
  Obstructive jaundice
Occasional
  Reticuloses*
  Sarcoidosis*
  Hepatitis (acute or chronic)
  Riedel's lobe
  Myelofibrosis*
  Rheumatoid arthritis*
  Diabetes mellitus
Rare
  Amyloidosis*
  Haemochromatosis*
  Wilson's disease*
  Storage diseases (e.g. Gaucher's)*
  Hydatid disease
  Primary liver neoplasm
  Budd–Chiari syndrome

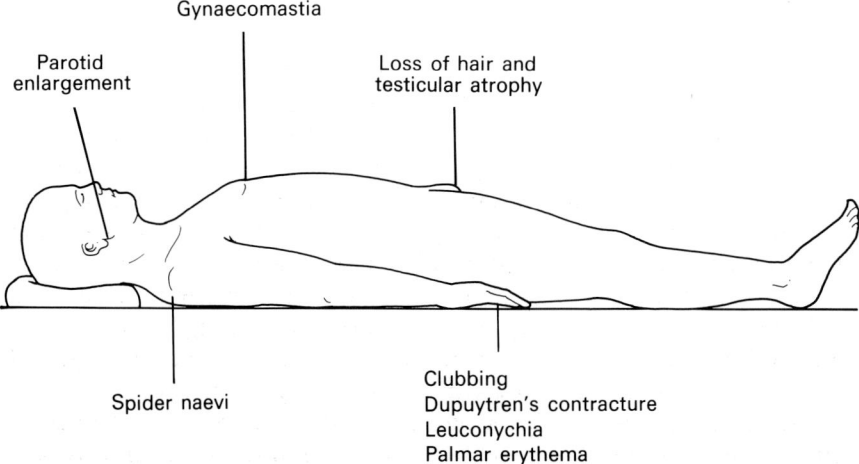

Gynaecomastia

Parotid enlargement

Loss of hair and testicular atrophy

Spider naevi

Clubbing
Dupuytren's contracture
Leuconychia
Palmar erythema

Fig. 2.4. Signs associated with liver disease.

Enlarged spleen

A palpable spleen is virtually always abnormal. Splenomegaly is sought during successive inspirations, again starting in the right abdomen but progressing diagonally towards the left costal margin across the umbilicus. Some find it best to place the left hand behind the lower rib cage to draw the spleen on to the examining hand by pulling the rib cage forward and down to the right, or in difficult cases, rotating the patient 45° to the right. If there is a definite mass under the left costal margin, the following signs separate the spleen from the left kidney or a mass:

	Spleen	Kidney
Is the edge sharp:	Yes	No
Is there a notch palpable on the medial border:	Maybe	No
Can you get above it:	No	No
Is it bimanually palpable:	No	Yes
Is there a band of resonance across it:	No	Yes

Slight splenomegaly occurs in infections such as glandular fever, Brucella abortus and infectious hepatitis, and in an early case of lymphoma. A moderately enlarged spleen (two to four fingers below the costal margin, 4–8 cm) occurs in cirrhosis with portal hypertension, chronic lymphatic leukaemia, and lymphoma like Hodgkin's disease. Very large spleens are usually due to myelofibrosis or chronic myeloid leukaemia and may reach to the right iliac fossa. In contrast to Britain, splenomegaly is so common in the tropics that the clinical aphorism is 'Most patients have enlarged spleens, some are just larger than others.' These and other causes are given in Table 2.3. A very large spleen of unknown origin occurs in various parts of the world and has been given different names, the commonest being tropical or non-tropical splenomegaly.

Ascites

Two or three litres of fluid can be present before it is detected clinically. Ascites can be confirmed by demonstrating shifting dullness on percussion: find the most lateral part of the abdomen resonant on percussion, then roll the patient to that side and percuss the same spot—a change from resonance to dullness strongly suggests free fluid. A search for a slight amount of fluid can be made by asking the patient to turn over on the knees and elbows; fluid collects around the umbilicus and this area becomes dull. The fluid thrill is more useful for testing a candidate's clinical ability in an examination than for diagnosis, as fluid is usually obvious already: an assistant's hand is placed sideways in the mid-line on the abdominal wall to prevent waves being transmitted and a flick of the finger on one side is sensed on the palm of the hand on the other side of the abdomen if ascites is present. Ballotting the liver and spleen is only possible when ascites is present and refers to the procedure of pushing the organ away firmly and feeling its return when it has floated back to strike the hand. Ascites may have to be distinguished from the large ovarian cyst

Table 2.3. Causes of splenomegaly.

Common
    Reticulosis (e.g. Hodgkin's disease)
    Portal hypertension
    Leukaemia
Occasional
    Sarcoidosis
    Rheumatoid arthritis
    Systemic lupus erythematosus
    Haemolytic anaemia
    Thrombocytopenia
    Polycythaemia rubra vera
    Myelofibrosis
    Subacute bacterial endocarditis
Rare
    Amyloidosis
    Storage diseases (e.g. Gaucher's)

Note: The biggest spleens occur in chronic myeloid leukaemia and myelofibrosis. Slightly enlarged spleens are found in glandular fever, infectious hepatitis and brucellosis. On a worldwide basis malaria and kalaazar are common.

(Fig. 2.5): the cyst can usually be felt and the dullness is in the centre and lower abdomen rather than in the flank.

Note whether the fluid retention is localized to the abdomen or is part of a generalized oedema as in congestive cardiac failure, renal disease or constrictive pericarditis—a transudate. Neoplasms or inflammation cause an exudate. The various causes are listed in Table 2.4. Analysis of fluid obtained by paracentesis may help in diagnosis. In theory, a protein content above 2.5 g/100 ml should indicate an exudate and below, a transudate, but in practice the level often is borderline and unhelpful. A bloody fluid strongly suggests neoplasm and an increased leucocyte count either neoplasm or infection; lymphocytes are increased in tuberculosis. A high amylase level may be found in chronic pancreatitis and the triglyceride level may confirm chylous ascites. Culture should be done if infection is suspected. Cytology often provides the most useful test and is positive in half or more patients with malignant ascites but this depends upon the expertise of the observer.

Miscellaneous abnormal findings
A *succussion splash* is usually audible without need of the stethoscope; it indicates

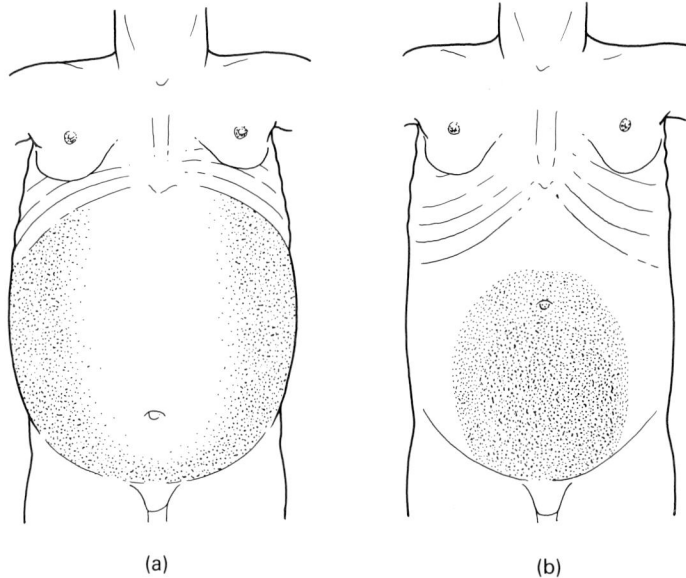

(a)   (b)

Fig. 2.5. (a) Ascites: dullness in flanks and umbilicus downwards. (b) Ovarian cyst: central dullness and umbilicus upwards.

Table 2.4. Causes of ascites.

Common
    Neoplasm
    Cirrhosis of the liver
    Congestive cardiac failure
Occasional
    Tuberculosis or other infection of the peritoneum
    Nephrotic syndrome
Rare
    Myxoedema
    Constrictive pericarditis
    Chronic haemodialysis
    Protein-losing enteropathy
    Inferior vena cava or hepatic vein obstruction (Budd–Chiari syndrome)
    Pancreatitis
    Chylous ascites (usually from a lymphoma with blockage of the lymphatics
      or thoracic duct)
    Malnutrition (common in underprivileged countries)

delayed gastric emptying unless a meal has been taken within 3 h beforehand. Finding a *palpable gallbladder* is highly significant: it is felt as a tense rounded or globular mass below the liver in the mid-axillary line and indicates obstruction of the bile duct below the entry of the cystic duct, usually by carcinoma of the pancreas (Courvoisier's law, Fig. 2.6). This law presumes that when gallstones are the cause of biliary obstruction, their formation has been associated with chronic inflammation and fibrosis which prevents the gallbladder distending. *Systolic murmurs* are

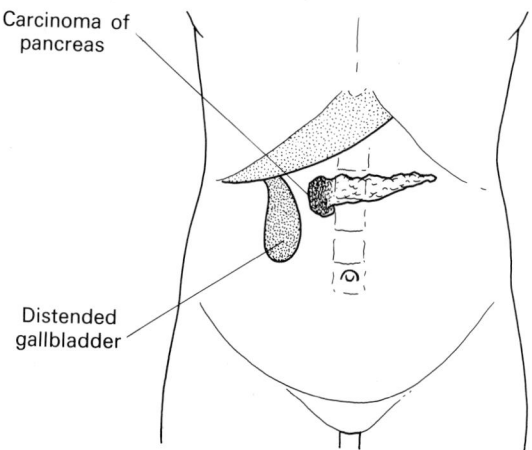

Carcinoma of pancreas

Distended gallbladder

Fig. 2.6. Courvoisier's law.

not uncommon and are usually of no significance, though they may indicate mesenteric atheroma or aneurysm; if however, they are heard over the liver, a primary liver cancer or alcoholic hepatitis may be present. A *venous hum* may be heard emanating from the umbilical vein in cases of portal hypertension; since the umbilical vein originates from the main left branch of the portal vein within the liver, this physical sign is helpful as it indicates patency of the portal vein and could therefore in theory abolish the need of splenic venography before a proposed surgical porto-caval anastomosis. A *rub over the liver or spleen* indicates abnormal friction of the parietal and visceral peritoneum: the commonest cause is after percutaneous puncturing of the liver capsule for biopsy or radiological studies, but it may indicate primary liver cancer or acute cholecystitis and, if over the spleen, an infarct.

Diagnosis of the 'acute abdomen'

The sudden onset of acute abdominal pain is often ominous. There are many causes (Table 2.5) and the diagnosis may be suspected by the previous history. However, eliciting the signs is critical for the survival of the patient and must be known by every doctor.

Table 2.5. Causes of acute abdominal pain.

Common
    Appendicitis
    Acute cholecystitis and gallstone colic
    Perforated peptic ulcer
    Intestinal obstruction (especially strangulated inguinal hernia)
    Non-specific abdominal pain (this accounts for many cases and nothing abnormal is
        found at laparotomy; sometimes irritable bowel is responsible)
Occasional
    Pancreatitis
    Diverticulitis
    Herpes zoster (for other medical causes see Table 8.16)
    Vascular: mesenteric thrombosis or embolism, sickle-cell crises in those of African or
        Mediterranean stock, aneurysm
Rare
    Perforated carcinoma or Meckel's diverticulum
    Primary peritonitis (more in children)
    Spinal conditions

Note: Possibilities in women are: ruptured corpus luteum cyst (at beginning of menses), ruptured Graafian follicle (midway between menses), torsion of ovarian cyst, ruptured ectopic gestation, and acute salpingitis.

Intestinal obstruction

Colic may imply the onset of intestinal obstruction (Table 2.6) and the cardinal signs of this are abdominal pain, vomiting and distension: vomiting occurs early with blockage of the upper gut and late from colonic obstruction—in the latter constipation occurs early. The patient with uncomplicated colic often moves around in the bed trying to find a comfortable position though these manoeuvres are usually unrewarding. The bowel sounds are often loud and increased with cramp-like pain. Faecal vomiting may come later and is characteristic of low gut obstruction. Failure to pass gas or faeces usually indicates complete small or large bowel obstruction.

At first, there may be no distension of the abdomen. Tenderness is not found unless the cause is inflammation or if gangrene of the gut has occurred; then peristalsis ceases and there are signs of peritonitis.

Diagnosis is confirmed by a plain X-ray of the abdomen (erect and supine) as this shows a 'step-ladder' appearance due to the transverse shadows of the valvulae conniventes of the small gut outlined by the dilated bowel. Fluid levels are also shown (Fig. 2.7). Sometimes the radiologist will give a micropaque meal if the obstruction is subacute or a barium enema. Usually, and especially in acute cases, operation is needed as soon as the patient's condition has been improved by fluid and electrolyte replacement intravenously, nasogastric suction and an antibiotic to

Table 2.6. Causes of intestinal obstruction.

Common
> Adhesions
> Carcinoma
> Hernia (often with strangulation)
> (Roundworms in the tropics)

Occasional
> Impacted faeces in the elderly
> Inflammatory: examples are Crohn's disease and diverticulitis
> Intussusception (often with strangulation and usually in a baby)
> Volvulus: this may occur from adhesions, from malrotation in infants, or sigmoid volvulus in adults (more likely in races eating high residue food)

Rare
> Strictures either congenital or from tablets like potassium chloride
> Ileus
> Meckel's diverticulum: this may present as volvulus, intussusception or band obstruction
> Gallstone ileus
> Food impaction
> Tumours outside wall of bowel (by pressure or invasion)
> Congenital intestinal obstruction: duodenal ileal atresia, imperforate anus, etc.

---

deal with bacterial overgrowth in the obstructed bowel. There is no method, apart from laparotomy, of diagnosing whether a strangulated loop of gangrenous intestine is present in patients with acute obstruction.

Peritonitis

In contrast to colic, the abdomen is tender and the patient lies still, as any movement, even coughing, increases the pain. Flexing the thighs helps to relax the peritoneum but any attempt to stretch the inflamed peritoneum may produce pain; for example, the peritoneum over the psoas muscle may be stretched by extending the thigh and the hip, and this sign may be positive in infections involving the psoas sheath as in a psoas abscess or inflammation extending from the pelvic appendix or ureter. Similarly, internal rotation of the thigh stretches the obturator fascia and may be a sign of appendicitis. Tenderness at the tip of the finger on rectal examination may indicate a pelvic abscess.

Generally, involuntary contraction of the abdominal muscle (guarding or rigidity) is a very reliable sign of intraperitoneal inflammation and is typical with perforated ulcer: the 'board-like' abdomen is diagnostic. Rebound tenderness is another way of stretching the peritoneum but is often best avoided as it causes unnecessary pain and is often falsely positive in nervous patients. Reflex intestinal inhibition occurs and bowel sounds disappear, indicating ileus.

Perforation of a viscus (e.g. peptic ulcer or colonic diverticulum) is proved by

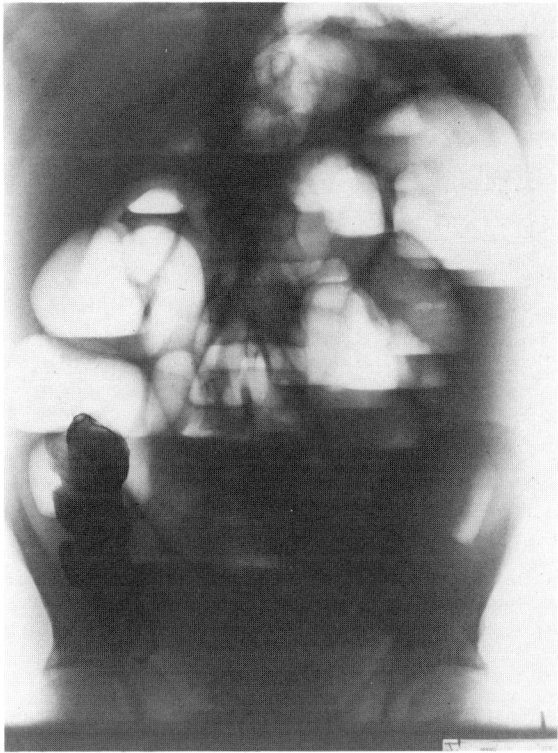

Fig. 2.7. Fluid levels and dilated small bowel in low intestinal obstruction.

detecting air in the peritoneum; an important clinical sign is finding resonance instead of dullness when percussing over the liver, providing that this is not due to emphysema or, rarely, to a loop of colon overlying it. The air or gas can sometimes, though not always, be seen on a plain film of the abdomen: subdiaphragmatic in upright views or along the lateral gutters in the decubitus position.

Traps for the unwary. Even the experienced can miss a perforation when, for example, it occurs in a patient already ill with ulcerative colitis and receiving corticosteroids; then the weakness and wasting of the abdominal muscles may explain the absence of rigidity and the steroids suppress inflammation—and analgesics obscure the pain. Appendicitis can be difficult to diagnose in pregnancy as the inflammation may not be localized; and with marked obesity, visceral inflammation may be protected from the overlying peritoneum by a greatly thickened omentum, apart from the diagnosis being more difficult because of the problem of palpating a fat belly. Whenever a surgical diagnosis of 'acute abdomen' is not obvious, a possible medical cause (p. 139) must be considered. Detailed history and examination with a test of the urine for sugar and protein are essential.

PART II
INVESTIGATIONS

Physicians think they do a lot for a patient when
they give his disease a name.

Immanual Kant

Use and abuse

Investigations must be ordered with care for they are often uncomfortable, sometimes painful, occasionally dangerous, costly—and may be misleading. Furthermore, advances in diagnosis have far exceeded those in treatment; so think whether the results of the tests could benefit the patient. Any investigations can be worrying and patients are less anxious if they know what to expect and what is expected of them. Doctors tend only to explain recent and complicated techniques, assuming the patient knows all about the barium meal, whereas most patients, especially those in hospital for the first time, need to be informed about even the simplest test, for it is the expectation of the unknown which is alarming.

Finally, decide whether the results are relevant or not to the patient's symptoms. There is truth in the aphorism, 'A healthy person is someone not fully investigated'.

Chapter 3
The Value of Blood Tests

The blood picture

Anaemia may be the first and only sign of many gastrointestinal disorders. The type of anaemia can usually be determined by examination of a blood film. Iron-deficient anaemia is often due to occult bleeding from the gut (Table 3.1) assuming that a common cause such as menorrhagia has been excluded. Anaemias of intestinal origin often result from more than one factor and a mixed or dimorphic picture may be seen when iron and vitamin B_{12} or folic acid deficiency occur together.

Iron deficiency anaemia (low Hb, low MCV, low MCHC, low MCH)
The blood film shows pale (hypochromic) small (microcytic) red cells which vary in size (anisocytosis) and shape (poikilocytosis). Serum iron concentration is low and usually less than 15% of the plasma total iron binding capacity (TIBC). The TIBC is raised in simple iron deficiency but may be lowered by chronic inflammation and protein-losing enteropathy. Iron stores are absent from the bone marrow.

Symptoms of anaemia may be accompanied by angular cheilitis, stomatitis, smooth tongue, brittle flattened or spoon-shaped fingernails, and (rarely) dysphagia.

Aetiology of iron deficiency:
1 Dietary lack.
2 Increased physiological demand (growth, menstruation, pregnancy, lactation).
3 Malabsorption.
4 Chronic blood loss (probably the commonest cause).

Rarer causes of hypochromic anaemia
Although usually due to iron deficiency, hypochromic microcytic anaemia may occur due to other disorders of haemoglobin synthesis (Table 3.2).

Megaloblastic anaemia
The appearance in peripheral blood of macrocytosis (Table 3.3) with hypersegmented neutrophils (containing more than five nuclear lobes) is usually indicative of megaloblastic anaemia (Table 3.4). Examination of the bone marrow shows megaloblasts, which are red cell precursors with a characteristic chromatin pattern of the nucleus despite normal cytoplasmic maturation. The nuclear changes reflect defective DNA synthesis. Other features often found on laboratory testing are raised serum levels of bilirubin and lactate dehydrogenase (LDH) due to premature destruction of large numbers of red blood cells. Megaloblastic anaemia is usually

Table 3.1. Causes of occult bleeding from the alimentary tract.

Common
>   Hiatus hernia
>   Peptic ulcer
>   Carcinoma of the stomach
>   Carcinoma of the large bowel
>   Drugs (aspirin, drugs for rheumatic diseases)
>   Haemorrhoids
>   Hookworm in tropical countries

Occasional
>   Crohn's disease
>   Ulcerative colitis
>   Diverticular disease
>   Oesophageal varices
>   Previous gastric surgery (part loss, part malabsorption)
>   Hereditary haemorrhagic telangiectasia
>   Polyps of the large intestine

Rare
>   Angiodysplasia, and other vascular malformations
>   Bleeding disorders; thrombocytopenic purpura,
>   polycythaemia rubra vera
>   Polyps of the stomach, or small bowel
>   (Peutz–Jeghers syndrome)
>   Meckel's diverticulum
>   Pseudoxanthoma elasticum
>   Ehlers–Danlos syndrome
>   Systemic sclerosis

Note: Hiatus hernia, colonic diverticulosis and haemorrhoids are common findings. It is risky to attribute chronic blood loss to them without visualization of the source or exclusion of more sinister co-existent pathology.

due to deficiency of folic acid or vitamin B_{12}; the causes are given in Tables 3.5 and 3.6.

Laboratory diagnosis
Deficiency of vitamin B_{12} or folic acid is usually confirmed by measurement of serum vitamin B_{12} (normal 160–900 ng/l) and both serum folate (normal above 3 ng/ml) and red blood cell folate levels (normal greater than 160 ng/ml of packed red cells). Serum folate levels are subject to rapid change so that true deficiency states may be masked by recent intake. Red cell folate gives a better index of the body's folic acid stores.

Table 3.2. Hypochromic anaemias not due to iron deficiency.

Cause	Haematological diagnosis	Gastrointestinal associations
Chronic infection Chronic inflammation Malignancy	Raised ESR, low serum iron and a low or normal total iron-binding capacity (TIBC)	
Thalassaemia	Increased HbF and HbA$_2$	Transfusional siderosis of the liver
Sideroblastic anaemia	Sideroblasts in the bone marrow	Pyridoxine (and folate) deficiency in some alcoholic patients
Lead poisoning	Basophilic stippling of erythrocytes	Abdominal (painter's) colic Blue line on gums

Table 3.3. Causes of macrocytosis (MCV raised).

Common
    Megaloblastic anaemia
    Alcoholism
    Reticulocytosis (due to haemolysis, blood loss etc.)
Rare
    Hypothyroidism
    Vitamin C deficiency
    Chronic liver disease

Table 3.4. Causes of megaloblastic anaemia.

Common
    Folic acid deficiency
    Vitamin B$_{12}$ deficiency
Rare
    Other defects in DNA synthesis

In the rare instances where vitamin B$_{12}$ or folic acid deficiency of dietary origin has caused megaloblastic anaemia, the diagnosis can be proven by showing an optimal haematological response to physiological oral doses of the vitamins given daily.

Deficiency of vitamin B$_{12}$ causes excess urinary excretion of methylmalonic acid, and deficiency of folic acid causes excess excretion of formininoglutamic acid

(FIGLU). Although these tests are seldom essential clinically, they may still be used rarely.

Metabolic pathway:

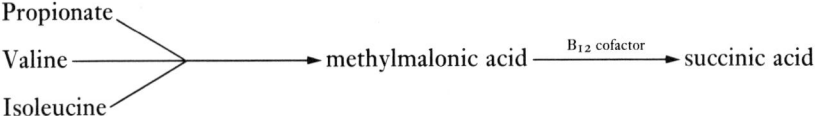

Propionate

Valine ⟶ methylmalonic acid $\xrightarrow{\text{B}_{12}\ \text{cofactor}}$ succinic acid

Isoleucine

Test. Give 10 g of L-valine or isoleucine by mouth. Measure 24-h urinary excretion of methylmalonic acid (normal up to 15 mg/24 h). In B_{12} deficiency urinary excretion of methylmalonic acid is increased.

Histidine ⟶ formininoglutamic acid (FIGLU) $\xrightarrow{\text{folic acid cofactor}}$ glutamic acid

Test. Give 15 g l histidine orally. Collect 8-h urine into acid. Estimate FIGLU excretion (normal up to 17 mg/8 h). In folate and B_{12} deficiency urinary FIGLU is increased.

Tests of vitamin B_{12} absorption. Vitamin B_{12} containing radioactive cobalt is given by mouth. In the Schilling test, following an oral 1 μg dose of vitamin B_{12} and an intramuscular flushing dose of 1000 μg of non-radioactive vitamin B_{12}, normal people excrete more than 10% of the oral dose in their urine during the following 24 h. For instance, in patients with pernicious anaemia low excretion when B_{12} is given alone is restored to normal when B_{12} is administered with intrinsic factor (IF) (Table 3.7).

Autoantibodies in pernicious anaemia. Patients with pernicious anaemia have a high incidence of autoantibodies to parietal cells (85%) and intrinsic factor (50%).

A dimorphic blood picture (mixed microcytosis and macrocytosis)
This results from combined deficiency of iron giving microcytosis, and folate or B_{12} deficiency giving macrocytosis. Coexistence of combined iron and folate deficiency suggest either a very poor diet causing nutritional deficiency or malabsorption from the proximal small intestine. When a dimorphic blood picture also shows features of splenic atrophy such as the presence of Howell–Jolly bodies or target cells the diagnosis is almost certainly adult coeliac disease (Fig. 3.1).

Table 3.5. Aetiology of folic acid deficiency.

Nutritional
    A poor diet especially lacking fresh green vegetables
Malabsorption from the proximal small intestine

Common	coeliac disease
	tropical sprue
Occasional	dermatitis herpetiformis
	Crohn's disease
	partial gastrectomy
	treatment with sulphasalazine or cholestyramine
Rare	specific congenital folic acid malabsorption

Increased requirements
    Rapid cell turnover e.g. haemolysis
    Pregnancy and lactation
Drugs
    Antimetabolites: methotrexate, pyrimethamine, trimethoprim,
                      phenytoin and phenobarbitone
                      alcohol

Table 3.6. Causes of vitamin B_{12} deficiency.

Common
    Pernicious anaemia
    Ileal disease or resection
    Gastrectomy (partial or total)
    Bacterial overgrowth of the small intestine
    Chronic tropical sprue
Rare
    Congenital deficiency of intrinsic factor
    Selective malabsorption with proteinuria
    Diphyllobothrium latum. Finnish fish tapeworm
    Dietary deficiency in vegans

Table 3.7. Urinary vitamin B_{12} excretion in the Schilling test.

Oral preparation	Normal	Pernicious anaemia	Bacterial overgrowth	Ileal disease
B_{12}	Normal	Low	Low	Low
$B_{12}+IF$	Normal	Normal	Low	Low
B_{12} after antibiotic therapy	—	—	Normal	Low

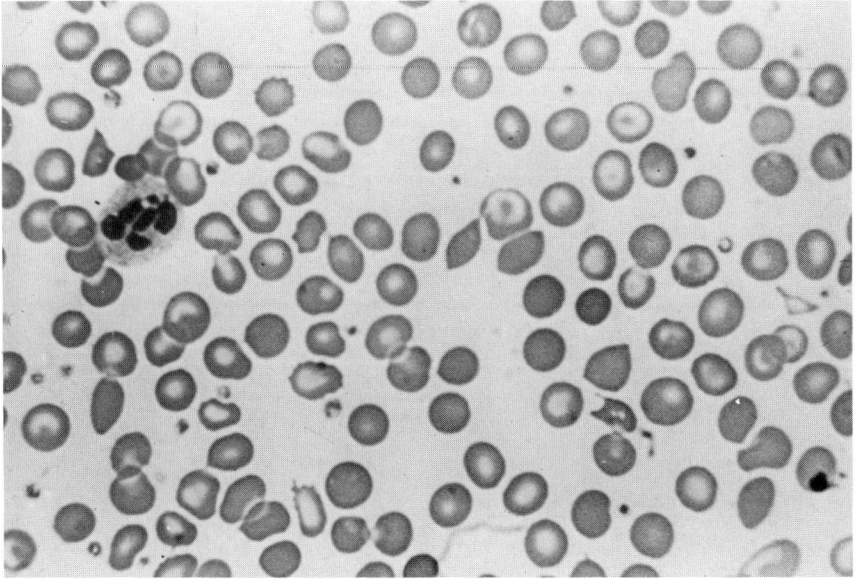

Fig. 3.1. Blood picture in a patient with adult coeliac disease. There is a dimorphic picture with mixed microcytosis and macrocytosis and hypersegmented neutrophils due to a combined deficiency of iron and folic acid. Howell–Jolly bodies are indicative of the splenic atrophy which can also be a feature of adult coeliac disease.

Other aspects of the blood picture

Red cell morphology
This may give other clues, e.g. spherocytosis may be associated with splenomegaly, jaundice and pigment gallstones in a patient with hereditary spherocytosis. Target cells, spur cells and burr cells are seen with liver disease (Fig. 3.2); acanthocytes are characteristic of abetalipoproteinaemia, a rare hereditary disorder which presents with fat malabsorption in childhood.

Fragmented red cells
These are seen on the blood film with intravascular haemolysis. This may be seen as part of:
1 Wilson's disease.
2 Zieve's syndrome. Haemolysis and massive lipaemia in patients with alcoholic liver disease.
3 Microangiopathic haemolytic anaemia may occur with mucin-secreting adeno-carcinoma, e.g. stomach.

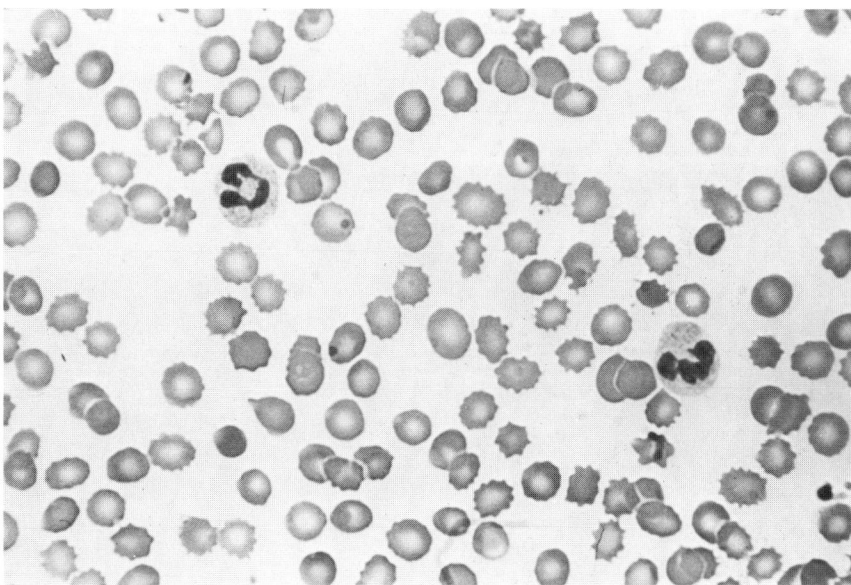

Fig. 3.2. Blood picture in a patient with severe alcoholic liver disease. Target cells are prominent and there are also bizarrely-shaped cells including spur and burr cells.

Raised haematocrit (Raised Hb, raised PCV)

Raised haematocrit may be due to:

1   Dehydration when a history of diarrhoea and vomiting, and signs of decreased skin turgor, tachycardia and postural hypotension may be found. The relative polycythaemia is corrected by rehydration.

2   Polycythaemia rubra vera in which an increased red cell mass is usually associated with leucocytosis and thrombocytosis. The patient may present with abdominal symptoms due to any of the following associated disorders:

    Peptic ulceration

    Splenomegaly

    Pruritus

    Venous thrombosis e.g. of the hepatic vein to cause the Budd–Chiari syndrome.

3   Rarely primary liver cancer produces polycythaemia analogous to the better known association with renal carcinoma.

Pancytopenia

Reduction in Hb, WBC and platelets may be due to:

1   Bone marrow suppression due to deficiency e.g. in severe megaloblastic anaemia or toxicity due to a variety of drugs or infections (e.g. viral hepatitis).

2   Hypersplenism of moderate severity is a common feature of portal hypertension.

Neutrophil leucocytosis
This occurs with:
1   Bacterial infection (usual).
2   Gastrointestinal haemorrhage (common).
3   Alcoholic hepatitis (common).
4   High-dose corticosteroid therapy (common).

A leucoerythroblastic picture
This consists of the presence on a blood film of immature cells of red and white cell series which are normally present in the bone marrow but not seen in peripheral blood (e.g. nucleated red cells). It is usually indicative of spread of carcinoma (e.g. of the stomach) to bone with replacement of the marrow.

Eosinophilia
Common:
1   Many helminthic infestations (e.g. trichinosis, ascariasis, strongyloidiasis, schistosomiasis, fascioliasis) are associated with eosinophilia of the peripheral blood during the phase of tissue invasion, but its absence later by no means excludes them.
Occasionally:
2   Inflammatory bowel disease.
3   Drug reactions, e.g. to sulphasalazine.
4   Hodgkin's disease.
Rarely:
5   Allergic or eosinophilic gastroenteritis.

Thrombocytosis (raised platelet count)
This occurs with increased risk of thrombosis in association with:
      iron deficiency
      carcinoma (e.g. of the stomach)
      bleeding
      inflammation
      hyposplenism (e.g. in coeliac disease).

Thrombocytopenia (reduced platelet count)
This may lead to purpura, bruising and haemorrhage and is caused by the following:
      portal hypertension
      megaloblastic anaemia
      alcoholism
      drug toxicity
      disseminated intravascular coagulation

Prolonged prothrombin time

This occurs in:

obstructive jaundice

hepatocellular disease

severe fat malabsorption from the intestine (rare)

disseminated intravascular coagulation

excess fibrinolysis

When a prolonged prothrombin time is the result of obstructive jaundice or severe fat malabsorption from the intestine, it corrects rapidly following parenteral administration of vitamin K.

Disseminated intravascular coagulation and excess fibrinolysis occur in association with Gram-negative sepsis, carcinoma of the gastrointestinal tract, fulminant hepatic failure.

Chapter 4
Blood Chemistry

Changes in plasma sodium and water

The interpretation of plasma Na^+ concentration should always be taken in conjunction with the patient's state of hydration. It is often important to know the sodium concentration of urine as well. Body weight is the most accurate measure of fluctuations in total body water. Dehydration due to combined Na^+ and H_2O deficiency is manifest as:

Early   loss of body weight

              orthostatic hypotension

              fast thready pulse and supine hypotension

Late   loss of skin elasticity

              reduced eyeball tension.

Dehydration due to water deprivation without salt depletion does not produce circulatory signs of tachycardia or hypotension at comparable degrees of weight loss. Overhydration is usually apparent as oedema or ascites, but considerable fluid retention detectable as increasing body weight has to occur before generalized oedema develops. A low plasma sodium may occur with no obvious dehydration or overhydration (Table 4.1).

Low plasma Na^+ with dehydration

Causes. Severe loss from diarrhoea, vomiting, sweating or gastrointestinal fistula. (The low plasma Na^+ is partly due to attempted rehydration with salt-poor fluids. The urine is concentrated and the urinary Na^+ concentration is less than 20 mmol/l unless dehydration has resulted in acute tubular necrosis of the kidney when plasma:urine osmolality is 1:1 and urinary sodium exceeds 20 mmol/l.)

Renal loss: Causes include adrenal failure, excess diuretic therapy and salt-losing nephropathy. (Urine sodium concentration is greater than 20 mmol/l.)

Treatment. The patient requires salt and water.

Low plasma Na^+ concentration with overhydration

The low (Na^+) merely indicates that the excess total body water is relatively greater than the excess of total body sodium. This is not an indication for administering sodium. Overhydration is apparent by oedema or ascites.

Table 4.1. Low plasma Na$^+$ with no obvious dehydration or overhydration.

Occasional

1 Diuretic therapy with K$^+$ depletion. Potassium supplements exchange for intracellular sodium which comes out of the cells to restore plasma Na$+$ to normal
2 Inappropriate ADH secretion

Rare

1 Myxoedema
2 Acute intermittent porphyria
3 Pseudohyponatraemia due to lipaemia or hyperproteinaemia, e.g. myeloma. The lipid or protein decrease plasma water per 100 ml of plasma so that the Na$^+$ concentration is low per 100 ml of plasma but normal per 100 ml of plasma water

Treatment. Restrict fluid intake to elevate plasma Na$^+$ concentration, restrict salt intake, promote salt and water loss by diuresis. Increase plasma osmotic pressure if hypoproteinaemia is severe.

Hypernatraemia

This usually indicates water deprivation (e.g. due to total dysphagia) but is rarely a feature of disease in adults. In babies hypernatraemia carries a serious risk of brain damage and can be caused by excess dietary sodium.

Changes in plasma potassium concentration (Tables 4.2, 4.3 and 4.4).

Plasma potassium is often a poor guide to total body potassium stores which may be depleted by several hundred millimoles before significant hypokalaemia develops. In most cases of K$^+$ depletion there is a metabolic alkalosis of ECF, and the rise of plasma HCO$_3^-$ may be a better indicator of total body K$^+$ stores. As K$^+$ ions are lost in diarrhoea, vomiting or diuresis, extracellular K$^+$ is replenished from the large intracellular stores of K$^+$ which diffuses out of the cells in exchange for hydrogen ions (Fig. 4.1). Significant symptoms of hypokalaemia develop when plasma K$^+$ is 2.0 mmol/l or less (normal 3.4–5.6 mol/l.). Severe hypokalaemia produces renal diabetes insipidus associated with polyuria. Paraesthesiae of the extremities progresses to tetanic carpopedal spasm and finally muscular paralysis. Paralytic ileus also occurs.

Changes in plasma chloride and bicarbonate concentration

The body regulates the acid base balance within close limits. Arterial plasma pH is normally in the range 7.36–7.44. Disturbances can be classified as:

1 Respiratory alkalosis, e.g. hysterical hyperventilation giving tetany.
2 Respiratory acidosis, e.g. CO$_2$ retention in lung disease.
3 Metabolic alkalosis.
4 Metabolic acidosis.

Table 4.2. Causes of hypokalaemic alkalosis.

Common
  1 Vomiting (The alkalosis is particularly severe due to loss of HCl from the stomach.
     Replenishment of both Na^+ and K^+ is most important when vomiting is due to
     pyloric stenosis. The same effect is produced by per nasal aspiration of gastrointes-
     tinal secretions, e.g. in paralytic ileus).
  2 Diarrhoea due to almost any cause (in diarrhoea due to malabsorption syndrome the
     hypokalaemic alkalosis often coexists with hypocalcaemia and hypomagnesaemia.
     This especially predisposes patient to tetany, and Chvostek's and Trousseau's signs
     may be positive).
  3 Diuretic therapy.
  4 Hyperaldosteronism, usually secondary as in cirrhosis (rarely primary).
Occasional
  1 Purgation due to laxative abuse.
  2 Corticosteroid excess, usually iatrogenic. Also Cushing's. Severe with ectopic ACTH
     production by tumours.
  3 Carbenoxolone therapy in the elderly
  4 Poor dietary K^+ intake, e.g. in anorexia nervosa.
  5 Alcoholism.
  6 Villous papilloma of the rectum or colon.
Rare
  1 Chloridorrhoea.
Treatment of K^+ deficiency in the usual hypokalaemic alkalosis is with potassium chloride.

Table 4.3. Causes of the rare hypokalaemic acidosis.

---

1 Pancreatic fistulae in which HCO_3^- rich fluid is lost.
2 Vipoma. Profuse watery diarrhoea simulating cholera results from excess production of
   the hormone vasoactive intestinal peptide (VIP).
3 Ureteric implants into the sigmoid colon (ureterosigmoidostomy) or ileal conduits.
4 Renal tubular acidosis.
Treatment of K^+ deficiency in the rare case of hypokalaemic acidosis is with a mixture of
   sodium and potassium citrate.

The sum of chloride + bicarbonate concentration normally approaches within
10 ± 2 mmol/l of that of sodium. In metabolic acidosis it is important to decide
whether:
1 There is increased chloride : bicarbonate ratio with a normal anion gap (Tables
4.5 and 4.6) e.g. Na^+ 140, Cl^- 115, HCO_3^- 15. Anion gap $= 140 - (115 + 15) = 10$
which is normal. There is hyperchloraemic acidosis.

Table 4.4. Causes of hyperkalaemia.

Common
1 Renal failure.
2 Therapy with potassium-conserving diuretics: spironolactone, triamterene or amiloride.

Occasional
1 Addison's disease. Hyponatraemia and hyperkalaemia may be the clue that weakness, weight loss, vomiting and diarrhoea are secondary to hypoadrenalism.
2 Hypoinsulinism in diabetic patients.

NB The commonest cause of a high K^+ concentration is probably a false value due to faulty techniques for venesection and handling of the blood sample, allowing leakage of K^+ from the cellular elements of blood into plasma prior to analysis.

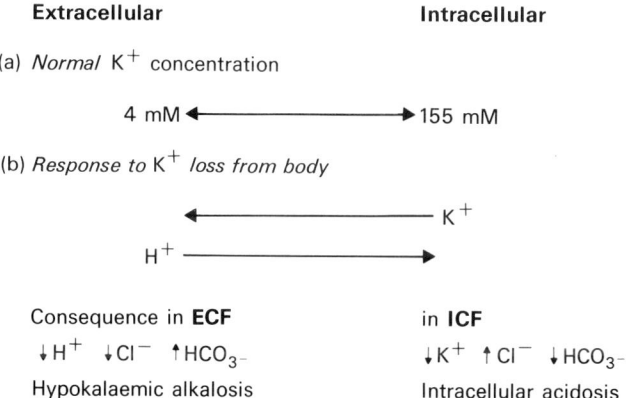

Extracellular   **Intracellular**

(a) *Normal* K^+ concentration

4 mM ⟵————————➤ 155 mM

(b) *Response to* K^+ *loss from body*

⟵———————————— K^+

H^+ ————————————➤

Consequence in **ECF**   in **ICF**
↓H^+ ↓Cl^- ↑HCO_3^- ↓K^+ ↑Cl^- ↓HCO_3^-
Hypokalaemic alkalosis   Intracellular acidosis

Approximation: for each pH 0.1 rise (alkalosis) there is a fall of 1 mmol/l of K^+ (hypokalaemia) in ECF.

Fig. 4.1. When the body is depleted of its potassium stores potassium moves from intracellular to extracellular fluid in exchange for hydrogen ions and usually produces an extracellular metabolic alkalosis.

Table 4.5. Causes of metabolic acidosis with normal anion gap.

1 Causes of hypokalaemic acidosis listed in Table 4.3.
2 Primary hyperparathyroidism.
3 Administration of ammonium chloride.
4 Anion exchange resins.

Table 4.6. Causes of metabolic acidosis with increased anion gap.

Common
1   Diabetic ketoacidosis, presence of β-hydroxybutyric acid.
2   Uraemia retention of sulphate etc.
Occasional
1   Lactic acidosis due to hypoxic shock, phenformin etc.
2   Salicylate overdose.
3   Ketoacidosis of the alcoholic. There is no hyperglycaemia. Excess production of β-hydroxybutyric acid is occasionally seen in chronic alcoholics after binge drinking.
4   Liver failure. Severe lactic acidosis is an occasional feature of terminal liver failure.
5   Fructose and sorbitol administration as intravenous calorie source has been largely discontinued due to their potential for precipitating severe lactic acidosis, especially in patients with liver disease.
6   Methanol ingestion. Metabolism to formic acid may produce a fatal metabolic acidosis
7   Self-poisoning, e.g. with ethylene glycol.

---

2   There is an increased anion gap, e.g. Na^+ 140, Cl^- 100, HCO_3^- 15. Anion gap $= 140 - (100 + 15) = 25$ which is raised. This means that other anions must be present in excess.

Metabolic alkalosis
This occurs due to those conditions listed in Table 4.2. Blood pH exceeds 7.45. In contrast to respiratory alkalosis the PCO_2 of the blood is normal or slightly increased.

Metabolic acidosis
This is usually apparent from the patient's deep sighing respiration. (Kussmaul respiration).

Changes in plasma calcium concentration
Plasma calcium levels are best interpreted in conjunction with plasma phosphate and alkaline phosphatase levels. Occasionally it is important to determine plasma magnesium in addition. Acid base balance is also of vital importance.

About 40% of plasma calcium (normal 2.25–2.75 mmol/l) is normally bound to protein, mainly serum albumin. It is the ionized non-protein bound calcium concentration which influences neuromuscular excitability and generally produces symptoms of hypocalcaemia and hypercalcaemia. The calcium concentration should be 'corrected' for changes in serum albumin to give the calcium concentration equivalent to 40 g/l albumin. Approximately, plasma calcium falls 0.2 mmol/l for each 10 g/l fall in serum albumin. Ionized calcium falls with a rise in

Table 4.7. Causes of hypercalcaemia.

Common
  1 Malignant disease either by directly involving bone or by ectopic hormone production. Ectopic production of parathyroid hormone or prostaglandin E_2 occurs rarely with primary liver cancer and other primary intra-abdominal malignancies but is commonest with bronchial cancer.
  2 Primary hyperparathyroidism. Hypercalcaemia is usually associated with a raised serum alkaline phosphatase and a low fasting plasma inorganic phosphate and high renal clearance of plasma phosphate. Primary hyperparathyroidism may cause abdominal pain due to associated: (a) Peptic ulceration which has an increased incidence in hyperparathyroidism. Rarely a parathyroid adenoma may coexist with a gastrinoma (the Zollinger–Ellison syndrome) in the syndrome of multiple endocrine adenomatosis. (b) Acute pancreatitis. It is important to exclude hypercalcaemia when convalescence from acute pancreatitis is complete. During hospitalization for acute pancreatitis the serum calcium may be depressed to normal or low levels thus masking the primary abnormality. (c) Renal colic due to calcium-containing stones. (d) Constipation. This frequently accompanies the dehydrating effect of the hypercalcaemia in hyperparathyroidism.
Occasional
  1 Vitamin D intoxication.
  2 Sarcoidosis.
  3 Myeloma.
  4 Hyperparathyroidism.
  5 Immobilization in Paget's disease of bone.
Rare
  1 Hypophosphatasia—an inherited disease.
  2 Vipoma.
  3 Milk-alkali syndrome. This rarely occurs nowadays, but is formerly well described as a consequence of milk and alkali ingestion for relief of peptic ulcer pain.

plasma pH (alkalaemia) so that respiratory alkalosis induced by hyperventilation or metabolic alkalosis induced by vomiting or any other cause may produce tetany due to a low plasma *ionized* calcium concentration although total plasma calcium is normal. Conversely, tetany virtually never occurs in acidotic patients however low the total plasma calcium concentration goes.

Hypercalcaemia (Table 4.7)
This may cause polyuria, lethargy, constipation, dysphagia, nausea and vomiting or psychiatric disorders.

Hypocalcaemia
Hypocalcaemia (Table 4.8) causes neuromuscular irritability with positive

Table 4.8. Causes of hypocalcaemia.

---

1 Acute pancreatitis. Calcium is precipitated as soaps. A high serum glucagon may also contribute by stimulating release of calcitonin which lowers plasma calcium levels.
2 Vitamin D deficiency causing osteomalacia. It is important in patients with gastrointestinal disease and an isolated rise of plasma alkaline phosphatase to suspect osteomalacia. The classical biochemical finding is of low normal calcium or hypocalcaemia, with low fasting phosphate and high alkaline phosphatase. The tendency to hypocalcaemia may have been corrected by secondary hyperparathyroidism which tends to raise serum calcium levels by mobilizing it from bone (producing subperiosteal erosions on phalanges) and promoting its reabsorption from the kidney (coincidentally enhancing phosphate excretion).
3 Neonatal hypocalcaemia. Tetany and convulsions may occur following ingestion of cow's milk due to its high content of phosphate.
4 Magnesium deficiency produces resistance to the actions of vitamin D and parathyroid hormone. In some instances hypocalcaemia only responds to vitamin D therapy after replenishment of plasma magnesium
5 Hypoparathyroidism. In primary hypoparathyroidism there is hypocalcaemia with a high plasma phosphate and low urinary phosphate excretion. Patients often have moniliasis affecting the oro-pharynx and causing nail dystrophy. Steatorrhoea may be present which resolves following correction of calcium metabolism.

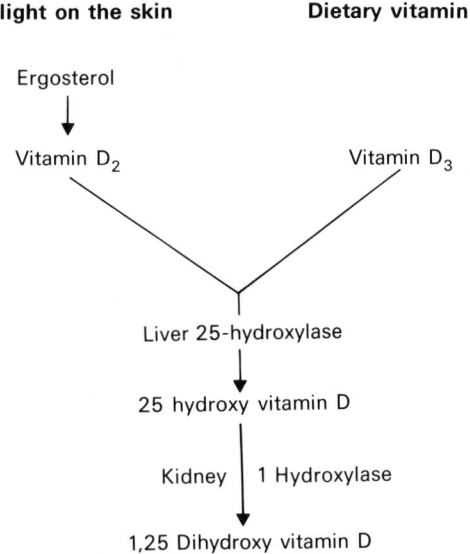

Fig. 4.2. Metabolism of vitamin D.

Chvostek's and Trousseau's signs. Later carpopedal spasm, convulsions and laryngeal stridor may occur.

Osteomalacia. This may present clinically with:

1   Spontaneous bone fractures—this usually occurs in the elderly in whom osteoporosis coexists.

2   Proximal myopathy. Difficulty climbing stairs or getting out of low chairs.

3   Tetany. This rarely occurs unless there is both steatorrhoea causing marked hypocalcaemia and diarrhoea or vomiting to give hypokalaemic alkalosis.

The diagnosis may be confirmed clinically by:

4   Biochemical analysis of the blood. In order of development the fasting plasma phosphate level is low relative to urea, alkaline phosphatase is raised, and finally plasma calcium level lowered despite correction for serum albumin.

5   Radiological evidence of pseudofractures (also known as Looser's zones) often seen in the pubic rami or ribs, but also in the humerus or femur. X-ray of the hands may show subperiosteal erosions involving the phalanges, evidence of the hyperparathyroidism which usually occurs secondary to osteomalacia.

6   Measurement of vitamin D or its metabolites in serum. 25-hydroxycholecalciferol is produced by the liver from cholecalciferol (vitamin D_3) and is the usual metabolite measured (Fig. 4.2).

1,25 Di-hydroxy cholecalciferol is an extremely powerful humoral agent, promoting calcium absorption from the intestine. The hormone enters the intestinal cell nucleus and induces synthesis of calcium binding protein, as well as stimulating mineralization of bone.

Changes in plasma concentrations of alkaline phosphatase and transaminase

Raised AsT, Raised Alk Phos

A combined disturbance of the enzymes aspartate aminotransferase, a transaminase (AsT) and serum alkaline phosphatase (SAP or Alk Phos) is strongly suggestive of liver disease. Sometimes liver disease produces an elevation of one without the other but much more commonly both are disturbed and it is the relative change in each which helps biochemically to differentiate hepatitis from cholestasis. If the transaminase is greater than 1000 (normal less than 35 iu/l) then significant hepatitis exists. If the alkaline phosphatase is more than three times the upper limit of normal (greater than 1000 if normal is less than 350 iu/l or greater than 39 King–Armstrong units with normal < 13) then cholestasis is usually the dominant clinical problem and attention should be focused on the biliary system.

Raised AsT, Normal Alk Phos

A hepatic origin of the aspartate aminotransaminase needs to be confirmed by collateral evidence, e.g. bilirubin, gamma glutamyl transpeptidase. Other origins can be sought by alternative enzyme determinations, e.g. creatine kinase will usually be elevated if the hypertransaminasaemia is a consequence of muscle damage.

Raised Alk Phos, Normal AsT
Most often the origin is liver or bone, but alkaline phosphatase may also originate from the intestine, leucocytes or placenta. A hepatic origin is confirmed by iso-enzyme electrophoresis or by elevation of other hepato-biliary enzymes in the blood, (5′nucleotidase, γ-glutamyl transpeptidase). A bony origin is suggested by abnormalities of serum calcium or phosphate and confirmed by radiology or scintigraphy (e.g. hyperparathyroidism, osteomalacia, Paget's disease, metastatic carcinoma).

Plasma albumin and globulin concentrations
A low serum albumin (Table 4.9) may be the result of
1   Underproduction by the liver.
2   Dilution or redistribution of a normal albumin pool.
3   Leakage of albumin from the body at rates in excess of the liver's ability to compensate by increased synthesis.

Albumin : globulin ratio
Raised globulins are characteristic of many inflammatory disorders, and may be used as an index of disease activity, e.g. in 'lupoid' chronic active hepatitis, disease activity is reflected by a raised gamma globulin and low albumin. Successful therapy suppresses the globulin and raises the albumin (Table 4.10).

Acute phase proteins
C-reactive protein, seromucoids (or orosomucoids), α_1 acid glycoprotein. The concentration of many serum proteins fluctuates according to the activity of many diseases. When there is active inflammation their concentration tends to increase. Their reaction is not specific to any disease; rather they may react in a similar way to

Table 4.9. Aetiology of hypoalbuminaemia.

---

1   Underproduction by the liver. (a) Lack of amino acid substrates due to: (i) Poor dietary intake: malnutrition; (ii) Maldigestion of dietary protein in pancreatic insufficiency; (iii) Malabsorption in severe intestinal disorders; (iv) Bacterial degradation of dietary protein in the presence of bacterial overgrowth producing deficiency of tryptophan and other essential amino acids. (b) Poor liver function.
2   Haemodilution: expansion of ECF is common with cirrhosis.
3   Redistribution: e.g. loss into the peritoneal cavity with ascites.
4   Excessive loss: in the urine (nephrotic syndrome), into the gut (protein-losing enteropathy), from the skin (exfoliative dermatitis; burns).

Table 4.10. Laboratory tests for investigation of liver disease.

A. Routine screening and monitoring

Blood	*Urine*
Bilirubin	Bilirubin
Aspartate aminotransferase (AsT or SGOT) or Alanine aminotransferase (ALT or SGPT)	Urobilinogen
Alkaline phosphatase	
Albumin	
Globulin	
Prothrombin time	

B. Searching for a cause

Test	*Condition*
Blood ethanol $\left.\begin{array}{l} \\ \\ \end{array}\right\}$ γ Glutamyl transpeptidase Mean corpuscular volume	Alcoholism
Hepatitis A $\left\{\begin{array}{l}\text{IgM anti-HAV} \\ \text{IgG anti-HAV}\end{array}\right.$	Recent hepatitis A infection Long-standing immunity to hepatitis A
Hepatitis B $\left\{\begin{array}{l}\text{HBsAg} \\ \text{anti-HBc} \\ \text{anti-HBs} \\ \text{HBeAg} \\ \text{anti-HBe}\end{array}\right.$	Hepatitis B infection Exposure to hepatitis B at some time Immunity to hepatitis B Marker of infectivity and herald of chronicity
Paracetamol	Acute self-poisoning
Serum iron $\left.\begin{array}{l} \\ \end{array}\right\}$ Total iron binding capacity and saturation index Ferritin	Screening for haemochromatosis
Caeruloplasmin	Wilson's disease
Alpha₁ antitrypsin deficiency	
Alpha fetoprotein	Screening for primary liver cancer
Mitochondrial antibodies	Screening for primary biliary cirrhosis
Smooth muscle antibodies $\left.\begin{array}{l} \\ \end{array}\right\}$ Antinuclear factor	Screening for chronic active hepatitis
IgG, IgA, IgM	

Other more specialized investigations (e.g. serum bile acid estimation) are described in Chapter 8.

---

a wide variety of conditions, e.g. Crohn's disease of the intestine, chronic active hepatitis, rheumatoid arthritis, and many other disorders involving other body systems. Their measurement may be useful, (a) to screen for organic disease in new patients, and (b) to follow disease activity in patients with chronic disease whose activity classically fluctuates.

Lipaemia

A comment from the haematologist or biochemist noting that the patient's serum was lipaemic (milky) should not be ignored. Fasting blood should be tested to exclude a significant hyperlipidaemia which may be related to the patient's symptoms.

1   Type I hyperlipidaemia: hyperchylomicronaemia causing pancreatitis in: (a) children with severe deficiency of lipoprotein lipase, and (b) women prone to the hyperlipidaemic effects of oestrogenic contraceptive steroids.

2   Type IV or type V hyperlipoproteinaemia may also be seen with pancreatitis or liver disease in the alcoholic patient. In Zieve's syndrome severe hyperlipidaemia of the alcoholic is associated with haemolysis.

Chapter 5
The Upper Alimentary Tract

The oesophagus

The oesophagus can be studied directly so easily that exact diagnosis is usually possible. Most patients with oesophageal symptoms have a barium swallow and a plain chest X-ray. If a structural lesion is seen suggesting peptic or malignant stricture, endoscopy is essential for histological and cytological diagnosis. Manometry, pH monitoring and the acid perfusion test are reserved for the relatively few patients where difficulties occur in diagnosing reflux oesophagitis or a motility disorder.

Radiology

Chest X-ray may reveal

1 Pulmonary shadowing due to aspiration of oesophageal contents. Severe pneumonitis may be caused by acid gastric contents and by the laxative liquid paraffin.
2 An air-fluid level behind the heart within a hiatus hernia.
3 Widening of the mediastinum due to a sigmoid oesophagus in achalasia.
4 Absence of a gastric air-bubble below the diaphragm in achalasia.

Barium swallow

This is usually performed both with the patient upright and lying down; the latter is needed to demonstrate hiatus hernia and gastro-oesophageal reflux. However, reflux of barium from the stomach to oesophagus is reported in only a third of patients with apparent reflux oesophagitis and in an only slightly smaller proportion of patients with no symptoms or other signs of reflux. The patient may be tilted in a head-down position with pressure applied to the abdomen, but reflux under these conditions need not imply any abnormality. In scleroderma involving the oesophagus, the patient is unable to swallow against gravity in the head-down (Trendelenberg) position. Late films taken after a swallow performed with a small amount of thick barium which coats the oesophagus often outlines oesophageal varices clearly but is less reliable than oesophagoscopy if they are small or temporarily underfilled. When there is no apparent structural lesion, various additional manoeuvres may help demonstrate the rarer disorders of motility seen in diffuse oesophageal spasm, achalasia and scleroderma; this may be the use of a 'bread bolus' when a mouthful of barium and partly chewed bread is swallowed. Cinéradiology has also been used to assess oesophageal motility disorders.

Oesophagoscopy

Direct inspection of the oesophagus is easily done through the forward-viewing flexible fibreoptic panendoscope (Fig. 5.1). This has virtually replaced the rigid oesophagoscope, except when a thorough inspection of the postcricoid region is needed or taking of larger biopsy specimens.

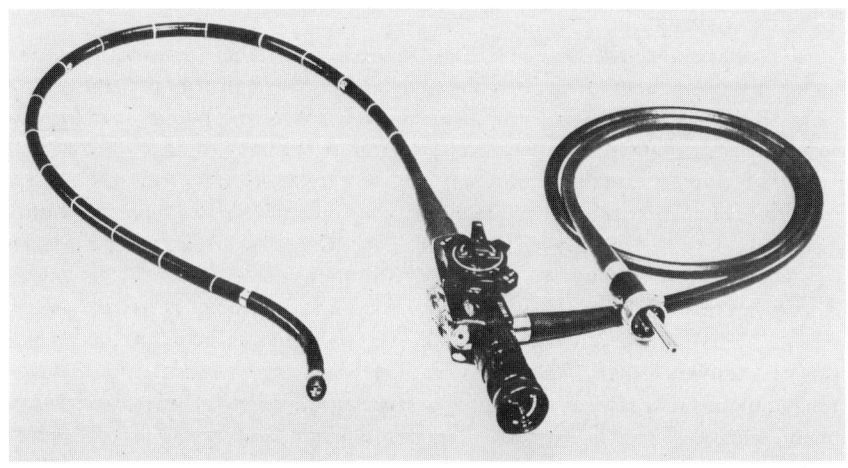

(a)

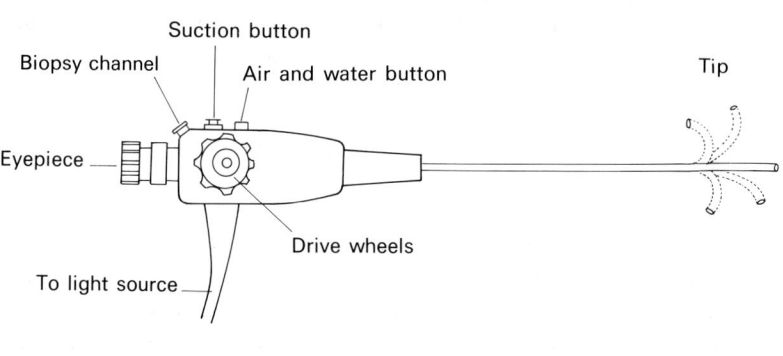

(b)

Fig. 5.1. (a) Forward-viewing fibreoptic endoscope; (b) diagram to show control.

Biopsy and cytology

Biopsies are taken through the endoscope and also cytology brushings if cancer is suspected. This is invaluable in differentiation of benign and malignant strictures. Unfortunately histological changes do not correlate well either with symptoms or with the naked-eye appearance at endoscopy where benign oesophagitis is suspected; changes in the distal oesophagus compatible with oesophagitis occur even in normal individuals, and some may lead to a false diagnosis. Histological changes in oesophagitis include infiltration by inflammatory cells, increase in length of the dermal papillae, and basal cell hyperplasia.

Special tests usually needing an oesophageal laboratory

Acid perfusion test

This is not a test of reflux but aims to detect sensitivity of the distal oesophagus to acid. It is the best of the available tests for evaluation of patients without abnormality on barium swallow who complain of symptoms possibly due to reflux oesophagitis. Solutions of isotonic sodium chloride and of 0.1 N HCl are put in separate bottles; the saline is run in first and then, without the patient's knowledge, it is changed to the HCl for 15 min at a rate of 10–20 ml/min; if pain occurs the solution is changed to 0.1 N sodium bicarbonate which should relieve the pain. The patient may be asked whether the symptoms experienced are the same as those being investigated. Although false positive results may occur in normal subjects, the effects are seldom so immediate as in those with oesophagitis. Oesophageal pain may be similar to that of cardiac origin. An ECG may be run during the test to detect the rare occasion when the procedure induces an attack of angina pectoris.

Manometry

Manometry may help in the early diagnosis of achalasia of the cardia, scleroderma and other motor disorders. An expensive multichannel pressure recorder and several pressure transducers are needed and intraluminal pressures are recorded either by water-filled polyvinyl tubes with lateral holes or by balloon-tipped tubes. Pressure recordings are taken in the stomach, gastro-oesophageal junction and oesophagus both during and between swallowing. On slow withdrawal of the tube from the stomach to the oesophagus there is a pressure reversal, the positive intra-abdominal pressure changing to the negative intrathoracic pressure. The normal resting oesophageal pressure is +2 to −20 cm water and the lower oesophageal sphincter is shown by a zone of increased pressure 2–3 cm above that of the gastro-oesophageal junction which relaxes during swallowing, the relaxation preceding arrival of the peristaltic wave. When the patient swallows, a positive peristaltic wave of 40–80 cm water develops.

pH studies

Continuous measurement can be made by an electrode placed 4–5 cm above the gastro-oesophageal sphincter in the lower oesophagus and connected to a variety of recording devices some of which are portable in normal daily activities. This provides hard data as to whether vague symptoms of belching, bloating or heartburn are likely to be due to reflux or merely incidental. Continuous pH monitoring can be performed for 24 h (usually 12–16 h) and episodes of discomfort or heartburn are then correlated with the number of times that oesophageal pH has fallen below 4 and also the mean duration of those episodes. It is generally believed that peptic oesophagitis can only occur when the pH is below 4. However, alkaline bile and pancreatic juice may also be important in producing oesophagitis, e.g. in postgastrectomy patients. In the interests of speeding up the test, some have monitored oesophageal pH during bouts of exercise designed to induce reflux, but such provocation tests are not thought to be as reliable diagnostically as monitoring during normal activity.

The stomach and duodenum

Barium meal
The term is a euphemism and it needs no gourmet to detect the difference from a meal; the X-ray examination is carried out in the semi-dark in an anxious person who swallows an indigestible tasteless potion. A single contrast X-ray shows only profile views of the barium-filled stomach to outline ulcers or growths, though in the duodenum the thinly barium-coated mucosa is seen *en face* through bowel distended with gas. Greater accuracy is obtained with the double-contrast barium meal where effervescent tablets or carbonated drinks are used so that mucosal lesions can be identified more easily.

The stomach must be empty and the patient laid prone or slightly inverted to study lesions at the cardia and hiatus hernia. Gastric stasis, usually from pyloric obstruction, is diagnosed when fluid and food residue forms a layer above the barium or when the stomach is not empty at 4 h.

'Gastrografin', an iodinated water-soluble opaque medium, is used in an emergency when perforation of an ulcer is suspected. Because it is hypertonic it promotes fluid secretion and therefore is not used if oesophageal obstruction or broncho-oesophageal fistula is suspected, with their attendant risk of aspiration. A dilute barium suspension is then to be preferred.

Upper gastrointestinal endoscopy
Fibreoptic endoscopy (Figs 5.1 and 5.2) allows direct inspection of the oesophagus, stomach and duodenum and lesions can be photographed in colour and biopsies taken. A forward or oblique viewing instrument is usually used but for a full view of the lesser curve of the stomach, the duodenal bulb and the ampulla of Vater, a side viewing instrument may be necessary.

The procedure must be explained fully to the patient beforehand as cooperation is so important. Sedation is usually given with benzodiazepines but is by no means essential and is often best avoided in bleeding patients because of the risk of inhalation, or in alcoholics who may go beserk and bite the instrument. Some spray the throat with local anaesthetic. The patient has to swallow and then the instrument is guided by direct vision. A change from the pale pink to the orange red mucosa of the stomach is seen at the gastro-oesophageal junction though this does

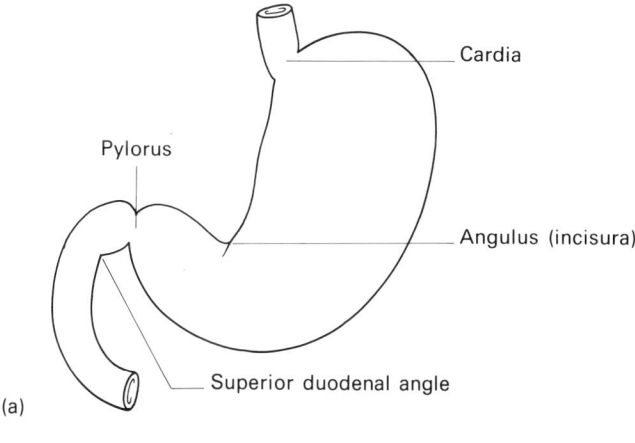

Cardia

Pylorus

Angulus (incisura)

Superior duodenal angle

(a)

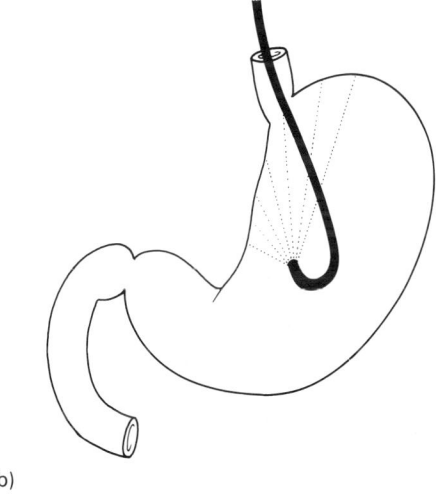

(b)

Fig. 5.2. (a) Landmarks at endoscopy; (b) retroversion.

not always correlate with histological changes in the epithelium. The greater curve and antrum of the stomach are viewed with air insufflation and the cardia can be viewed by looping older endoscopes or merely by fully flexing the tip of the most modern instruments (Fig. 5.2).

Risks involve a slight possibility of perforation, usually in the hypopharynx. Pneumonia may occur especially in ill patients due to inhalation of gastric contents. Cardiac arrest and respiratory depression have been reported, so methods of resuscitation should be available.

Endoscopy has not only improved diagnosis, but also opened the door to new forms of treatment:

1   Removal of foreign bodies from the stomach.
2   Dilatation of oesophageal strictures.
3   Injection of oesophageal varices.
4   Control of upper gastrointestinal haemorrhage by diathermy with contact electrodes, lasers or other methods.
5   Polypectomy.
6   Sphincterotomy and removal of gallstones.

Should the patient have an X-ray or an endoscopy?

1   Indications for barium meal are strongest when an oesophageal lesion is suspected. Because of the risk of perforation during endoscopy it is almost mandatory to have a barium swallow performed before endoscopy in the investigation of dysphagia.
2   Endoscopy is most strongly recommended for biopsy and cytology of oesophageal strictures and gastric ulcers shown on barium meal when malignancy requiring surgery needs to be ruled out before commencing medical ulcer-healing treatment.
3   Endoscopy is generally regarded as preferable to barium meal in the investigation of upper gastrointestinal bleeding. Small mucosal lesions, such as erosive gastritis, may be overlooked in radiological studies but can be clearly identified endoscopically provided the procedure is within 24–48 h of presentation. If bleeding is occurring distal to the stomach, endoscopy has the additional advantage over barium studies that vascular radiographic studies are still possible.
4   Barium meal or endoscopy may be advocated for the initial investigation of dyspepsia. First choice will depend on local factors such as expertise, availability, waiting list length etc. The double contrast barium meal carries almost no discomfort or hazard. Endoscopy is a little more accurate, and allows definitive diagnosis by biopsy, but is more uncomfortable and slightly hazardous, and experts are not always available.
5   Endoscopy is sometimes the method of choice because it has been anticipated that endoscopic therapy may be appropriate, following confirmation of the diagnosis.

Measurement of hydrochloric acid secretion

Assessment of the acid response either to histamine or preferably the synthetic gastrin-like pentapeptide pentagastrin (peptavlon) has replaced former tests of acid secretion using substances like gruel or alcohol. Administration of histamine 0.04 mg/kg must be preceded by injection of an effective H-1 histamine antagonist 30 min previously. Although this theoretically blocks all histamine receptors outside the stomach patients may still experience unpleasant side-effects.

With a gastric aspiration tube carefully positioned, all fluid secreted by the stomach is collected. Total acid secretion in the first hour is termed basal acid output (BAO). At the end of this collection period, pentagastrin is injected (6 μg/kg bodyweight) subcutaneously or intramuscularly and all gastric secretion collected for another hour, usually in 10 or 15 min aliquots. The total amount of acid secreted in the second hour is called the maximal acid output (MAO) and the mean of the two highest consecutive 10 or 15 min collections is peak acid output (PAO).

1   Endoscopy has virtually replaced the need for acid secretion tests in diagnosing peptic ulcer and anyway there is much overlap between normal and abnormal; an acid output greater than 50 mmol/h strongly favours duodenal ulcer. Some believe that choice of ulcer surgery between operations such as highly selective vagotomy or partial gastrectomy can be made rationally according to the patient's preoperative acid studies. However, as yet there is no convincing evidence that this approach reduces postgastrectomy problems or recurrent ulcer risk.

2   Although it may be difficult to collect gastric juice after operations on the stomach, the insulin test (Hollander's test) is used to assess the completeness of vagotomy. Insulin 0.1–0.2 μg/kg is injected intravenously and the resultant hypoglycaemia acts centrally to stimulate gastric secretion through the vagus nerve. Blood is taken at 30 and 45 min to ensure that an adequate hypoglycaemic stimulus has been produced. This may be unpleasant for patients and can also be dangerous unless someone is available to inject glucose if necessary.

3   The pentagastrin test is used to confirm diagnosis of Zollinger–Ellison (ZE) syndrome; BAO is greater than 10 mmol/h in 70% of patients with ZE but in only 10% of other duodenal ulcer (DU) patients. A ratio of BAO : MAO greater than 0.4 is found in more than 50% of ZE patients but in only 5% of DU patients.

4   If the only information needed is whether hydrochloric acid is secreted or not, as in the diagnosis of pernicious anaemia, a single sample of gastric juice collected after an appetising meal may provide the answer.

Serum gastrin

There are various circulating gastrins but the three biologically active forms are known as G34, G17 and G14 as they contain thirty-four, seventeen and fourteen amino acids each. Most radioimmunoassays measure G17, small gastrin. The normal range in fasting serum is 5–50 pmol/l. Measurement of fasting serum gastrin levels is usually reserved for patients with a severe ulcer diathesis suspected of having the ZE syndrome. It is indicated in patients with multiple ulcers, ulcers at unusual sites, ulcers recurring after gastric surgery, aggressive bleeding and those with associated hyperparathyroidism. Patients must not be taking H_2 receptor antagonists.

Causes of hypergastrinaemia

1   Producing hyperacidity. Proven: (a) ZE syndrome, (b) isolated retained antrum (see Fig. 5.3). Possible: (c) antral G-cell hyperplasia.

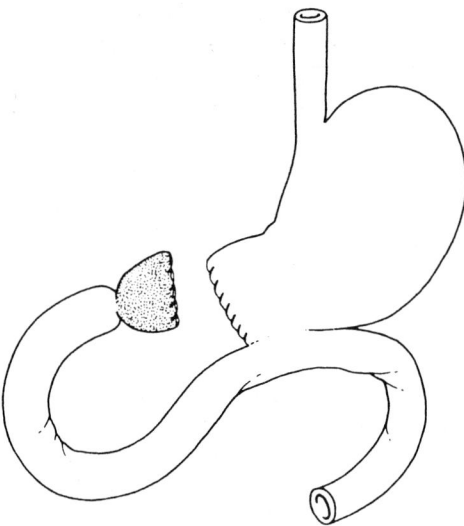

Fig. 5.3. The isolated retained antrum. A rare cause of hypergastrinaemia leading to peptic ulceration occurs when a portion of gastric antrum has been left at Polya gastrectomy. As this part is not acidified, there is no inhibition of its gastrin secretion.

2   Response to hypoacidity. (i) Antral achlorhydria or hypochlorhydria, e.g. atrophic gastritis of pernicious anaemia, and (ii) chronic renal failure.

Diagnosis of the ZE syndrome
1   Gastric acid secretion studies (see above).
2   Measurement of fasting serum gastrin: A fasting gastrin greater than 1000 pmol/l with hyperacidity is diagnostic of the ZE syndrome provided the isolated retained antrum syndrome is excluded. Many ZE cases have intermediate levels of fasting gastrin and in them stimulation tests with secretin or calcium are helpful.
3   Measurement of serum gastrin during stimulation tests: Secretin, 3 units/kg, given as an intravenous bolus produces a paradoxical rise of serum gastrin with an increment of greater than 100 pmol/l over basal in nearly all patients. In other causes of hypergastrinaemia, secretin usually causes a fall in gastrin levels. Similarly intravenous infusion of calcium 12–15 mg/kg over 3 h causes only small increments of acid output or serum gastrin levels in normal subjects. In ZE patients serum gastrin levels increase two- to three-fold and gastric acid output approaches the levels obtained during a maximal response to pentagastrin or histamine.

Tests with limited clinical application

Gastric emptying
Tests are seldom of much use clinically except for the diagnosis of pyloric stenosis; then stomach emptying during a barium meal is usually the guide. Barium is

unphysiological for research purposes and other tests use liquid meals containing dyes like phenol red but require intubation which may affect the result. Isotopic labelling of a solid meal with technetium or chromium can also be used but further research validation is necessary before their clinical value can be assessed.

Bile reflux

Reflux of bile into the stomach may be of aetiological significance in gastric and oesophageal pathology. Scintigraphy with Tc-HIDA as a bile marker may be used to monitor bile reflux. The position of the stomach is usually marked by scanning a Tc-labelled drink.

Non-endoscopic intubation of the upper gastrointestinal tract

The passage of various types of nasogastric, duodenal and intestinal tubes is necessary for certain diagnostic procedures (Table 5.1). Intubation is less unpleasant for the patient when done by an experienced person who has an understanding and confident approach. Cooperation of the patient is essential, so he must be told about the object and what will happen beforehand; often the patient reaches the laboratory knowing virtually nothing about it.

Equipment and connections must first be checked. In certain circumstances the

Table 5.1. Indications for non-endoscopic intubation of the upper gastrointestinal tract.

Oesophagus
    pH monitoring
    Motility studies
    Dilatation of strictures
    Tamponade of bleeding varices (Sengstaken tube Fig. 14.4)
Stomach
    Washout of gastric contents after deliberate or accidental poisoning (wide bore tube)
    Diagnostic aspiration to detect and monitor bleeding
    Acid secretion studies
    To obtain culture material for tuberculosis
Duodenal and gastric
    Decompression of intestinal obstruction e.g. ileus after laparotomy
    Aspiration for parasites e.g. hookworm, strongyloides
    Pancreatic function tests
    Bile collection to test lithogenicity
Small bowel
    Instillation of dilute barium for a small bowel enema X-ray
    Mucosal biopsy
    String test or tube aspiration for detection of bacterial overgrowth and ova, cysts or
        parasites e.g. strongyloides, giardia
    Segmental perfusion studies

pharynx can be anaesthetized by lozenge or spray. Tubes are best passed with the patient sitting up and the head slightly forward as this makes swallowing easier and guides the tube into the oesophagus. Most patients prefer the tube going through the mouth, but passage through the nose is indicated when the patient is unconscious, cannot coordinate swallowing or refuses to open his mouth.

To pass the tube through the nose, first lubricate the nose with lignocaine jelly and lubricate the tube. Sit the patient up and introduce the tube along the floor of the nose. Resistance may be felt when the tube reaches the naso-pharynx; the patient is then asked to swallow (with water if this is not contraindicated), and the tube is advanced. It should pass down the oesophagus without resistance and the gastro-oesophageal junction is reached at about 40 cm.

The risk of passing a nasogastric tube is minimal. If it enters a bronchus coughing or cyanosis may occur but this is usually quickly recognized and can be confirmed by holding the end of the tube against the cheek or ear to feel if air is being exhaled or the position of the tube in the stomach confirmed by auscultating over the stomach for a bubbling sound during injection of 2–3 ml of air and testing any aspirated material for acidity. Prolonged intubation produces a sore throat, and carries the risk of oesophagitis leading to stricture formation.

For acid secretion the position of the tube in the stomach is checked by giving the patient 20 ml water to drink after passing the tube 50–60 cm; this is aspirated and the tube withdrawn 2.5 cm, and the manoeuvre repeated—and continued until the highest level at which water can be aspirated is found and the tube taped (preferably on to the cheek) in position. For more complex positioning, e.g. for pancreatic function tests or jejunal biopsy, it is necessary to check with an X-ray image intensifier that the radio-opaque tube has the correct configuration. When continuous aspiration is needed during an investigation the strength of suction applied should be controlled at low levels and ideally alternated with short periods of insufflation to prevent the mucosa being sucked into the tube due to excessive sustained negative pressure.

Applied negative pressure should not exceed 7 mmHg relative to atmospheric pressure. Nurses and other assistants must be warned against aggressive suction on a syringe. Minimal suction drains gastroduodenal contents easily, provided the tube is correctly positioned and there is fluid present. Strong suction merely produces a row of circular bruises in the mucosa corresponding to the holes in the tube.

Chapter 6
The Liver, Biliary System and Pancreas

Although it is common parlance to describe various estimations of blood chemistry, including bilirubin, transaminase and alkaline phosphatase (Chapter 4), as liver function tests, in truth they generally tell one little or nothing about the way the liver is functioning. Rather they reflect some aspect of liver dysfunction or injury, and being non-specific may even be deranged when the liver is perfectly normal. Nevertheless they do focus one's attention on the liver and in conjunction with urine testing (page 136) give some clue to the nature of the problem.

The working of the liver is often well reflected by its ability to synthesize protein. Factor VII and other components of the blood's coagulation system have a half-life of only a few hours, so that *prolongation of the prothrombin time* is about the best index of the severity of liver damage in the early stages. *Serum albumin* has a much longer half-life so that hypoalbuminaemia due to poor liver function implies a longer duration of disease.

Serum bile acids
Measurement of *serum bile acids* provides a sensitive and specific test of liver function, but its clinical advantages over more traditional methods is unproven. Bile acids undergo an enterohepatic circulation (Fig. 6.1) which involves a highly efficient first-pass extraction from the portal bloodstream by the liver. A small drop in hepatic efficiency causes a proportionately much higher change in the amount of bile acids entering the systemic circulation. For example, a fall from 95 to 90% extraction for a conjugated primary bile acid will lead to a doubling (or 100% increase!) in the entry of that bile acid into the systemic circulation. Commonly serum bile acids are estimated in peripheral blood taken 2 h after a fatty meal. The meal ensures gallbladder contraction and delivers a large bolus of bile acids to the liver via the portal vein following their intestinal reabsorption. It is currently the most readily available bile acid test for clinical application.

Imaging techniques used routinely

Ultrasound
This is simple, cheap and safe. Its reliability depends to a large extent on the operator. In experienced hands it is highly reliable (greater than 90% accuracy) in detecting dilated bile ducts. It is therefore employed routinely in investigating *cholestatic jaundice* (Fig. 6.2.). When dilated bile ducts are shown (Fig. 6.3) the patients should be allocated theatre time for operative treatment but have a

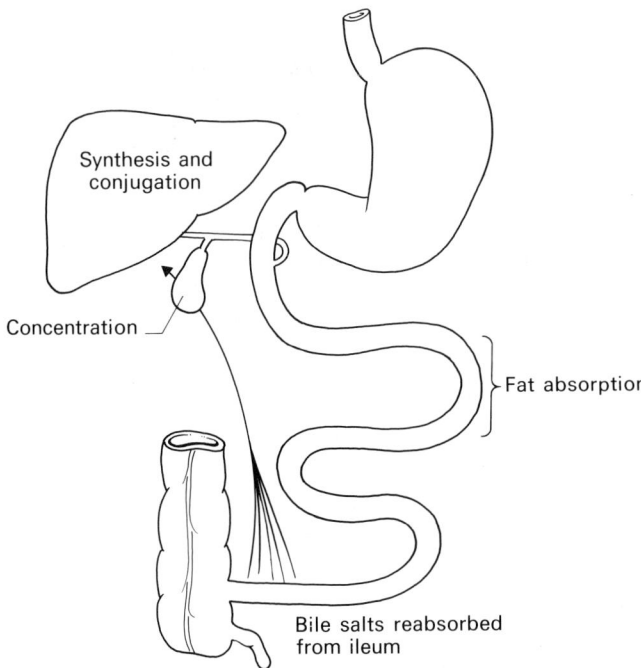

Fig. 6.1. The enterohepatic circulation. Bile acids are normally conserved within the enterohepatic circulation, about 95% being reabsorbed from the intestine. The total amount of bile acids within the body, known as the bile acid pool, circulates from six to ten times daily.

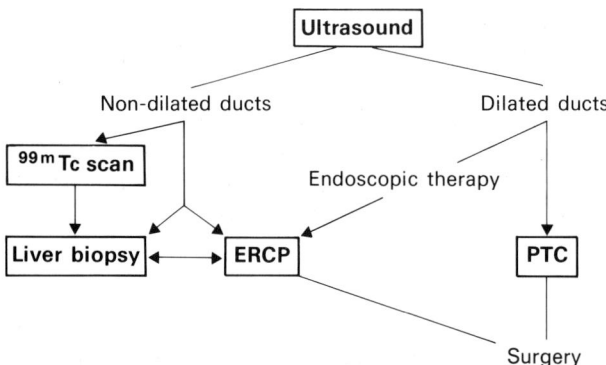

Fig. 6.2. Sequence of possible investigations in a patient with unexplained cholestatic jaundice. The flow chart shows a logical approach to the diagnosis of jaundice when an obstructive cause is possible.

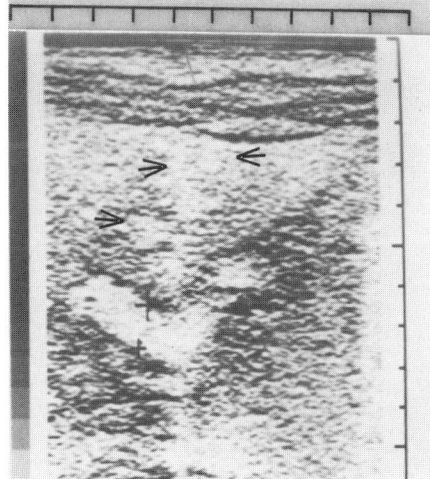

Fig. 6.3. Ultrasound examination of the liver. Dilated bile ducts are shown within the liver confirming that biliary obstruction is the likely cause of jaundice in this patient.

percutaneous transhepatic cholangiogram (PTC) prior to this to (a) confirm that the ducts are dilated and (b) give the surgeon extra information regarding the site and nature of the obstructing lesion. Ultrasound is also used to distinguish solid and cystic masses in the liver and can be used to guide needles precisely to intrahepatic lesions for biopsy or aspiration (e.g. drainage of an abscess cavity). For suspected *pancreatic disease* the technique is often less successful (about 50%). Bowel gas often interferes with the image and the patient must fast before imaging is attempted. When successful, ultrasound may reliably diagnose cysts in the pancreas, and is useful in monitoring changes in the size of pancreatic pseudocysts. Abnormal solid masses within the pancreas can also be detected, and the pattern of echoes may distinguish chronic pancreatitis from carcinoma with moderate reliability. Ultrasound may be used to guide a fine needle tip into the pancreatic mass to aspirate material for cytology. This technique represents a major advance in confirming the diagnosis of pancreatic cancer without laparotomy.

Ultrasound is efficient, and probably more sensitive than oral cholecystography at demonstrating *gallstones* within the gallbladder (Fig. 6.4). However, it is poor at detecting gallstones within the common bile duct, especially in its lower part.

Scintigraphic scanning

^{99m}Tc—*Technetium (tin or sulphur) colloid scan.* Following intravenous injection of ^{99m}Tc colloid, radioactivity is rapidly concentrated within the normal liver as a result of its removal by reticuloendothelial cells. A gamma camera image normally shows a homogenous dark image representing a normal-sized liver and spleen (Fig. 6.5a). Two major categories of abnormality are seen: (a) one or more focal filling

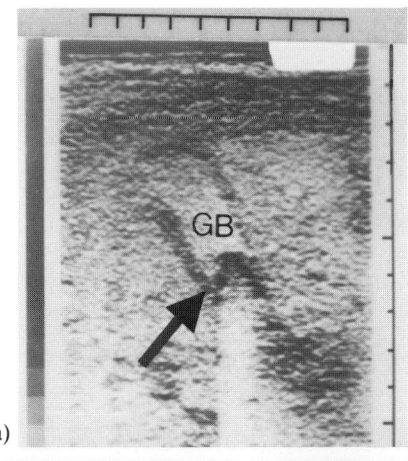

(a)

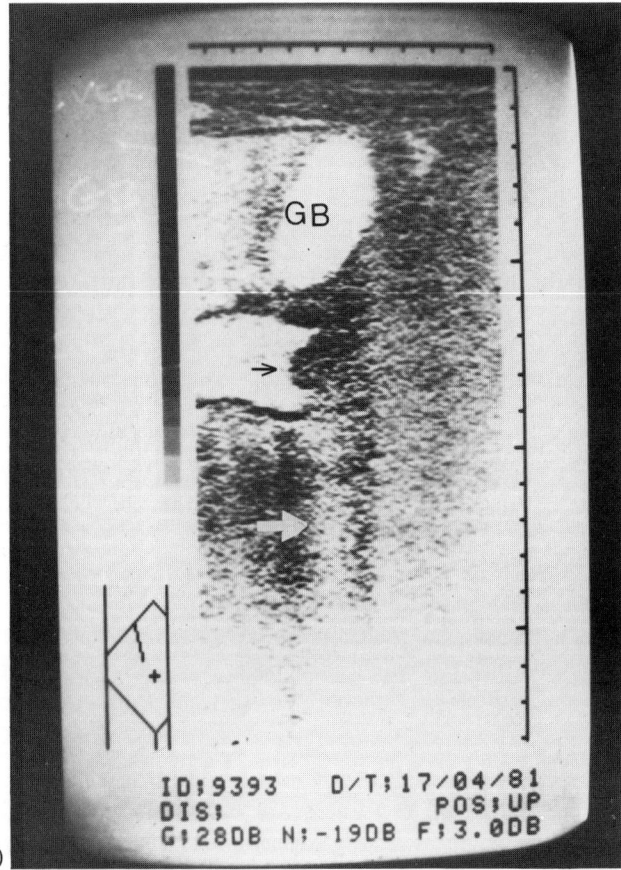

(b)

Fig. 6.4. Ultrasound demonstration of gallstones. (a) A gallstone (arrow) is shown within the gallbladder (GB). The stone is highly reflective and casts an acoustic shadow. (b) A rounded filling defect (black arrow) is shown within a dilated common bile duct and casts an acoustic shadow (white arrow). A part of the gallbladder (GB) is also visible.

defects within the liver, which may as a result be enlarged (Fig. 6.5b). This image is produced by space-occupying lesions, e.g. tumours, cysts or abscesses, and (b) diffuse decrease in density of the liver image due to generalized parenchymal disease. This is the usual finding in cirrhosis, when in addition the splenic image is often enlarged and porto-systemic shunting is apparent from uptake of colloid in the bone marrow of the spine (Fig. 6.5c). In severe alcoholic hepatitis there is, typically, almost no uptake of Tc colloid by the liver, and virtual absence of a liver image on a scan should suggest the diagnosis. Another characteristic though rare appearance is of selective uptake by an enlarged caudate lobe in the Budd–Chiari syndrome.

^{99m}Tc–*HIDA scan.* ^{99m}Tc–HIDA (a derivative of iminodiacetic acid) is normally excreted rapidly in bile. A clear image of the liver, bile ducts and gallbladder are obtained in rapid succession and progression of the ^{99m}Tc-HIDA to the bowel is seen. The test is useful for confirming gallbladder disease, such as acute cholecystitis. Non-opacification of the gallbladder is extremely strong evidence in favour of gallbladder disease (Fig. 6.6). HIDA scanning is of doubtful value in screening for extrahepatic biliary obstruction unless it is complete. Nevertheless it may be helpful in excluding mechanical obstruction in patients with hepato-jejunostomy, recent liver transplantation and other similar problems where more invasive forms of cholangiography are unsuitable. It is now the procedure of choice for separating neonatal hepatitis from extrahepatic biliary atresia.

Scanning methods used occasionally or rarely

^{75}Se-*selenomethionine scan.* A 'cold' area on ^{99m}Tc–sulphur colloid scan which appears 'hot' on ^{75}Se scanning is highly suggestive of a primary hepatocellular carcinoma. The radiolabelled amino acid is concentrated in tissues which are rapidly synthesizing new proteins including the pancreas. It is now seldom, if ever, used for imaging the *pancreas.* A normal pancreatic image is strong presumptive evidence that there is no significant pancreatic pathology, but the test involves a substantial dose of irradiation and false positive results are common. The test is also not applicable to many patients such as diabetics and post-gastrectomy patients, in whom a sensitive non-invasive pancreatic test is most desirable.

^{67}Ga–*gallium scan.* Radioactive gallium is concentrated in areas of acute inflammation such as a liver abscess and also, not infrequently, by primary liver cancer. The scan may be used for localizing an infection in a patient with pyrexia of unknown origin and a neutrophilia. Because the test is dependent on neutrophil migration there has to be a delay of 48–72 h between the Ga injection and scanning.

^{131}I-*Rose Bengal.* Like gallium this agent is concentrated within primary liver cancer and may be used following a ^{99m}Tc scan. A filling defect on the ^{99m}Tc scan

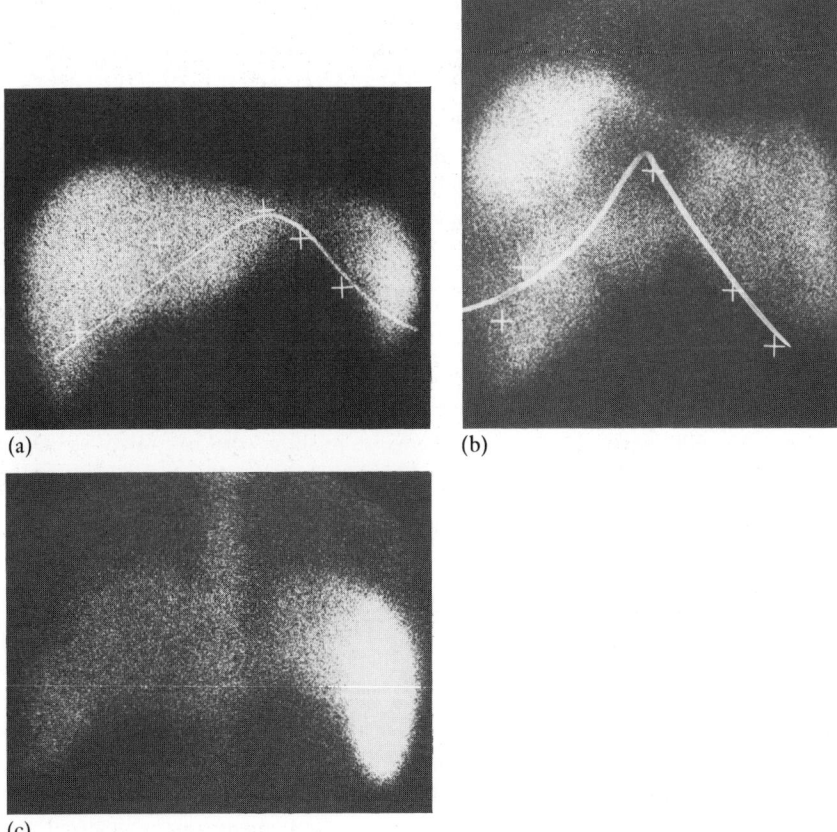

(a)

(b)

(c)

Fig. 6.5. Liver scanning with ^{99m}Tc colloid. (a) Normal appearance of liver and spleen. The costal margin has been marked in with a line and crosses for reference. (b) A space-occupying lesion is apparent in the midline as a filling defect within the liver. (c) There is poor uptake throughout the liver with spillover of the scintigraphic material into the bone marrow of the vertebral column and an enlarged spleen. This appearance is typical of cirrhosis with portal hypertension.

corresponding with an area in which Ga or Rose Bengal are concentrated is strong presumptive evidence for the diagnosis of primary liver cancer. It has also been used in neonatal jaundice when faecal excretion of ^{131}I-Rose Bengal was monitored for excluding biliary atresia. Because of the difficulties involved in separating faecal specimens from urine in neonates the test has largely been superseded by the ^{99m}Tc-HIDA scan for this purpose.

Computerized axial tomography (CAT scanning)
This is rarely indicated in investigating jaundice. It is not as effective as ultrasound

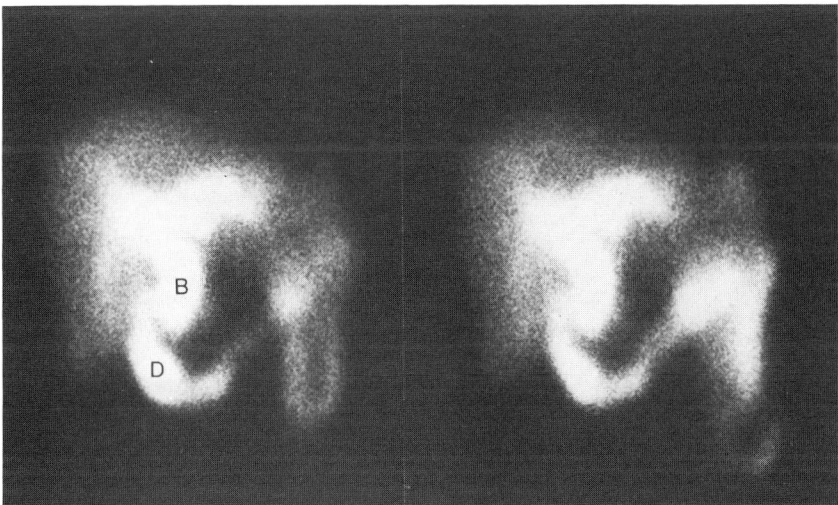

Fig. 6.6. HIDA Scan. ^{99m}Tc HIDA has been used to investigate the biliary tract.
Although the outline of the liver, bile duct (B) and duodenum (D) is clearly seen there has
been no filling of the gallbladder indicating disease of the gallbladder. The two scans were
taken 2 min apart, and it can be seen that more scintigraphic material has entered the
small intestine during that time.

for demonstrating dilated bile ducts, is also more expensive and involves
X-irradiation of the patient. Its use is best reserved for occasional puzzling cases of
hepatomegaly, for detecting liver involvement in lymphoproliferative disorders,
and of intrahepatic space-occupying lesions such as tumour, abscess or hydatid
disease (Fig. 6.7). Tumours as small as 1.5–2.0 cm diameter can be detected and
distinguished from cysts. It is occasionally helpful in diffuse disease of the liver such
as haemochromatosis where the density is increased or in fatty infiltration where
density is reduced but simpler methods usually suffice.

Pancreatic lumps of 3 cm or more can be detected though it is not always easy to
distinguish neoplasia from inflammatory disease. Diffuse enlargement, calcification
and duct dilatation can all be shown. (Fig. 6.8).

Computerized axial tomography scanning is of little use in finding masses inside
the alimentary tract, but it can help in assessing patients with cancer of the
oesophagus or rectum, because the extraluminal extent of the mass can be seen
better than with other methods. It is invaluable in spotting enlarged para-aortic and
other lymph nodes in suspected lymphoproliferative disorders.

Nuclear magnetic resonance (NMR)
This relatively new imaging technique produces images comparable to those
produced by CAT scanning. Nuclear magnetic resonance depends upon magnetic
fields and radiofrequency pulses, and may distinguish between tissues which are in

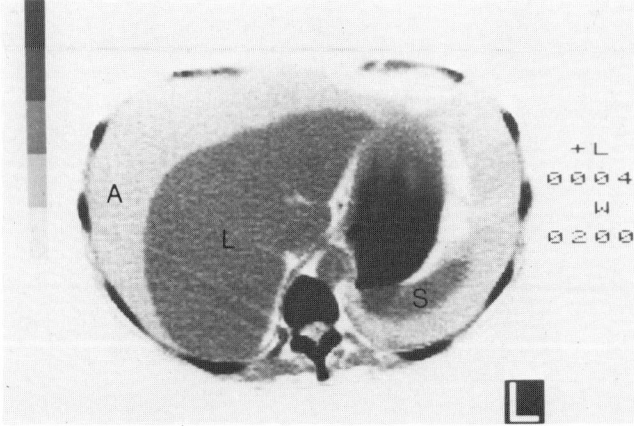

Fig. 6.7. CAT scan to demonstrate the liver. The liver (L) and spleen (S) are clearly shown in a patient with ascites (A).

differing states of metabolism (e.g. due to regional ischaemia) though they are indistinguishable by CAT scanning which depends on their radiodensity.

Radiology

Oral cholecystography
Usually on the evening before the examination, the patient swallows a radiodense iodine-containing material which is normally well absorbed and then excreted in bile. X-rays are taken of the gallbladder on the following morning before breakfast and again after a fatty meal. In non-jaundiced patients this is successful in providing an image of the gallbladder in more than 90%. If no image is seen, the attempt may be repeated giving a double dose of the cholecystographic material. Filling defects within the gallbladder can be shown to be mobile (stones) by taking films in the prone and upright position (Fig. 6.9). Jaundice is an absolute contraindication to oral cholecystography since competition for biliary excretion between accumulated bilirubin and cholecystographic agent prevents any possibility of the gallbladder filling.

Intravenous cholangiography
This technique is seldom required since the advent of ERCP and PTC. It involves intravenous infusion of a radiodense iodine-containing substance which is concentrated in bile. X-rays including tomography of the bile duct are taken. The technique does not work in jaundiced patients for the same reasons given for oral cholecystography. It may still be useful in patients with normal liver function tests and persistent pain after cholecystectomy in whom ultrasonography has not

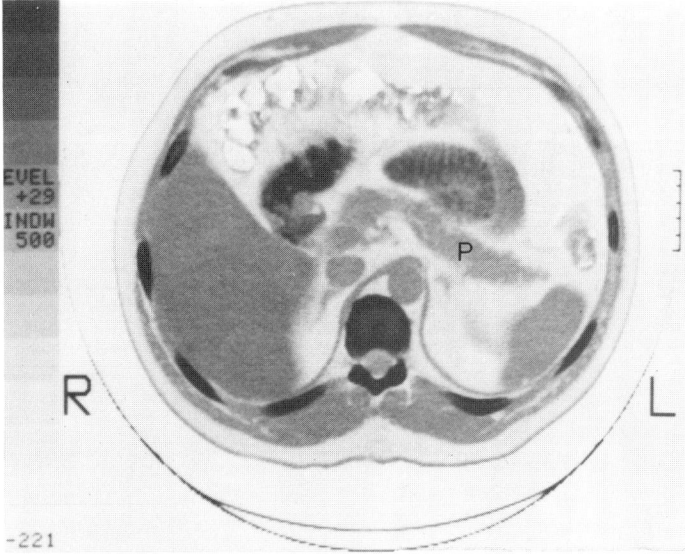

Fig. 6.8. CAT scan to demonstrate the pancreas. The body and tail of the pancreas (P) are clearly identifiable.

revealed a residual gallstone, but significant doubt remains. Infusions of the dye are occasionally associated with anaphylaxis.

Percutaneous transhepatic cholangiography (PTC)
PTC permits cholangiography in jaundiced patients in whom the intravenous technique is sure to fail. It is almost 100% successful if ultrasound has shown dilated ducts, but less so when bile ducts are not dilated. PTC is contraindicated if there is a prolonged prothrombin time, thrombocytopenia or a prolonged bleeding time. Recent cholangitis increases the risk of septicaemia following PTC which is therefore best avoided. Prophylactic antibiotic should be given routinely, and is essential in patients with a previous history of cholangitis.

Technique. PTC is performed under local anaesthetic. It requires radiological facilities for screening and taking X-ray pictures. With the patient lying flat on his back, a narrow stainless steel needle is inserted into the liver in the mid-axillary line and advanced as far as the spine, bisecting an imaginary line joining the dome of the diaphragm to the air bubble visible within the duodenal cap. Contrast is injected continuously as the needle is withdrawn and can be seen to enter radicles of the hepatic artery, portal vein, hepatic vein and biliary system and at a later stage the lymphatic system opacifies. The needle's position is maintained once a biliary radicle is opacified, and sufficient contrast to outline the biliary system is injected (Fig. 6.10).

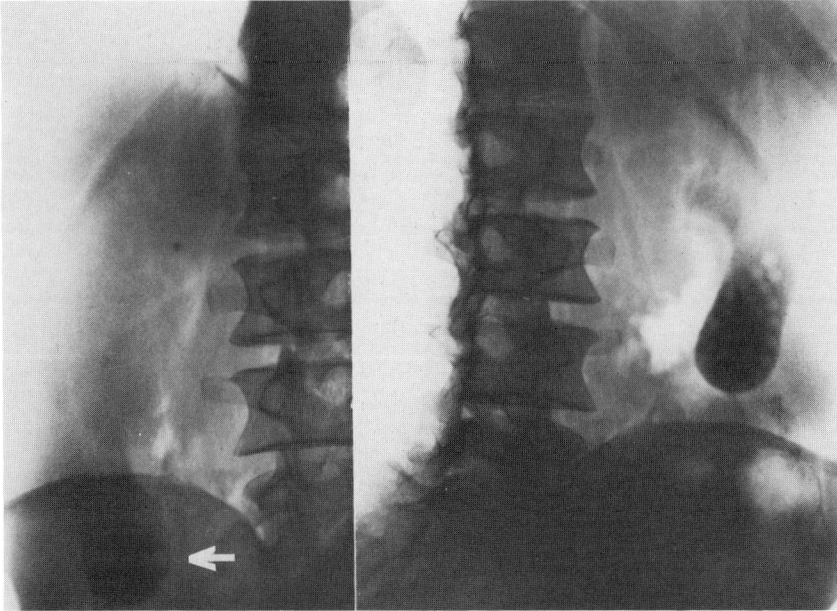

Fig. 6.9. Oral cholecystogram showing gallstones. Multiple radiolucent defects can be seen within the gallbladder in the erect position (on the left) and in the view taken with the patient lying on her side (right). Multiple small radiolucent stones which float as a layer in the erect position as shown here (arrow) are suitable for attempted dissolution therapy.

Complications. Bleeding into the peritoneum or intrahepatic haematoma; cholangitis with septicaemia. Provided the contraindications and precautions listed above are observed the complication rate is very low. Nevertheless it is advisable to time PTC to precede surgical intervention by as short a time as reasonable.

Endoscopic retrograde cholangiopancreatography (ERCP) (Fig. 6.11)
The endoscope is used to cannulate the papilla of Vater in the second part of the duodenum. This usually gives access to both the bile and pancreatic duct. Occasionally the major papilla allows cannulation of the bile duct and ventral pancreas only; then the main pancreatic duct can only be outlined via the accessory papilla.

Indications for retrograde cholangiography. These can be any of the following:
1 Diagnosis of cholestatic jaundice.
2 As a prelude to therapeutic procedures e.g. endoscopic papillotomy.
3 Cholangiography in patients allergic to contrast materials.
4 Investigation of post-cholecystectomy pain.

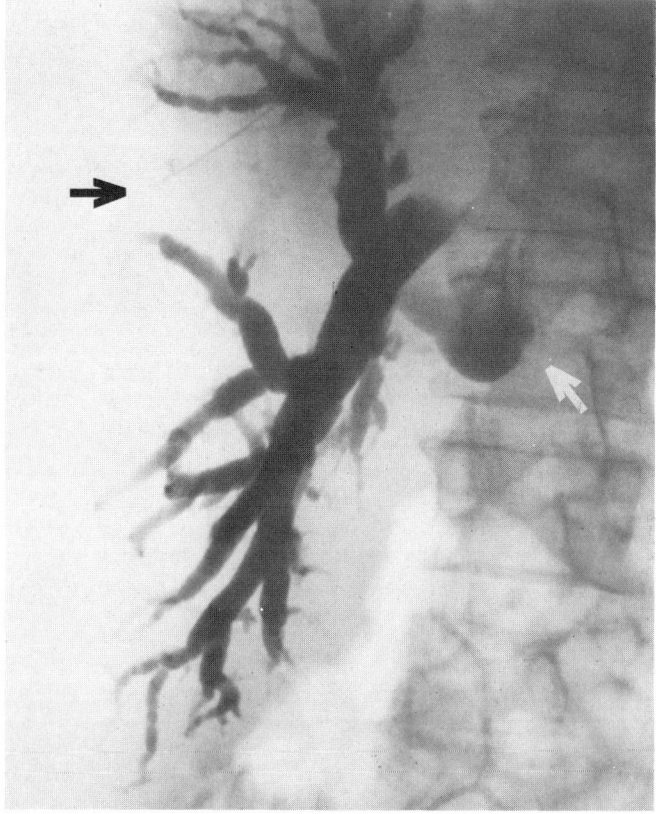

Fig. 6.10. Percutaneous cholangiogram. The 'skinny needle' (black arrow) has been inserted into the liver percutaneously. Contrast has been injected to outline the biliary tree and has shown a blocked common hepatic duct (white arrow). This was later shown to be caused by a cholangiocarcinoma.

Indications for pancreatography (Fig. 6.12). These can be any of the following:

1   To detect the presence of pancreatic disease.

2   To outline the pancreatic duct when a precise knowledge of its anatomy is needed when considering surgery.

3   To permit histological or cytological diagnosis of malignancy in patients with a known mass in the pancreas. Pancreatic juice is aspirated after the intravenous injection of the hormone secretin and the secretions are immediately processed to prevent degradation of the cytological material.

Complications. Infection is a very serious, potentially fatal complication of ERCP, and usually occurs after injecting contrast into a poorly draining, obstructed duct

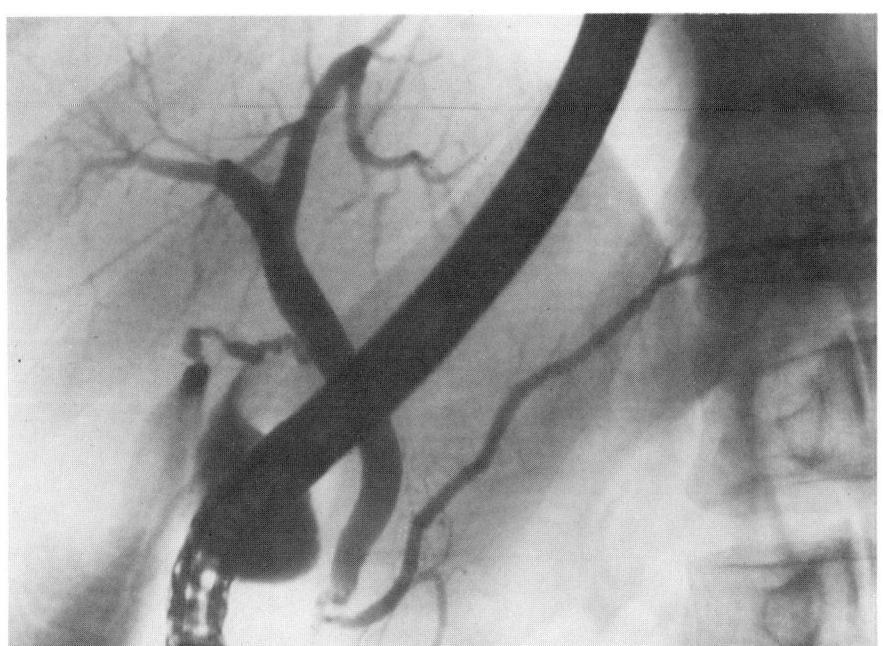

(a)

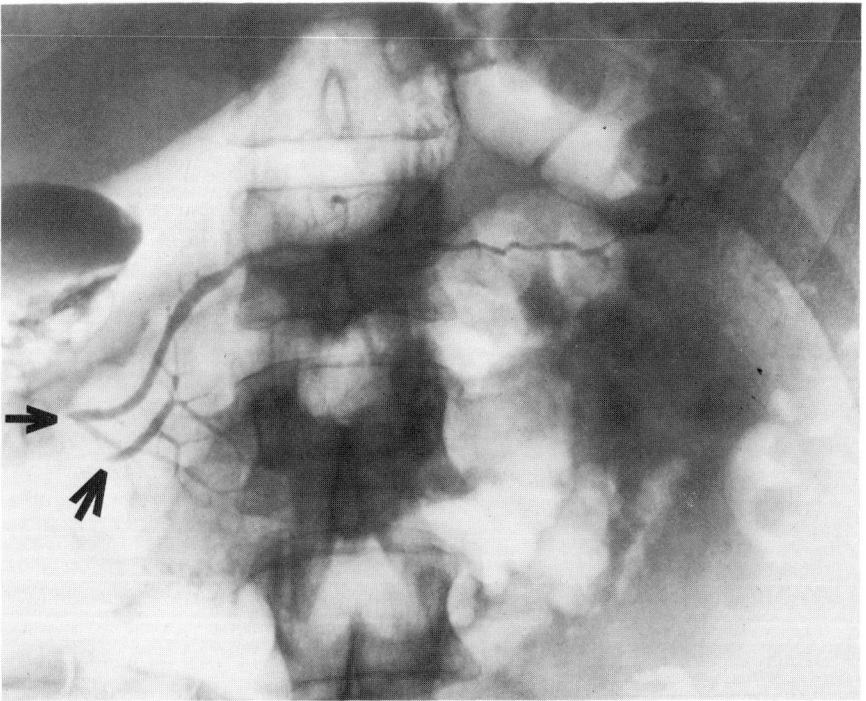

(b)

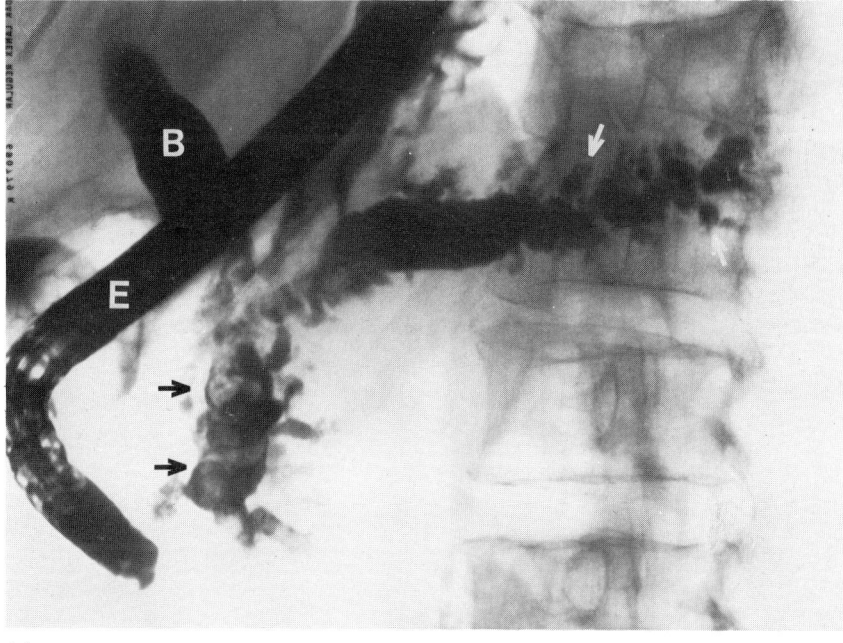

(c)

Fig. 6.11. ERCP. (a) This shows the normal anatomy of the biliary system with filling of the intra- and extrahepatic bile ducts as well as the gallbladder. (b) This shows a normal variant pancreatogram obtained by injecting into both the papilla of Vater and accessory papilla within the duodenum. Failure of fusion of embryologically distinct portions of the pancreas has kept the short ventral duct (lower arrow) and the long dorsal duct (upper arrow) separate. (c) A grossly abnormal pancreatogram has been shown by ERCP. The endoscope (E) is still present in the duodenum. The bile duct (B) is also shown. Several filling defects are present within the pancreatic duct (black arrows) and the main duct and its side branches (white arrows) are markedly dilated.

system. So a previously diagnosed pancreatic pseudocyst constitutes an almost absolute contraindication to ERCP.

Portal venography
The portal vein may be opacified directly by injection either into the spleen (Fig. 6.13) or via the percutaneous transhepatic route. This provides more detailed visualization of the portal venous system and its collateral channels than during the venous phase of superior mesenteric arteriography. Splenic pulp or portal venous

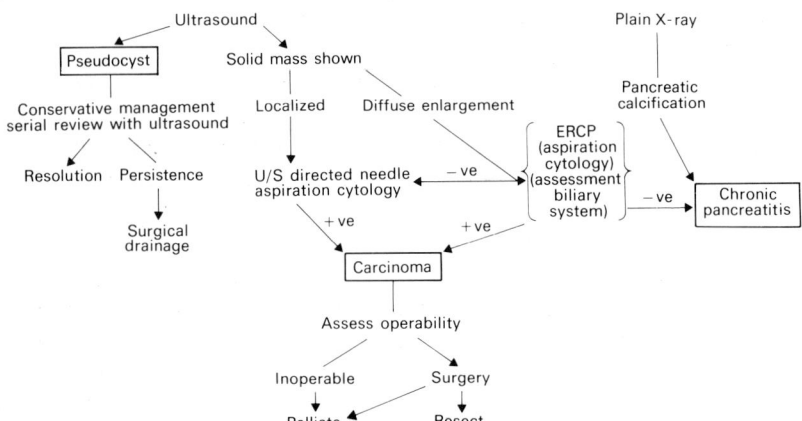

Fig. 6.12. Imaging techniques in pancreatic investigation and treatment. A logical sequence of tests is suggested to arrive at a diagnosis of pancreatic disease.

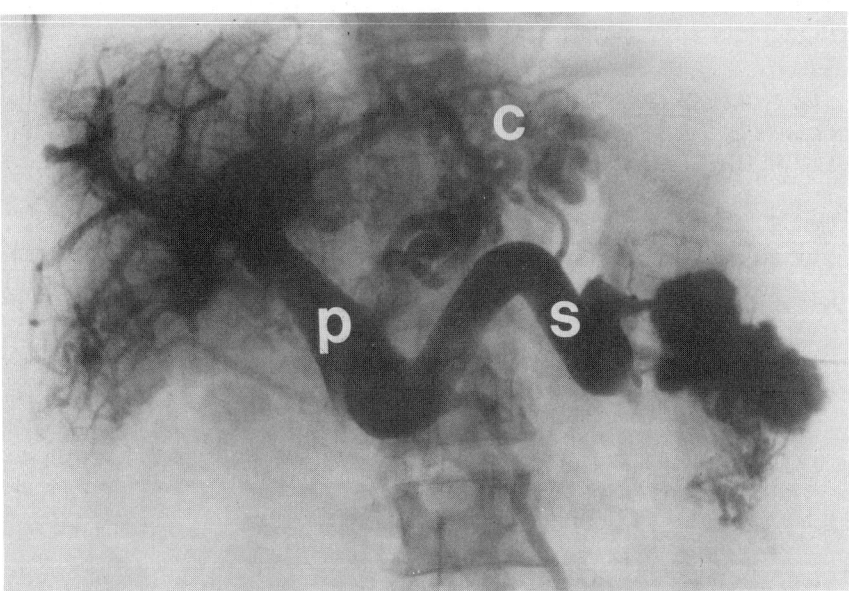

Fig. 6.13. Portal venography. Contrast has been injected into the spleen via a needle introduced percutaneously. Contrast is seen to flow via the splenic (S) and portal (P) veins towards the liver. Collateral veins (C) are seen flowing towards oesophagogastric varices.

pressure can be measured directly at the time by connecting the needle to a pressure manometer.

Transhepatic portal vein catheterization provides an approach for the sclerosis of veins which are flowing towards bleeding varices. The transhepatic approach also permits blood sampling from multiple sites within the portal, splenic and mesenteric veins in an attempt to localize endocrine tumours, e.g. gastrinoma or insulinoma.

Hepatic venography

A catheter is passed via a peripheral vein (usually brachial or femoral; rarely jugular) into the hepatic vein. It is particularly useful in assessing post-sinusoidal portal hypertension (Budd–Chiari syndrome) but also permits measurement of the wedged hepatic venous pressure (WHVP) which correlates closely with portal vein pressure in cirrhosis. In pre-sinusoidal portal hypertension portal pressure exceeds WHVP. The catheter is pushed until it becomes firmly lodged (wedged) within the liver substance or the hepatic vein can be occluded by a balloon. Because flow is arrested in that tributary of the hepatic vein the pressure measured is the same as that on the portal side of the liver. (No flow ≡ no fall in pressure.) The catheter is then connected to a manometric pressure measuring device to read WHVP and then withdrawn a little to give free hepatic vein pressure (FHVP). The difference between these two measurements (WHVP–FHVP) is the pressure gradient across the liver. Pressure is also measured in the inferior vena cava (IVC) at the level of the hepatic·vein and below the level of the liver. In the Budd–Chiari syndrome enlargement of the caudate lobe often constricts the IVC so that venous pressure is high below that level. Detection is important since any attempt to reduce portal pressure by a side-to-side porto-caval shunt into this high pressure portion of the IVC will probably be unsuccessful.

Hepatic arteriography

This is performed by selective catheterization of the hepatic artery or by injection into the coeliac axis. It is most useful for investigating tumours and other space-occupying lesions when assessing operability. In a patient with primary liver cancer it is of vital importance to know if the tumour is confined to either the right or left lobe, in which case it is potentially curable by partial hepatectomy (Fig. 6.14).

On occasions, following selective arteriography to show tumour circulation, embolization of the artery may be performed to reduce tumour bulk by ischaemic necrosis. This may also reduce symptoms due to an incurable malignancy e.g. carcinoid metastases.

Superior mesenteric arteriography

The venous phase of splenic or superior mesenteric arteriography gives information regarding the patency of the portal vein (Fig. 8.14b). The superior mesenteric artery frequently supplies a part of the liver, as a congenital anomaly.

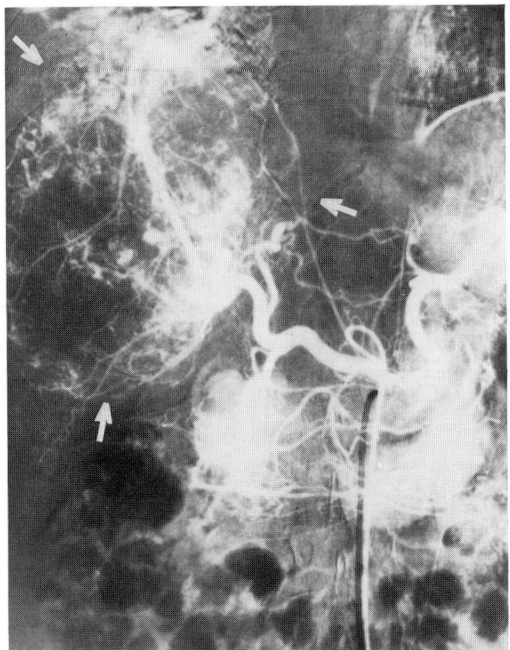

(a)

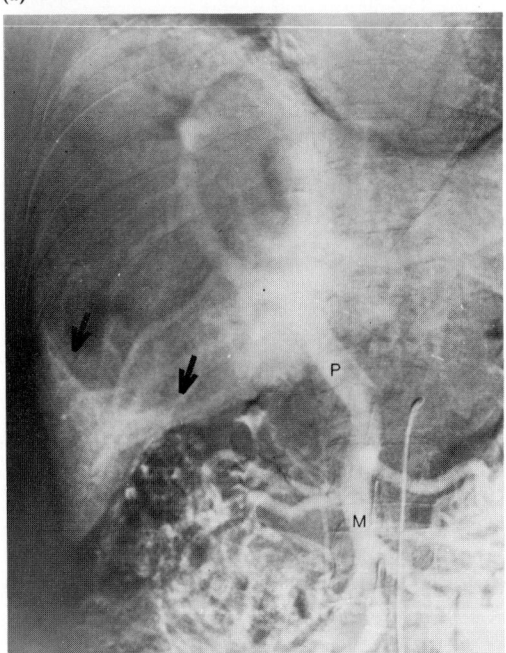

(b)

Liver biopsy

Percutaneous needle liver biopsy is frequently performed when investigating unknown liver disease and can also be helpful for monitoring the progress of chronic liver disease.

You should anticipate the uses for which a biopsy may be required. Frequently the entire biopsy is fixed for (a) histology, but this is inappropriate if tissue is required for (b) bacteriological culture e.g. in a patient with fever of unknown origin, (c) chemical analysis (e.g., of Cu, Fe in storage diseases) or of enzymes in hereditary metabolic disorders, or (d) other occasional requirements e.g. electron-microscopy.

Check that coagulation is within normal limits; prothrombin time and a platelet count are the minimum. The following are contraindications:

1 Bleeding tendency.
2 Vascular hepatic lesions, e.g. haemangioma.
3 Hydatid disease.

If a biopsy is essential and the coagulation state is unsatisfactory despite parenteral vitamin K therapy, the risk of a biopsy by the percutaneous route after infusion of fresh frozen plasma and platelets may be acceptable. Alternatively the biopsy may be done internally by a transjugular approach. The latter is also preferred when there is a strong indication for liver biopsy in the presence of much ascites.

Technique (Fig. 6.15)

The patient is put at ease whilst practising breath-holding after maximal expiration. An entry point over liver dullness in an intercostal space just anterior to the mid-axillary line is marked. Lignocaine hydrochloride 1% is infiltrated into the skin and along the biopsy route. The skin is punctured by a narrow sharp scalpel blade. The biopsy needle is introduced until the needle is fixed in the diaphragm when there is paradoxical upward movement of the doctor's hands as the diaphragm descends during inspiration. The patient stops breathing after full expiration during the remainder of the biopsy manoeuvre.

Menghini technique

The needle is evacuated by injecting saline; it is then plunged into the liver

---

Fig. 6.14. (*opposite*) Hepatic arteriography. This patient had a histologically proven primary liver cancer and was being investigated during consideration for surgical treatment. The coeliac axis angiogram (a) shows a profuse, disorganized tumour circulation (arrows) derived from the hepatic artery, (b) the late venous phase of a superior mesenteric arteriogram in the same patient shows normal filling of the superior mesenteric vein (M) and portal vein (P). The tumour is now apparent only as a filling defect surrounded by liver which show a normal sinusoidal pattern (arrows). This examination is typical of most liver tumours which derive their blood supply from the hepatic artery but not the portal vein. The increased flow which occurs with primary liver cancer often produces an audible bruit.

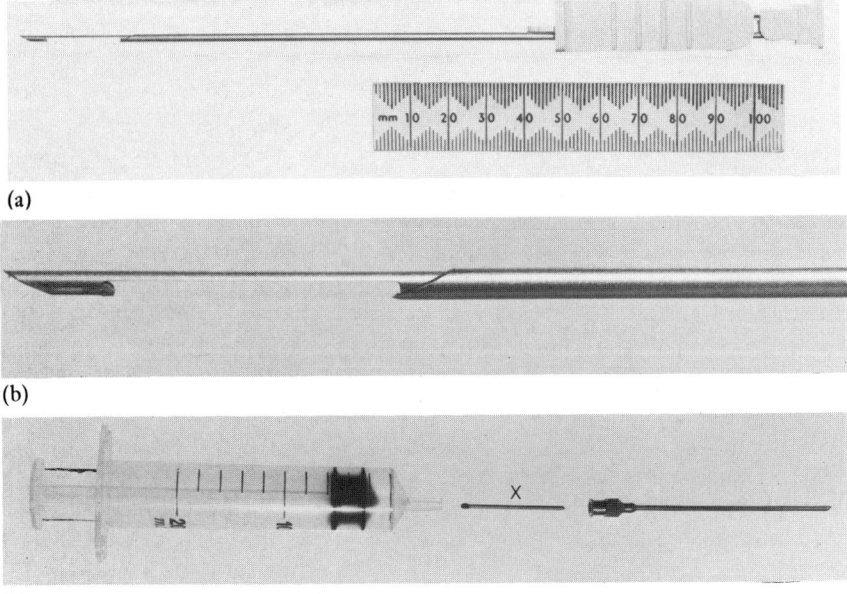

(a)

(b)

(c)

Fig. 6.15. Liver biopsy. Two percutaneous liver biopsy needles are shown. The Trucut needle (a) has a bevelled trocar (b). Withdrawal and advancement of the outer cutting sheath within the liver provides a core of liver tissue along the bevelled section. The Menghini needle (c) depends upon suction being applied via a syringe as the needle is plunged into the liver and during its withdrawal. The insert (x) must be inserted into the needle prior to the procedure in order to prevent disintegration of the biopsy due to suction.

substance whilst suction is applied to the syringe and maintained during its withdrawal.

Tests which quantitate aspects of liver function

The following tests are examples of true liver function tests and, as such, are useful for research into liver disease. Although rarely used clinically, they may, by indicating the amount of functional liver tissue, provide a useful prognostic indication and thus influence patient selection for certain forms of therapy.

[14]C-aminopyrine breath test. This test is probably the best currently available for estimating functional liver cell mass in jaundiced patients. It is relatively easy to perform and analyse. The patient ingests 1.5 μCi ^{14}C-aminopyrine and breath CO_2 is collected and analysed as described on page 99. ^{14}C-methyl groups of aminopyrine are metabolized to [14]CO_2 in the hepatic microsomes, and low rates of [14]CO_2 production have been shown to indicate a poor prognosis in alcoholic liver disease and following paracetamol self-poisoning.

Bromsulphthalein excretion. Bromsulphthalein (BSP) is extracted by the liver which conjugates it to glutathione and then excretes it in bile. BSP competes with bilirubin for uptake into the hepatocyte so that it is only helpful diagnostically in patients with a normal serum bilirubin and when jaundice is due to the rare Dubin–Johnson syndrome.

(i) *Bolus injection*: In normal subjects less than 5% of the injected dose (5 mg/kg b.w.) remains in the circulation after 45 min but this retained fraction is increased in most forms of liver disease. Though it has been largely superseded by the estimation of serum bile acids, BSP clearance remains a sensitive index of liver dysfunction. In the Dubin–Johnson syndrome a specific abnormality is found; initial clearance is normal so that the 45 min value is unremarkable but there is a later rise in blood levels at 90 and 120 min due to reflux of the bromsulphthalein–glutathione conjugate into blood.

(ii) *Infusion test*: Continuous intravenous infusion of BSP and frequent blood sampling permit estimation of hepatic storage capacity and transport maximum (Tm). The BSP Tm is probably one of the best tests of liver functional capacity but is difficult and therefore seldom used (note that anaphylactoid reactions to BSP may occur so that intravenous hydrocortisone should always be at hand when BSP is being administered).

Galactose elimination test. The liver alone removes galactose from the blood. The rate of fall of serum galactose concentration after a load therefore depends on how much liver there is and how well it is working.

Laparoscopy

Laparoscopy permits views of the liver and gallbladder as well as the peritoneum, spleen and other intra-abdominal organs. Retroperitoneal organs such as the pancreas are only partially seen with some difficulty. The procedure is particularly useful in assessing malignancy because dissemination to the liver or peritoneum can be seen, and the patient can be spared a futile laparotomy with its accompanying morbidity. Primary liver cancer can be assessed for its operability. Biopsy of focal liver lesions can be guided under direct vision. Cirrhosis of the liver can usually be appreciated by its macroscopic appearance and biopsy during laparoscopy generally avoids the misdiagnosis due to sampling error which occurs with blind percutaneous biopsy.

Abdominal paracentesis

A diagnostic tap for aspirating ascites is performed with a sterile hypodermic needle and syringe by inserting the needle through the anterior abdominal wall at a point which is dull to percussion due to fluid. The patient first empties his bladder and then lies supine while fluid is aspirated from either iliac fossa or from the midline below the umbilicus. If a little fluid only is present aspiration may only be possible through a peri-umbilical approach with the patient kneeling on 'all fours'. About 50 ml of fluid is aspirated, inspected and then sent for biochemical, cytological and bacteriological studies.

Tests of exocrine pancreatic function

Physiology: Acid in the duodenum causes release of the hormone secretin. Secretin(S) stimulates the pancreas to produce a watery secretion rich in bicarbonate.

Proteins and products of their digestion within the duodenum cause release of the hormone cholecystokinin–pancreozymin (CCK–PZ). CCK–PZ stimulates the pancreas to produce a viscid secretion rich in digestive enzymes including trypsin, amylase and lipase.

Intubation tests

S/CCK–PZ test. The duodenum is intubated after an overnight fast. Parenteral injections of secretin and CCK–PZ are given and duodenal juice is aspirated. It is necessary to have a separate nasogastric tube continually aspirated to avoid entry of gastric acid into the duodenum. This would otherwise neutralize duodenal alkali and result in a falsely low estimation of pancreatic bicarbonate secretion. Duodenal juice is analysed for HCO_3^- concentration; HCO_3^- output and trypsin activity. Less often lipase or amylase activity is assayed.

Lundh test meal. This test depends upon endogenous secretin and CCK–PZ release in response to a specially constituted meal. The Lundh meal consists of 500 ml of a mixture of 6% fat, 5% protein and 15% carbohydrate. It is introduced into the stomach and duodenal contents are continually aspirated for measurement of trypsin.

The S/CCK–PZ test and Lundh test meal may occasionally produce a differing result. In disease of the duodenal and jejunal mucosa such as adult coeliac disease, pancreatic response to a test meal may be defective due to inadequate hormone release in the absence of any pancreatic disease, as confirmed by a normal response to the S/CCK–PZ test.

Tubeless (oral) pancreatic function tests

BT–PABA test. N-benzoyl-L-tyrosyl-p-amino-benzoic acid (BT–PABA) is digested by the pancreatic enzyme chymotrypsin to release p-amino benzoic acid (PABA). The released PABA is absorbed and the proportion of administered PABA which is excreted in a 6-h urine collection reflects the adequacy of pancreatic exocrine function. False positive results (low urinary PABA despite normal exocrine pancreatic function) are produced by small bowel malabsorption of PABA, e.g. in coeliac disease and by chronic liver disease or renal insufficiency. These may be corrected for by administering a separate dose of PABA on another occasion (or ^{14}C-PABA at the same time) and determining its urinary excretion. Several drugs including paracetamol, frusemide, thiazides and sulphonamides interfere with analysis of urinary PABA.

Fluorescein dilaurate test. Hydrolysis of the synthetic diester by pancreatic esterase releases fluorescein which is absorbed and excreted in the urine. Administer either fluorescein dilaurate or unesterified fluorescein orally on consecutive days. Measure urinary fluorescein excretion. This test is subject to similar drawbacks as the BT-PABA test (i.e. dependence on gastric emptying, intestinal absorption, renal excretion).

Dual-labelled Schilling test. Vitamin B_{12} (cyanocobalamin) bound to R factor requires digestion by a pancreatic protease prior to transfer of the vitamin B_{12} to intrinsic factor which facilitates its absorption. Simultaneously administered IF-B_{12} theoretically permits correction for non-pancreatic causes of low excretion, e.g. pernicious anaemia, intestinal malabsorption and renal failure. Administer orally IF-(^{57}Co) B_{12} and R protein (^{58}Co) B_{12} complex. Measure the ratio of ^{57}CoB$_{12}$; ^{58}CoB$_{12}$ in urine.

Current clinical status of pancreatic function tests
Tubeless tests appear reliable in distinguishing pancreatic disease from other causes when it is sufficiently advanced to produce steatorrhoea. Their reliability in detecting lesser degrees of pancreatic insufficiency needs further evaluation, but they do not appear to be as sensitive as duodenal intubation tests. A practical guide to follow is given in Fig. 6.16.

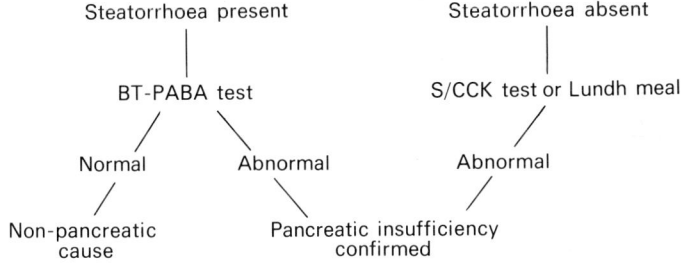

Fig. 6.16. Pancreatic function tests. The schema suggests a logical use of pancreatic function tests when a measure of pancreatic exocrine activity is required.

Chapter 7
The Small Intestine, Colon and Rectum

(A) The small intestine
The small intestine has, because of its distance from the mouth and anus, eluded the routine endoscopist so far. Nevertheless, tubes can be passed into it to sample its contents and collect specimens of the mucosa by suction biopsy.

Investigation of small intestinal disease falls under three headings:
1 Detection of nutritional deficiency.
2 Morphology—radiology and histology.
3 Function—tests of absorption.

Radiological examination
The small bowel is the most difficult section of the alimentary tract to X-ray. Its length, the series of superimposed coils, and the lack of any landmarks to guide the radiologist as to whether the barium has passed any particular segment are obvious difficulties. If too much barium is given, superimposed coils of flooded intestine cause hidden areas. During a *barium follow-through* examination, frequent screening of barium as it passes along the bowel with appropriate films using pressure techniques is better than spot films taken at routine intervals. The transit time from stomach to caecum in normals varies from 30 min to 4 h or more, but estimation of rate of passage of barium has little or no value in diagnosis except with obvious intestinal obstruction.

If the barium follow-through series is unsatisfactory a *small bowel enema* can be done (Fig. 7.1). A tube has to be passed through the duodenum and large volumes of dilute barium are infused.

Angiography where a catheter is introduced into either the coeliac or superior or inferior mesenteric artery, can be used to show vascular lesions, sometimes neoplasms, and the site of active bleeding.

Lymphangiography can demonstrate abnormal lymphatics as are found in intestinal lymphangiectasia, and also retroperitoneal lesions though the last can be seen by a non-invasive technique using the *CAT body scanner*.

Intestinal biopsy
A per-oral jejunal biopsy tube such as the Crosby–Kugler or Watson capsule (Fig. 7.2) is swallowed and guided through the pylorus under screening. Biopsies are usually taken just beyond the duodeno-jejunal junction. A small fragment of mucosa is sucked into the aperture in the side of the capsule and snipped off by a knife. This specimen is examined through a dissecting microscope or hand lens and

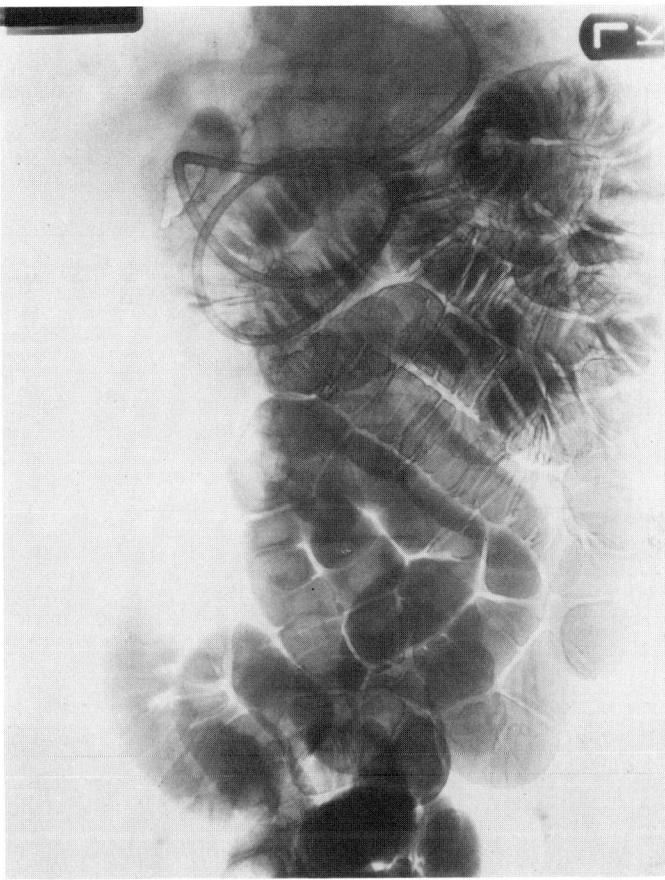

Fig. 7.1. Small bowel enema. A tube is positioned in the upper jejunum and dilute barium is poured rapidly into the small intestine. This displays fine detail even where loops of bowel overlap.

an immediate diagnosis is often possible (Fig. 7.3); it is then sent for histological section and, in special cases, for examination under the electron microscope. The risk of perforation is remote though greater in children. Haemorrhage from the biopsy site occasionally occurs and sometimes the knife fails to cut a piece of mucosa completely and gets stuck but it frees itself within a day or two. Some patients refuse or cannot swallow the capsule; then it can be passed under sedation fixed to the tip of the endoscope. It is sometimes possible to see the villi and to suspect the flat mucosa of coeliac disease through the endoscope. Taking duodenal biopsies endoscopically is quicker and simpler than jejunal biopsy. Normal finger-like villi on endoscopic duodenal biopsies effectively exclude coeliac disease. However,

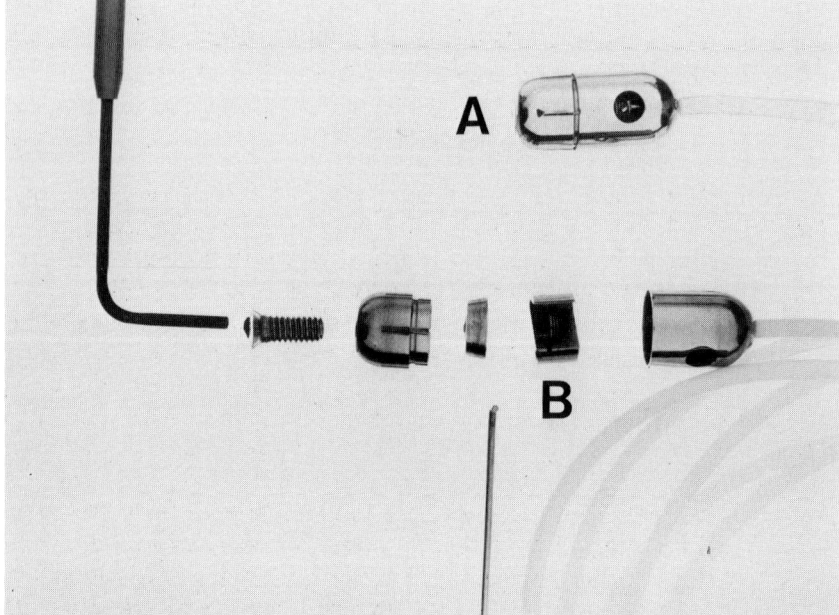

Fig. 7.2. Jejunal biopsy capsule. A jejunal biopsy capsule is shown in its assembled (loaded) form (A) and in its separate component parts. The spring-loaded knife (B) is fired by suction on the tube when the side opening is occluded by jejunal mucosa.

because of the smallness of endoscopic biopsies and the normal tendency for duodenal villi to be shorter than those in the jejunum the converse is not true and a firm diagnosis of coeliac disease should probably not be made without confirmation by jejunal biopsy. Biopsy specimens must be carefully spread flat on to card for fixation and subsequent sectioning so that tangential cutting, which gives a false impression of villous shortening and blunting, can be avoided.

Scintigraphy

Leucocyte scans
Recently, isotopically labelled white cells or platelets have been re-injected into the patient for the localization of intra-abdominal inflammatory lesions. They may be used as an alternative to gallium scanning for diagnosis of subphrenic or pelvic abscess. They may also prove useful in showing the extent of active inflammation in Crohn's disease.

Antibody scans
Radioactive antibodies to carcinoembryonic antigen (CEA) or alpha fetoprotein have been injected to show the presence and extent of tumour recurrence or

metastasis. They obviously depend upon the exhibition of the appropriate antigen on the cell surface of the malignant cell. Para-aortic node involvement by alpha fetoprotein positive testicular tumour or hepatic metastases of CEA-positive colonic cancer may be shown in this way.

Tests of absorption

A simple, reliable test of intestinal function would enable patients to be selected for faecal fat studies or even avoid the need for this. The large number of test substances proposed such as butter, fat, olive oil, glycerine, vitamin A and sugars is a sign that none carries the stamp of certainty. Optimistic early studies with new tests are often followed by reports showing less and less distinction between normal and abnormal, so the test becomes valueless—not surprising when urinary excretion or blood levels of a substance used in any oral tolerance test is the result of several factors: thus a flat blood curve cannot prove that a substance was not absorbed for it may signify rapid utilization or speedy removal to the tissues or in the urine or be due to slow gastric emptying with complete absorption over a longer period. For example, the *glucose tolerance test* may separate pancreatic steatorrhoea where high curves are common from adult coeliac disease where flat curves are more likely, but it is seldom used for this purpose for reasons of non-specificity outlined above. For this reason many investigators now bypass these functional studies in the diagnosis of small intestinal disease (Fig. 7.4).

Xylose absorption test

The xylose absorption test can be used to detect defective absorption from the proximal small intestine and an abnormal result is expected in coeliac disease. Xylose is a pentose (5-carbon sugar) which is absorbed by the jejunum but not metabolized by the body so that the absorbed sugar should appear quantitatively in the urine. A 5 g load is preferred to 25 g, since the larger dose may have marked osmotic effects. Normally 4 g appears in the urine over the 5-h collection period. False positive results (low urinary excretion despite a normal jejunal mucosa) occur due to renal impairment, dilution in the extracellular fluid of overhydrated patients and overgrowth of the proximal intestine by bacteria which metabolize xylose. Some have shown the test to have better discriminatory value if a 2-h urine collection is used, or if a 1-h blood xylose level is measured and expressed as blood xylose concentration per unit body surface area.

Vitamin B_{12} absorption test (cf. Table 3.7)

Vitamin B_{12} absorption is a function of the terminal ileum which can be assessed by the Schilling test. Ileal disease must be differentiated from other possible causes of B_{12} malabsorption (cf. Table 3.6).

Collection and analysis of faeces

In the investigation of weight loss and diarrhoea, faecal fat estimation should always

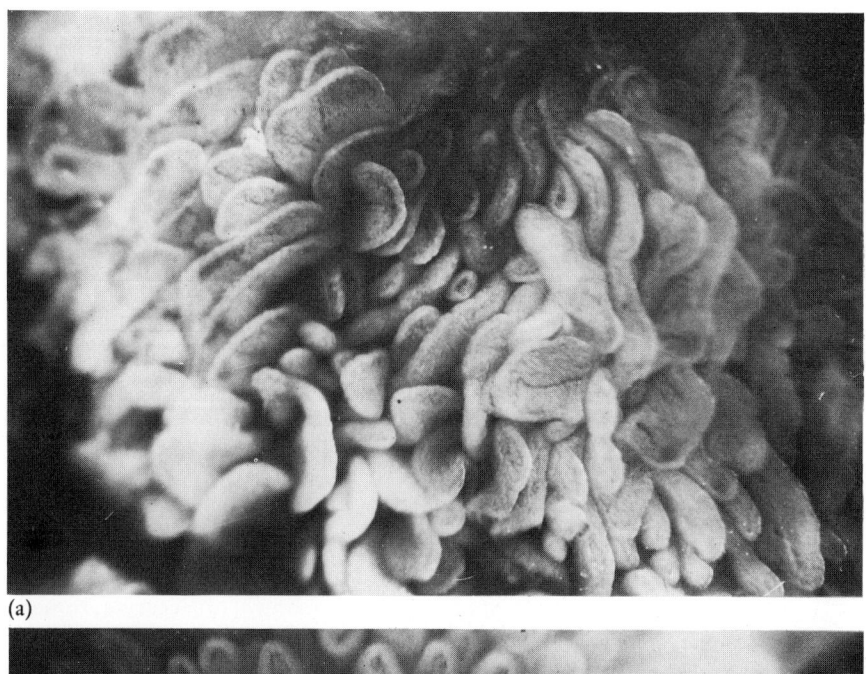

(a)

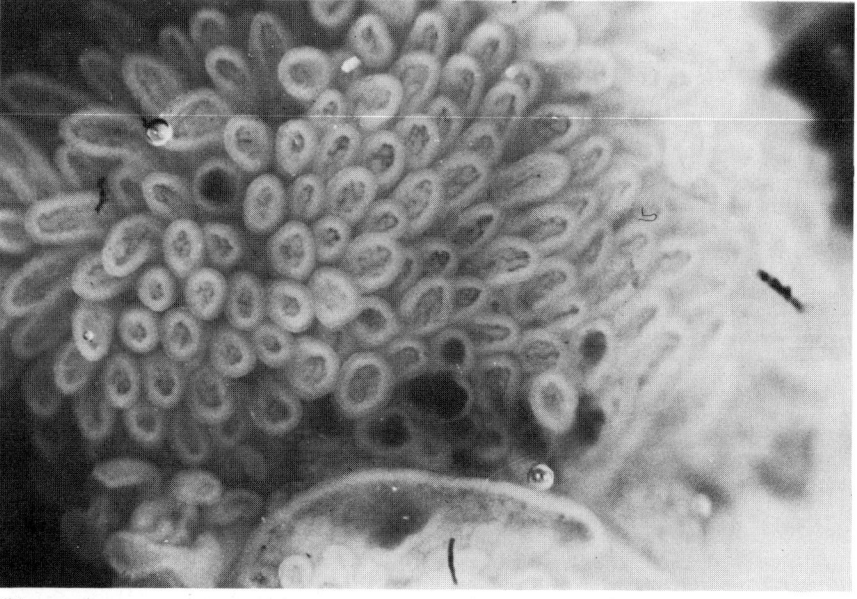

(b)

Fig. 7.3. The villus appearances in a jejunal biopsy viewed by dissecting microscopy. (a) Broad leaves and fingers; (b) fingers; (c) ridges or convolutions; (d) flat. (a) and (b) are compatible with normality but do not exclude a more subtle abnormality seen on histological examination. (c) and (d) are abnormal. (c) corresponds to severe partial villous atrophy graded histologically. It was taken from a patient with tropical sprue and is typical of that condition. (d) corresponds to subtotal villous atrophy seen histologically and is typical of untreated coeliac disease. The black orifices represent the openings of the crypts of Lieberkühn which are visible due to the complete absence of villi from this specimen.

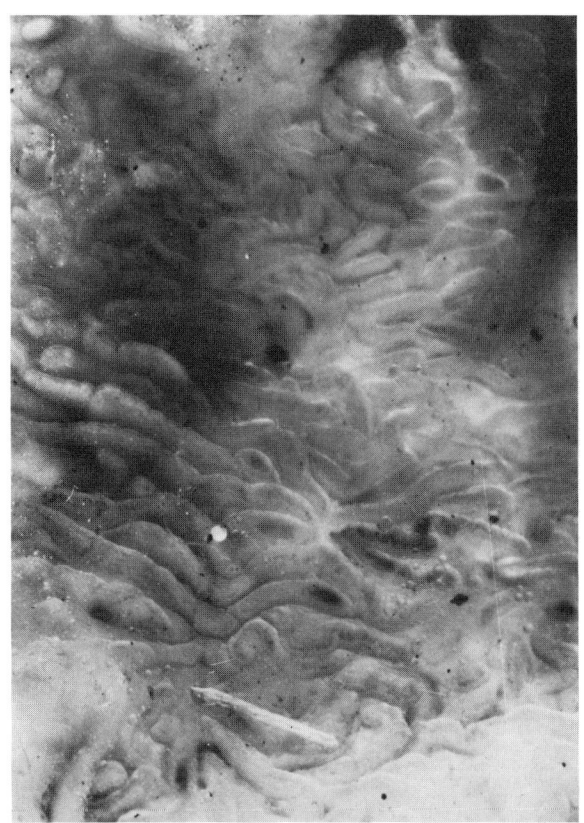

(c)

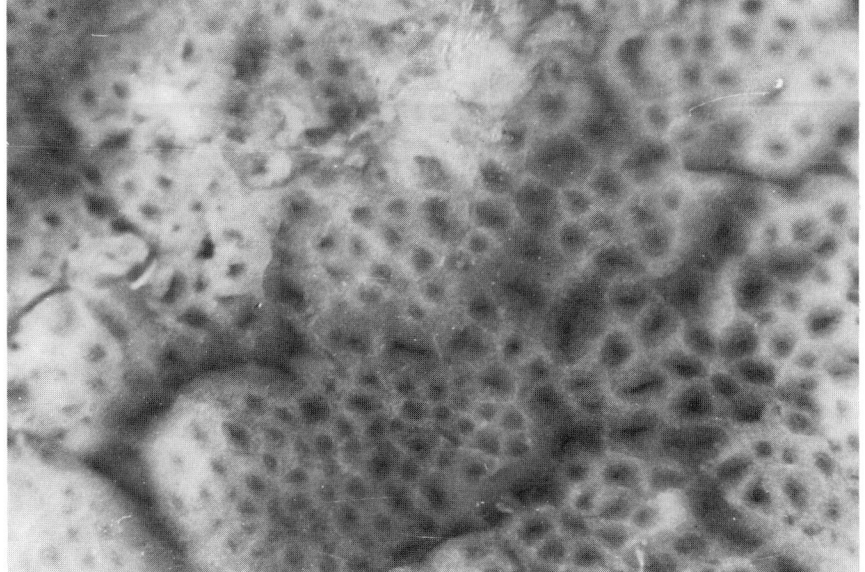

(d)

Disease of the jejunum e.g. adult coeliac disease

Screening test	Blood film (features of iron and/or folate deficiency ± hyposplenism), serum and red blood cell folate levels

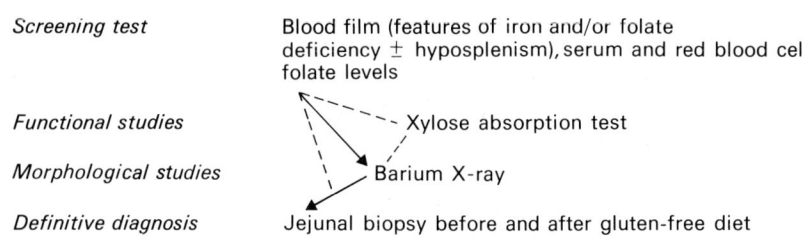

Functional studies	Xylose absorption test
Morphological studies	Barium X-ray
Definitive diagnosis	Jejunal biopsy before and after gluten-free diet

Disease of the ileum e.g. Crohn's disease

Screening test	ESR, C reactive protein or other acute phase reactant Serum albumin Blood picture

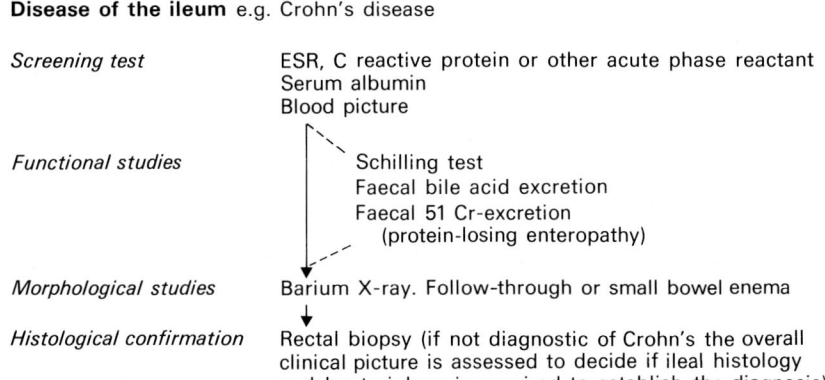

Functional studies	Schilling test Faecal bile acid excretion Faecal 51 Cr-excretion (protein-losing enteropathy)
Morphological studies	Barium X-ray. Follow-through or small bowel enema
Histological confirmation	Rectal biopsy (if not diagnostic of Crohn's the overall clinical picture is assessed to decide if ileal histology and bacteriology is required to establish the diagnosis)

Fig. 7.4. Approach to the diagnosis of small intestinal disease. This schematic approach to the diagnosis of adult coeliac disease and Crohn's disease illustrates how absorption studies may be bypassed in favour of more precise radiological and histological studies.

be paired with (daily) weighings of stool to give total wet weight. This enables the doctor to distinguish between stool frequency and diarrhoea with or without steatorrhoea and can be invaluable in the monitoring of therapeutic manoeuvres (Fig. 7.5). Don't forget to inspect the stools directly yourself (cf. p. 320).

Estimation of faecal fat excretion

Chemical analysis. A small amount of fat is excreted in the stool normally, such as 2 or 3 g daily (7–12 mmol); part comes from the food but most is endogenous from cellular debris. Causes of an excess are listed in Table 7.1. *All* stools passed by the patient must be collected over 3 days and longer in doubtful cases. The total fat present is measured; on an ordinary ward diet which contains approximate 70 g fat, this should average less than 7 g (25 mmol)/day. To assess the effects of therapy it is preferable to use a diet of known fat content. The minimum should be 50 g daily and borderline abnormalities may be revealed by increasing dietary fat to 100 g daily or more. Measurement of split and unsplit fat in stools is valueless, for, although fat passed in pancreatic disease should be mainly neutral and unsplit, it is often split by lipase produced by colonic bacteria. In practice, therefore, total fatty acids are estimated to include faecal free fatty acids and those derived *in vitro* by hydrolysis of glycerides. Errors in determining faecal fat excretion are due to the following:

1   Imperfect collection of stools—(specimens are easily missed by busy nursing staff).

2   Inadequate dietary intake—less than 50 g fat/day.

3   Constipation, so often the result of putting the patient to bed.

The errors are reduced in patients with a rapid intestinal transit time and rapid rectal emptying time. In those with slow bowel movements several methods have been attempted to mark stool collections for periods of 3, 4 or 5 days. These include the use of:

1   Chromium sesquioxide (Cr_2O_3). A standard dose is taken orally each day for the period of the collection. Analysis of chromium in the stool is troublesome.

2   Radio-opaque pellets are taken with the food for the duration of the test. Stool collections can be X-rayed to determine their relationship to food ingestion.

3   Coloured markers such as carmine may be given prior to the collection period and again at the end to help identification of the 3- or 5-day stool.

In practice the errors involved in faecal collections are usually ignored, and these more sophisticated techniques are reserved for balance studies which are part of a precise scientific protocol.

Radioactive techniques. These are less sensitive than stool fat determination.

1   One method is by giving the fat triolein, labelled with [131]iodine, and then measuring radioactivity in the serum urine and stool. The test has many pitfalls; in particular it is known that iodinase activity in the gut mucosa may release ^{131}I and thus invalidate the results.

2   A second radioactive test involves administration of [14]-carbon-labelled triglyceride. Absorbed triglyceride is metabolized to CO_2 and H_2O. After collection of expired air, the specific activity of [14]CO_2 can be determined by radioactive counting. Although errors can be introduced if CO_2 production from other sources is highly variable (e.g. in thyrotoxicosis or obesity), the test does appear to correlate well with chemical analysis of faecal fat excretion.

Technique for measurement of [14]CO_2 in breath tests

The patient exhales through a straw into a solution of hyamine hydrochloride which traps CO_2. When 1 mmol of hyamine has taken up 1 mmol of CO_2 the colour of the solution changes due to an acid-base indicator, and the patient stops blowing. The proportion of radioactive [14]CO_2 contained in 1 mmol of expired CO_2 (specific activity) is then determined by liquid scintillation counting.

This aspect of the technique is the same for ^{14}C-triolein, ^{14}C-glycocholate and ^{14}C-aminopyrine tests.

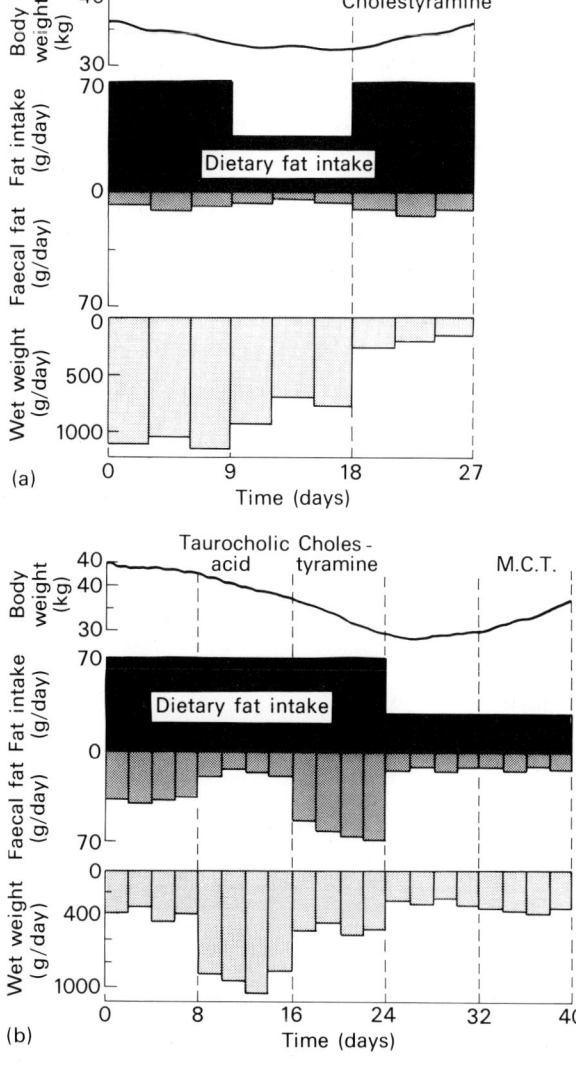

Fig. 7.5. Fat balance studies. (a) *Patient 1*. Limited ileal resection. Days 0–9: the patient has severe diarrhoea (stool wt 1 kg/day) and is continuing to lose weight. Days 9–18: withdrawal of dietary fat has only a marginal effect, if any. Days 18–27: cholestyramine given with meals abolishes diarrhoea, though increasing faecal fat excretion slightly. The patient begins to regain his lost weight. Note that this patient's diarrhoea was largely due to the effects of bile acids in the colon—cholerrheic diarrhoea.

(b) *Patient 2*. Extensive small bowel resection. Days 0–8: The patient has massive steatorrhoea (30–40 g/day faecal fat) and is losing weight. Days 8–16: A misguided attempt at treatment with oral bile acid supplements with meals diminishes faecal fat excretion

Table 7.1. Pathogenesis of steatorrhoea.

Luminal	Lipase deficiency	Pancreatic disease
		Inactivation by acid (ZE syndrome)
	Bile acid deficiency	Biliary obstruction and liver disease
		Ileal malabsorption
		Degradation by bacterial overgrowth
		Precipitation by acid (ZE syndrome)
	Poor stimulation of gall bladder and pancreas. Poor mixing of duodenal secretion with food.	Gastro-jejunostomy
Mucosal	Inadequate surface area	Intestinal resection or by-pass
	Disease	Coeliac disease
		Tropical sprue
		Crohn's disease
		Whipple's disease
		Hypogammaglobulinaemia
		Amyloidosis
		Lymphoma
	Defect in fat transport	Abetalipoproteinaemia
Lymphatic	Lymphatic insufficiency	Lymphangiectasia
		Lymphoma
		Tuberculosis
Mechanism unknown		Hypoparathyroidism

Detection of bacterial overgrowth

To diagnose malabsorption syndrome secondary to bacterial overgrowth of the small intestine you must show:

1 An anatomical lesion capable of producing stasis.
2 Metabolic consequences (see below).
3 Resolution of metabolic consequences following appropriate antibiotic therapy.

Causes. Typical causes of small bowel bacterial overgrowth include:
1 Surgical short circuit operations, e.g. Polya gastrectomy.

significantly, but exacerbates (cholerrheic) diarrhoea and the patient loses weight faster. Days 16–24: Cholestyramine abolishes cholerrheic diarrhoea but exacerbates steatorrhoea. The patient continues to waste away. Days 24–32: At last! the patient is put on a low fat diet. This limits steatorrhoea and diarrhoea and the patient begins to regain metabolic balance. Days 32–40: The additional calories derived from medium chain triglycerides (MCT) supplements to the diet help the patient regain weight.

2 Jejunal diverticulosis.
3 Systemic sclerosis.
4 Colonic fistula into the stomach or small bowel.

Methods of detection

Direct methods

Aspiration of small intestinal juice. This is the most direct way of detecting overgrowth. The juice can be used for:
1 Bacteriological culture under aerobic and anaerobic conditions with quantitative bacterial counts.
2 Demonstration of secondary bile acids. Deconjugation and dehydroxylation of primary bile acids by bacteria produces secondary bile acids (Fig. 7.6).
3 Detection of acetate, propionate or butyrate. These short-chain fatty acids are produced by bacterial metabolism. Their production during chewing the cud allows cattle to derive nutritional benefit from the cellulose they eat.

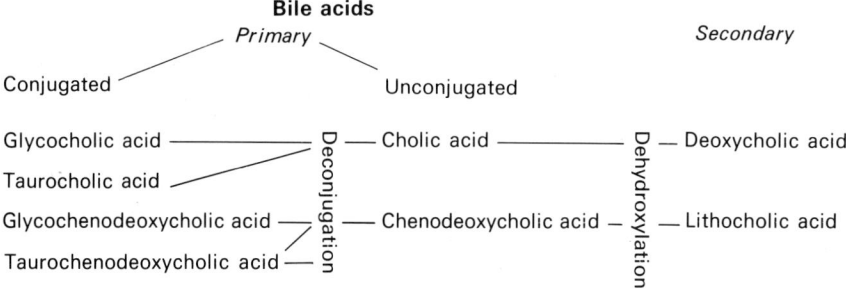

Fig. 7.6. Metabolism of bile acids. Primary bile acids may be conjugated with glycine or taurine or unconjugated. Bacterial dehydroxylation of bile acids produces secondary bile acids which may also be conjugated with either glycine or taurine as they pass through the liver.

Indirect methods

Breath tests. We here consider two types of test, as follows:
1 Breath H_2 test. The human body does not normally produce H_2, which is, however, a normal by-product of bacterial carbohydrate metabolism. The fasting patient should have a very low baseline concentration of expired H_2. Breath H_2 is monitored following ingestion of a sugar, e.g. xylose or lactulose. Lactulose is a non-absorbable disaccharide. Its ingestion will therefore normally produce a sharp

increase of breath H_2 when it arrives in the caecum, and is sometimes used in this way to estimate the transit time from stomach to caecum. An earlier peak of breath H_2 following lactulose ingestion suggests bacterial overgrowth within the small bowel.

2   ^{14}C-glycocholic acid breath test. Bacterial deconjugation of bile acids produces ^{14}C-glycine which is metabolized to $^{14}CO_2$ and then exhaled (Fig. 7.7). Normally very little $^{14}CO_2$ is released in the breath since the ^{14}C-glycocholic acid has been conserved within the bile salt pool and is undergoing an enterohepatic circulation. An early peak of breath $^{14}CO_2$ is typical of a patient with proximal small bowel

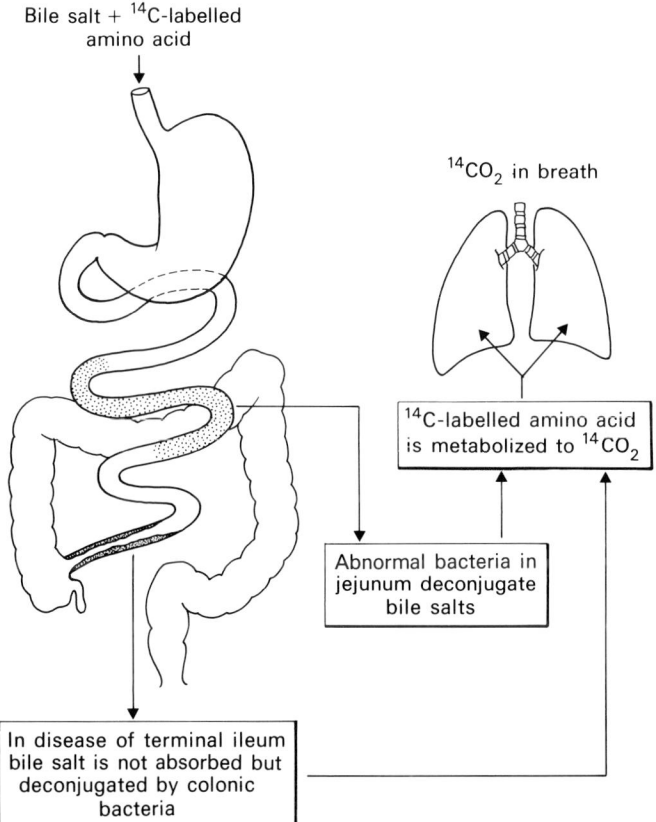

Bile salt + ^{14}C-labelled amino acid

$^{14}CO_2$ in breath

^{14}C-labelled amino acid is metabolized to $^{14}CO_2$

Abnormal bacteria in jejunum deconjugate bile salts

In disease of terminal ileum bile salt is not absorbed but deconjugated by colonic bacteria

Fig. 7.7. The ^{14}C bile acid breath test. Carbon-14 labelled glycocholic acid is given by mouth. Normally it is absorbed intact and undergoes enterohepatic circulation. If it is degraded by bacteria the ^{14}C is metabolized and eventually exhaled at $^{14}CO_2$. Measuring the specific activity of breath $^{14}CO_2$ provides a useful measure of bacterial contamination of the small intestine, though raised levels also occur with bile salt malabsorption as a result of degradation by colonic bacteria.

bacterial overgrowth. A late peak is typical of a patient with a distal blind loop but cannot be differentiated from results with ileal malabsorption in which malabsorbed bile acid is deconjugated by normal colonic flora. This problem can be overcome if the glycocholic acid has a dual label, ^{14}C in the glycine and a bacterial resistant ^{3}H in the cholic acid moiety. Bacterial overgrowth of the ileum produces increased breath CO_2 but normal faecal ^{3}H. Colonic deconjugation of bile acids is accompanied by an increase of both breath CO_2 and faecal ^{3}H excretion.

Not all bacteria which colonize the small bowel give positive breath tests with either method e.g. deconjugation of ^{14}C-glycocholate occurs in about two-thirds. The two breath tests can be thought of as complementary since one or other or both tests will be positive in nearly all cases of bacterial overgrowth.

Schilling test (Table 3.7). Vitamin B_{12} is removed by anaerobic bacteria. Malabsorption of B_{12} is not affected by the addition of intrinsic factor but is abolished by antibiotics.

Faecal fat estimation. Malabsorption of fat may occur as a consequence of bacterial metabolism of bile acids. Abolition of steatorrhoea by antibiotic therapy thus confirms the diagnosis of bacterial overgrowth.

Urinary indican excretion. Indicans, e.g. indoxyl sulphate, are produced by bacterial metabolism of protein. Abnormally raised amounts of indican excretion therefore indicate either bacterial overgrowth of the small intestine or protein malabsorption giving colonic bacteria access to dietary protein.

Diagnosis of hypolactasia

Of the disaccharidase deficiencies, hypolactasia is by far the most common. The following methods may confirm the diagnosis:

Direct methods
Estimation of lactase activity in a jejunal biopsy sample of mucosa. The enzyme activity is usually expressed as units per gram of protein in the specimen.

Indirect methods
1 Lactose breath test. Fifty grams of lactose is given by mouth and breath hydrogen excretion is monitored. In a normal test all the lactose is absorbed and, in the absence of bacterial overgrowth of the small intestine, breath hydrogen does not increase significantly. Malabsorption of lactose produces high peaks of hydrogen excretion due to colonic fermentation.
2 Lactose tolerance test. Fifty grams of lactose is taken orally. Blood glucose is monitored as in the glucose tolerance test. Malabsorption of lactose is accompanied by a flat blood glucose curve and the patient frequently complains of bloating, wind and diarrhoea due to the unabsorbed osmotic load.

3 Lactose barium meal. Fifty grams of lactose is taken with barium. A plain abdominal X-ray is taken 1 h later. If the result is negative the appearances are those of a normal barium follow-through. A positive test shows large volumes of dilute barium in the caecum and adjacent bowel.

Tests of small bowel permeability

Altered small bowel permeability can be shown in several diseases, and can be detected by non-invasive tests which may have a future role in screening for disease or monitoring response to therapy, e.g. in screening for adult coeliac disease and monitoring response to a gluten-free diet. Normally monosaccharide-sized molecules such as xylose and mannitol are efficiently absorbed from the jejunum but very little disaccharide-sized molecules such as lactulose and cellobiose penetrate the mucosa. In disease states absorption of xylose and mannitol is decreased but mucosal leakiness permits absorption of the larger molecules. The patient drinks a (preferably hypertonic) mixture of two or more sugars and their relative absorption is determined from their concentrations in a urine collection. The ratios xylose:lactulose or mannitol:cellobiose is high in normals but low in diseases which increase intestinal permeability.

Gastrointestinal bleeding of obscure origin

Occasionally patients may have episodes of major gastrointestinal bleeding whose origin is undetermined following gastroscopy, sigmoidoscopy and colonoscopy. Causative lesions are usually not apparent to the surgeon's eye at laparotomy, since they may be small mucosal lesions which are not palpable and do not alter the serosal surface of the bowel. The following procedures may help to localize the source of bleeding in these rare cases.

Scintigraphy

1 ^{99m}Tc-colloid scan. This technique is recommended for localization of active (especially lower) gastrointestinal bleeding. Following intravenous ^{99}Tc sulphur colloid, extravasated blood gives an area of high radioactivity whereas background activity falls rapidly due to its removal by the liver (Fig. 7.8a). Liver activity obscures lesions in the right upper quadrant. If scintigraphy gives a positive result, subsequent arteriography focusing on the same region has a high probability of demonstrating (and localizing more precisely) the bleeding source.

2 ^{99}Tc pertechnetate. Unlike ^{99}Tc colloid, this agent is concentrated within gastric mucosa. It is very useful in the diagnosis of haemorrhage from a Meckel's diverticulum. Heterotopic gastric mucosa is found in one-third of asymptomatic Meckel's but is nearly always present when bleeding is a problem (Fig. 7.8b).

Arteriography

Arteriography is most valuable if performed during an episode of brisk bleeding when extravasation of contrast can be seen with losses of 0.5 ml/min or greater.

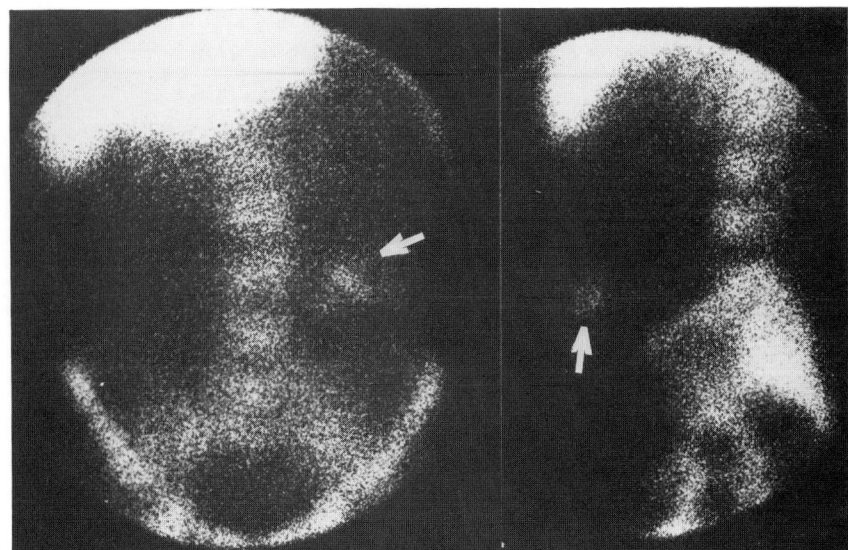

(a)

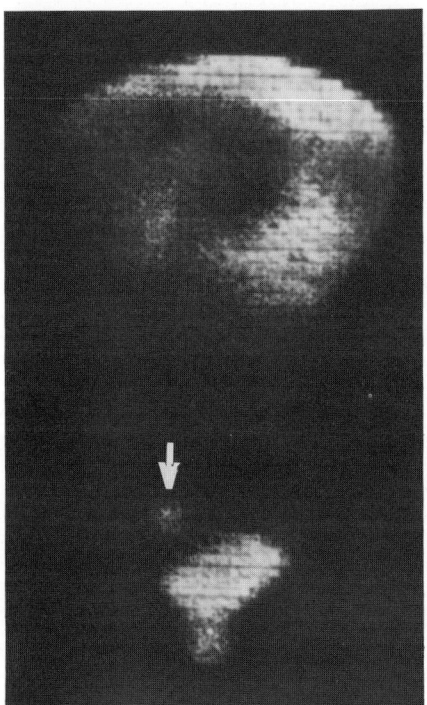

(b)

Other signs which may indicate the site of the bleeding lesion include a tumour blush, vascular malformation, pooling of contrast and an early filling vein. In a patient with upper gastrointestinal bleeding, especially variceal bleeding, the arteriography catheter may be sited within the superior mesenteric artery and left there for a few days to allow *local intra-arterial infusion of vasopressin*. This is effective in reducing portal pressure and is less likely to produce cardiac ischaemia than peripheral administration of vasopressin. However, there is a significant risk of ischaemic necrosis of the bowel.

The string test
This is a simple device for sampling upper gastrointestinal contents. The Entero-test device consists of a silicone rubber-lined gelatin capsule containing a nylon string. It can be passed to the upper small intestine and samples, uncontaminated by organisms from the mouth or oesophagus can be analysed for bacteria (either in stagnant bowel syndrome or to find a typhoid carrier), for pH, enzymes, or possibly blood.

Radiotelemetry
The radio pill has been used to measure temperature, pressure and pH changes as it passes through the alimentry tract, so avoiding psychological stress and other changes resulting from intubation. A radio receiver with aerial is placed on the bedside table. It is a research procedure and might be used in the future to study motility changes in patients with the irritable bowel syndrome.

(B) The colon and rectum

Examination of the stools (for rectal examination see Part I)
Looking at a stool can make a diagnosis obvious and save numerous investigations, but actually seeing a stool can be difficult as the nursing staff are trained to throw them away.

Fig. 7.8. (*opposite*) Scintiscanning in diagnosis of gastrointestinal bleeding of obscure origin. (a) ^{99m}Tc-colloid scan: Technetium colloid was given to a patient with cirrhosis during gastrointestinal haemorrhage when the stomach and duodenum had been shown to be free of blood. The scintigraphic material has been taken up by the liver and bone marrow after 20 minutes but bleeding into the gut has produced a hot spot (arrowed) visible on antero-posterior and lateral views.

   (b) ^{99m}Tc-pertechnetate scan: This examination was performed in a child who had suffered several episodes of acute gastrointestinal bleeding. Pertechnetate is normally localized within the gastric mucosa. It can be shown to have outlined the stomach and bladder. In addition there is a 'hot spot' just above the bladder (arrowed) indicating the presence of gastric mucosa within a Meckel's diverticulum which had caused the bleeding.

Macroscopic

The reader should know what a normal stool looks like. Its shape varies greatly and is of little help diagnostically, and the small rabbit-like stool may be passed by the healthy as well as by those with irritable colon. Blood from anorectal disease is seen as streaks on the surface of the stool, whereas blood from lesions higher will be mixed as is typical in ulcerative colitis. Passage of pure blood occurs with haemorrhoids, polyps, diverticulitis, cancer, intussusception and infarction of the colon. Patients with bleeding peptic ulcers occasionally pass red blood, but usually melaena. Reddish stools occur after eating beetroot or drinking claret.

Tarry black melaena stools indicate partial digestion of blood, especially by hydrochloric acid in the stomach, so usually point to bleeding in the upper gut. If in doubt mix the stool with a small volume of water which may appear red, and chemical tests for blood can be done. Oral iron makes stools a grey-black colour which can mimic melaena. Black stools are also caused by the ingestion of charcoal, bismuth compounds and liquorice in large amounts. Large, pale stools point towards steatorrhoea.

Pallor is not usually due only to fat but to alteration in bile pigment, probably due to reduction by bacteria; the surface may darken after exposure to light or air. Bulkiness results from failure of absorption both of food and water. Bacterial metabolism produces hydroxy-fatty acids such as ricinoleic acid, the active ingredient of castor oil, which activate adenyl cyclase in the colonic mucosa to promote salt and water secretion. The smell is foul and rancid from fermentation of undigested food products. In pancreatic steatorrhoea, blobs of unsplit fat like butter may be seen. Stools may contain excess of fat though their appearance and colour are normal. The unsavoury use of epithets related to food is illustrated by the rice water stools of cholera and the pea soup ones of typhoid.

Microscopy of the stool

This may show abundant fatty acid crystals which suggest steatorrhoea, though do not indicate its cause. Globules of neutral, unsplit fat together with an excessive quantity of striated meat fibres point to pancreatic steatorrhoea; the globules can be distinguished from those of liquid paraffin or cooking oil by special stains.

Some bacteria cause diarrhoea by releasing an exotoxin which stimulates intestinal secretion. Cholera toxin and the heat-labile exotoxin of *E. coli* stimulate adenyl cyclase in the small intestine resulting in profuse secretion for which the colonic reabsorption capacity is insufficient; microscopy of the stools shows virtually no red blood cells nor white cells. This is in marked contrast to diarrhoea caused by organisms which invade the gastrointestinal mucosa, in which large numbers of erythrocytes and leucocytes usually abound. Generally speaking, diarrhoea is most profuse when of small intestinal origin and patients may be in danger from dehydration. Colonic diarrhoea may also be profuse, but more commonly involves rectal pain known as tenesmus associated with frequent passage of small stools composed mainly of blood and mucus.

Biochemical analysis of stools

In the investigation of diarrhoea of obscure origin it may be useful to measure stool electrolytes and osmolality. Sodium and potassium concentrations are summed and doubled. In secretory diarrhoea (e.g. chlorridorrhoea, vipoma, *E. coli* exotoxin or *V. cholerae*) the answer is within 40 mmol/l of stool osmolality. In osmotic diarrhoea (e.g. hypolactasia, purgative abuse) the answer falls well short of stool osmolality minus 40 mmol/l. In the most devious purgative abusers, it is helpful to alkalinize the urine which may turn pink due to the presence of phenolphthalein in many laxative preparations.

In carbohydrate intolerance, the stool can be shown to be highly acid due to bacterial fermentation products.

Analysis of stool enzyme activity has been used to screen for pancreatic insufficiency in the investigation of young children who fail to thrive.

Diagnosis of enteric infection and infestation (Table 7.2)

Protozoa and helminths

Tapeworms and threadworms can easily be seen, but microscopy of a stool suspension is needed to diagnose pathogenic protozoa and helminthic ova.

Table 7.2. Infectious causes of diarrhoea.

Protozoa and helminths
Entamoeba histolytica
Giardia lamblia
Strongyloides stercoralis
Trichuris trichuria
Fasciolopsis (intestinal fluke)
Schistosoma (blood fluke)
Bacteria
Shigella
Salmonella
Campylobacter jejuni
Clostridium perfringens (food poisoning);
C. difficile (antibiotic-induced enterocolitis)
Vibrio cholerae
Eschericha coli
Yersinia enterocolitica
Staphylococcus aureus
Viruses
Rotavirus
Parvovirus

Repeated examinations may be needed and ideally stools should be taken immediately to the laboratory when, for example, amoebiasis is suspected. *Giardia lamblia* and the ova of *Strongyloides stercoralis* may be found in the stool, but often stool examination is negative despite symptoms due to infestation of the small intestine by these parasites. If their presence is strongly suspected despite negative stool microscopy, duodenal sampling is recommended. Threadworms (*E. vermicularis*) are often not diagnosed by examining the stool as the adult female parasite is seldom longer than 10 mm and the stool contains ova in only 10% of infected patients. The usual way of diagnosis is to obtain ova from the peri-anal skin using the transparent adhesive tape test. Parents do the test on their children preferably in the early morning. A centimeter of transparent adhesive tape is pressed on one end of a microscopic slide and the tape is folded backward so that the sticky surface faces outwards. The slide is then put gently onto the anal verge so that the sticky surface touches the anus and immediate peri-anal area; the tape is then flipped over so that the adhesive surface attaches to the slide and this is examined under the microscope.

Bacteria

Special containers are usually provided and the stool should reach the laboratory on the day that it is passed. Salmonella, shigella, and campylobacter are important causes of acute diarrhoea.

Nearly 2000 serotypes of Salmonella have been described, so it is not surprising that they cause a spectrum of conditions including gastroenteritis, enteric fever, septicaemia, focal infections such as osteomyelitis and are also secreted by healthy carriers. Some strains of *E. coli* have also been shown to be pathogenic but their identification requires serological testing.

Many non-pathogenic *E. coli* inhabit the normal gut. Some pathogenic strains of *E. coli* adhere to small intestinal villi and produce diarrhoea by elaboration of exotoxin, but others invade the mucosa. Pathogenic *E. coli* commonly cause infantile diarrhoea and probably account for about 75% of traveller's diarrhoea.

Recently the exotoxin of *Clostridium difficile* has been accepted as a cause of antibiotic-induced enterocolitis. In patients in whom profuse diarrhoea follows antibacterial therapy, a stool sample may be analysed for the enterotoxin. Tubercle bacilli may be found in intestinal tuberculosis or cases of open pulmonary tuberculosis.

Viruses

These are being increasingly recognized as causes of infective diarrhoea, especially in children, though a viral infection is rarely proved. Rotavirus infection is the commonest cause of infantile diarrhoea, and results in massive morbidity and mortality worldwide, especially in undernourished infants with restricted medical care. The virus can be recognized in the stool by electron microscopy. Parvoviruses (e.g. the Norwalk agent) may affect all ages.

Radiology

Plain abdominal X-ray

This is especially helpful for diagnosing acute toxic dilatation of the colon in ulcerative colitis; the air outline of the colon can be seen with loss of haustrations and pseudopolyps. Cancer may be suspected if there is an abrupt end to the shadow. Volvulus of the sigmoid colon is also apparent as a massively dilated air-filled loop which occupies the whole abdomen. Rarely the caecum is on a mesentery and can undergo volvulus to produce obstruction. Other possible radiological signs are shown in Table 7.3.

Table 7.3. A plain film of the abdomen: this quick and non-invasive investigation can be of considerable help—providing that the radiologist is told exactly what is the object.

'Acute abdomen'
    Obstruction: dilated bowel and fluid levels
    Perforation: air under the diaphragm or elsewhere in peritoneum
    Sub-phrenic or other intra-abdominal abscess: gas/fluid collection
    Volvulus
    Intussusception
    Toxic dilation of colon in ulcerative or Crohn's colitis
Chronic conditions
    Gallstones
    Calcification of pancreas (in alcoholic pancreatitis)
    Calcification in aortic aneurysm or slow-growing tumours

Barium enema

Give the radiologist plenty of information because the method of preparation and examination may have to be altered. For example, the risk of perforation is present in acute ulcerative colitis or acute diverticulitis. The air-contrast barium enema (double contrast) is more time-consuming but gives better results as the mucosa is clearly outlined, and it leaves fewer cases of doubt to be resolved by colonoscopy.

Arteriography

This method can diagnose tumours of the colon, especially if vascular, but has largely been replaced by colonoscopy. It is necessary to diagnose angiodysplasia of the right side of the colon which causes rectal bleeding in the elderly (and is associated with aortic valve disease); there are small clusters of arteries on the anti-mesenteric border of the caecum and ascending colon.

Endoscopy

Proctoscopy
This can be done by the inexperienced in contrast to sigmoidoscopy which carries a
risk of perforation. If cold, the instrument is warmed and is pointed towards the
symphysis pubis to go through the anus then pointed towards the sacrum for the
rectum. If the patient is encouraged to bear down as though he is opening his bowel
during the introduction of the proctoscope or sigmoidoscope, relaxation of the anal
sphincter occurs, making instrumentation easy and free of discomfort. The mucosa
of the anus can be inspected for a fissure and a good view can often be obtained of
the rectum. A normal rectal mucosa virtually excludes ulcerative colitis. This is the
best way for diagnosing internal haemorrhoids—the patient strains while the
proctoscope is slowly withdrawn and the purplish veins will be seen to bulge in the
left lateral, right posterior and right anterior positions. Rectal biopsy can be done
and specimens of stool taken for further examination.

Sigmoidoscopy
This technique is rapid, safe and informative and should be part of routine
out-patient investigation of diarrhoea, tenesmus and other lower abdominal
complaints. It allows direct inspection of the rectal mucosa. Biopsies can be taken to
provide histological diagnosis of rectal neoplasms, and the ulcerative or inflammatory colitides.

Position. Left lateral: the patient lies on a couch in the left lateral position with the
knees drawn up and the buttocks just protruding over the edge. Elevation of the
pelvis by some 10–15 cm (with a sandbag or suchlike) increases the possibility of
passing beyond the recto-sigmoid junction. Knee-chest: the thighs are vertical and
the chest is close to the examination table. The bowel tends to fall away from the
pelvis, thus facilitating advancement of the instrument.

Colonoscopy
Fibreoptic colonoscopy permits direct inspection of the entire large bowel, and on
occasions, the terminal ileum.

Patient preparation. For satisfactory examination to occur it is essential to prepare
the patient to obtain a clear bowel. This includes use of aperients (2 days), avoidance
of oral iron therapy (5 days), a liquid diet (1–3 days) and a liquid purge on the day of
the examination (either administered orally, e.g. mannitol, or rectally, e.g. warm tap
water).

Indications. The technique is particularly useful in:
1   Lower gastrointestinal bleeding for (a) detection of its source and (b) possible
electrocoagulation.

2 Inflammatory bowel disease for (a) diagnosis when sigmoidoscopy and rectal biopsy is not diagnostic, (b) assessment of the extent and distribution of disease, (c) cancer surveillance in extensive (total) colitis of more than 10 years' duration.

3 Colonic polyposis for (a) detection of polyps and differentiation of benign v. malignant, (b) their removal by colonoscopic polypectomy when suitable.

4 Follow-up investigation of abnormalities, e.g. polyps, strictures, seen on barium enema.

Flexible fibreoptic sigmoidoscopy

This is a safe, quick and useful addition to rigid sigmoidoscopy. A single enema is usually all that is needed for preparation and, when used as an out-patient investigation, could reduce the number of barium enema examinations. Since most colonic neoplasms occur on the left side of the colon, they can be diagnosed and treated by this technique which allows rapid inspection of the rectum, sigmoid and descending colon up to the splenic flexure. It spares the patient the rigorous preparation required for total colonoscopy, and is much less time-consuming for the endoscopist.

Detection of chronic gastrointestinal blood loss

Stool testing for occult blood

The test depends on the pseudo-peroxidase activity of haemoglobin which produces a blue colour from impregnated guaiac on addition of peroxidase developer solution. Degradation of peroxidase activity during intestinal transit makes the test less sensitive to bleeding lesions high in the gastrointestinal tract (20–40 ml/day) compared to recto-sigmoid sources (1–2 ml/day).

A true positive result therefore depends on the rate of faecal daily blood loss, the location of its source and the timing of the test in relation to bleeding since many lesions bleed intermittently. False negative results will be reduced by increasing the number of tests (usually 3 on consecutive days).

During the period of testing the patient is not allowed to eat red meat, raw vegetables high in peroxidase activity (radish, cauliflower) or receive oral iron therapy, since all of these can produce false positive results.

Use of faecal occult blood tests in mass population screening for colonic neoplasms is currently under evaluation. Highly sensitive tests yield large numbers of false positive results and an unnecessarily heavy resource requirement for invasive follow-up investigation. Low sensitivity tests will inevitably miss many colonic neoplasms (false negatives) which bleed only a little or infrequently.

Tests are convenient for sampling at home and mailing to the laboratory.

Radioisotope detection of occult gastrointestinal bleeding

^{51}Chromium-labelled erythrocytes. The patient's own red cells are labelled *in vitro* with sodium (^{51}Cr) chromate and then re-injected. By serial determination of radioactivity in blood and total daily stool collections, daily gastrointestinal blood loss can be determined precisely since the isotopic label is neither secreted nor reabsorbed from the gut.

^{59}*Iron.* When ^{59}Fe is administered to the iron-deficient patient, it is almost entirely incorporated into red cell haemoglobin. Counts of whole body ^{59}Fe or of the ^{59}Fe concentration in blood samples remain virtually constant for 100 days in the absence of bleeding.

PART III
ESSENTIAL BACKGROUND INFORMATION

Knowledge is of two kinds. We know a subject
ourselves, or we know where we can find the
information about it.

Dr Samuel Johnson

Chapter 8
General Problems

The spectrum of gastrointestinal disorders seen in hospital wards bears little relation to that in general practice, for hospital patients are a selected group. The two main causes for patients consulting their general practitioner (Table 8.1) are acute 'infections' (usually diarrhoea with or without vomiting) and functional disorders (vague symptoms sometimes of undetermined origin). Consultants tend to concentrate their attention more on specific disorders like peptic ulcer and Crohn's disease which are rare in general practice and so more easily missed by the family doctor. However, at the out-patient clinic, there is seldom any lack of those with vague complaints—especially belly ache—which are not of organic origin, such as nervous dyspepsia and the irritable bowel syndrome (Table 8.2)

Chronic abdominal pain

Chronic abdominal pain is a common problem and up to 50% of patients in some gastrointestinal clinics suffer from it. It can be defined as pain continuing longer than 3 months; physical signs are usually absent and investigations negative apart from incidental findings which confuse the issue. Pain is subjective and no-one but the patient knows its intensity; nor is there any method of measuring it. Often patients appear after years of uncertainty—the victims of numerous erroneous diagnoses, unnecessary investigations and even fruitless operations. The longer the duration, the less likely is organic disease; yet even when time has excluded any reasonable possibility of malignancy, fear of this, both in the mind of the patient and of the doctor, may linger and the longer the duration of the trouble, the more difficult it is to cure.

No age is exempt. Ten per cent of children suffer from it and some continue with it as adults. Adults may present with symptoms that mimic peptic ulcer, gallbladder disease, or carcinoma; some are even admitted as an 'acute abdomen'. Three questions must be answered when a patient presents with pain of undetermined origin:

1 Does the pain resemble any known disorder?
2 Have investigations been carried out satisfactorily and relevant diseases excluded?
3 Do the description of the pain and any associated symptoms indicate either an organic or psychosomatic disorder?

Methods of diagnosis
Diagnosis depends upon pattern matching and this causes error; for the stereotypes

Table 8.1. Annual consultation rates for patients with gastrointestinal diseases attending General Practitioners (RCGP/OPCS 1974).

Disease	Annual consultation rates (per 1000)
Acute gastrointestinal infections	66
Functional disorders and symptoms	62
Peptic ulcers and oesophagitis	21
Neoplasms	10
Acute abdomen (appendicitis etc.)	4
Herniae	11
Piles, etc.	15
Gallbladder, etc.	10
Others	11
Total	240

(From *Common Diseases: the Nature, Incidence and Care*, John Fry.)

of disease used for teaching can be wrong, and though chronic abdominal pain is so common in practice the subject is often missing from books.

Importance of the history

A detailed history often gives the clue to diagnosis. Yet it is easy for the family doctor, instead of listening, to write a prescription for tablets to keep the queue of patients moving, or for the hospital doctor to fill up a form for yet another X-ray. Too much depends upon the patient's lucidity and the doctor's ability to interpret lay words. Indigestion, acidity, and heartburn may mean almost anything and wind often implies epigastric discomfort or pain.

A detailed analysis of the pain is essential:

Character. Organic pain is often described as aching, boring or gripping and not called pricking or stabbing.

Severity. Exaggerated descriptions such as 'like a two-edged sword being plunged around my belly' are unlikely to be used by those with organic disease and seldom have been experienced.

Situation. Organic disease is usually localized to one area, and the more diffuse the pain, especially if in upper and lower abdomen, the less likely is disease.

Table 8.2. Number of patients suffering from dyspepsia and colorectal disorders amongst 483 referrals to a combined medicosurgical gastroenterology clinic (Salter *et al.*, 1975) to show high incidence of disorders not of organic origin.

Disorder	No. of patients
Dyspepsia	
Gastric ulcer	24
Carcinoma stomach	7
Duodenal ulcer	90
Nervous dyspepsia	51
Colorectal disorders	
Carcinoma	8
Diverticular disease	18
Ulcerative colitis	16
Irritable bowel syndrome	52
Simple constipation	17

Frequency. Organic pain fluctuates in severity whereas *continuous* pain perhaps present day and night for weeks or years is probably psychosomatic.

Any special times of occurrence. For example, whether the pain is related to or follows stress.

Factors that aggravate or relieve the pain. Important clues can be obtained from the effect of food, drink, alkali, defaecation and so on.

Associated symptoms may be important:

1 Abdominal symptoms which seldom have an organic basis are feelings of fullness and bloating, continuous nausea, belching and prolonged burning sensations.

2 Complaints which are usually psychogenic are tiredness, headache, dizziness, depression, sexual difficulties and insomnia.

The previous or family history may be important. There may have been operations for removal of normal viscera like the appendix or gallbladder; some say 'I've had everything taken away' or 'Oh yes, I've had all the 'ectomies'. A nervous breakdown or other psychiatric illness may have occurred. Occasionally the pain is familial and a reaction to stress which is part of the family pattern.

Clinical examination

Examination should be considered as a therapeutic measure. It must be painstaking and thorough—indeed unnecessarily so—for this can do much to reassure and cure.

Complete examination is always necessary but now the focus will be on the abdomen. Some prod themselves to find areas of tenderness and others lie on the couch with the eyes closed—as if brave sufferers of pain; both are unlikely with organic disease. Tenderness is often misleading. True tenderness is a useful index of inflammation as in acute appendicitis; it is not a particularly helpful sign of peptic ulcer unless this is penetrating, nor of malignant disease. Organic tenderness is usually localized and constant in position whereas tenderness from anxiety is diffuse and may change during the examination, or disappear when the patient's mind is diverted. Exquisite pain even with light touch is of no organic significance and tenderness in one spot, often superficial, virtually excludes intra-abdominal disease; for example a doctor when trying to prove disease of the gallbladder by Murphy's sign may cause a tender area on a rib or produce an anxiety pain.

Beware of mistaking structures that can be felt in a normal abdomen for disease (Fig. 2.1). Tell the patient whether anything relevant is found. Or reassure completely.

How far to investigate

The reasons for investigating these patients are: *fear* (often dispelled if a careful history is taken) of missing organic disease, to *reassure with a normal result* or the *urge to do something*—the 'desperation test'. Many will have been investigated already so X-rays and other results should be seen and not repeated unless necessary.

Routine tests will have included the following:

Blood count. The presence of anaemia implies alimentary disease. A raised ESR suggests inflammatory bowel disease or connective tissue disorder perhaps causing vasculitis, though it can be due to unrelated causes. A normal ESR makes organic disease unlikely though does not exclude it.

Serum biochemistry. A biochemical profile is often available with results of ten or twelve routine tests. The serum calcium occasionally suggests something missed by the clinician: hypocalcaemia points towards adult coeliac disease which can be painful whereas hypercalcaemia, perhaps from hyperparathyroidism or sarcoidosis, causes vague abdominal symptoms. The serum amylase is usually normal in chronic pancreatitis unless done during an episode of pain. Rarely, hyperlipaemia may resemble pancreatitis because of pain; inspection of serum stored overnight in the refrigerator may show it to be milky and the level of fasting triglycerides may be high. Porphyria, though also rare, causes psychiatric symptoms and unnecessary laparotomy because of abdominal pain—it can easily be excluded by testing the urine with Ehrlich's aldehyde reagent.

Complicated and expensive tests should not be ordered without good reason. The final investigation—direct inspection by laparotomy—is sometimes advised

Table 8.3. Disorders which are often incidental and symptomless.

Chronic gastritis
Duodenitis
Hiatus hernia
Gallstones
Cyst on the ovary
Diverticulosis

---

but carries the risk of the surgeon blaming the pain upon some irrelevant finding (Table 8.3) like an adhesion, because motility defects like irritable bowel cannot be seen.

Admission of patient to hospital
Admission is often preferable to trying to solve a long-standing case at out-patients, and watching and talking to the patient in the ward is more rewarding than an expensive 'work-up' of tests, and a psychiatric assessment can be done.

Observation during an attack is invaluable. Sometimes hysterical features are prominent, and organic pain often causes an increase in pulse or sweating. Examination then may, though rarely, reveal a lump due to intermittent intussusception and the stethoscope may reveal loud peristalsis when colic is suspected, perhaps due to subacute obstruction. A sample of blood is taken for the serum bilirubin and amylase, and urine examined for evidence of renal disease and to exclude porphyria. Temperature is taken and (rarely) a plain radiograph may show a dilated loop of gut due to obstruction by volvulus or internal hernia. When psychogenic pain is suspected, an injection of saline sometimes stops it immediately though up to 20% of those with organic disease could be placebo reactors.

Disorders causing chronic abdominal pain
In the past, various labels (Table 8.4) have been used but these are now obsolete. Today the term functional is often used, but this can have two meanings: psychogenic—or a disturbance of the physiological function—both of which may

Table 8.4. Diagnoses previously used to explain abdominal pain, though now obsolete.

Adhesions (without evidence of intestinal obstruction)
Chronic appendicitis
Chronic cholecystitis
Displaced uterus

---

be present in patients with irritable bowel. Most can be fitted into one of the following conditions though there is much overlap.

Worry pain

Transient aches and pains are common in the healthy, but may persist in someone with an emotional problem or who unduly fears cancer.

Worry pain perpetuated by non-disease

This happens when a normal or irrelevant finding is wrongly regarded by the doctor as significant. Findings (Table 8.3) which are often symptomless, can only too easily be accepted as the cause instead of being coincidental.

Abdominal neurosis

The abdomen often acts as a sounding-board for the emotions, so symptoms may be part of a psychoneurosis. This is easily overlooked for it is a common idea that pain means physical illness. Surgeons can be unaware that neurosis exists and surgical books—including monographs about abdominal pain—even fail to mention it. Yet several studies have shown that psychiatric factors are a common cause of abdominal pain.

Support for a psychogenic disorder may be provided by the patient's personality. An exaggerated description of symptoms is common: the patient who smilingly and even laughingly says that the pain is making life unbearable. Weeping during a consultation indicates depression and seldom occurs even with terminal organic disease. Patients vary strikingly in their complaint threshold, some first visiting their doctor when their disease is advanced, whereas others notice sensations which would pass unobserved by the average person; then symptoms pour out and the greater the number the less likely is organic disease. Sometimes examination becomes impossible because of continuous talking; then the clinical thermometer comes in useful as it induces silence when placed under the tongue. The complaint of other bodily feelings likely to be psychosomatic provides positive evidence for diagnosing neurosis. Psychological factors superimposed upon organic disease provide a snare for the unwary. Also neurotic patients are not immortal and develop organic disease. Caution is necessary in those over 50 years who have never suffered from nervous illness before as organic disease is then likely. However, although a wrong diagnosis of neurosis can be bad for the doctor's reputation, an unjustified organic diagnosis may be disastrous as it can cause invalidism, unnecessary operations and deprivation of much of the enjoyment of eating. Treatment is most effective when carried out before patients have been confused by doing the rounds of various hospitals and different specialists.

An occasional patient makes a career of suffering and as Szasz (1968) wrote, 'in the game of painsmanship, the patient's aim is to produce undiagnosable pain and unrelievable suffering. This creates meaning for his life and power to control his human environment ... such persons crave medical and surgical (and *not* psychiatric) intervention to make their role as sick patients legitimate'.

Irritable bowel
This explains much abdominal pain and is due to a disturbance of motility which can affect any part of the alimentary tract from oesophagus to anus (p. 318).

Nervous dyspepsia
Dyspepsia often arises from problems in the psyche; pain or discomfort may be localized to the epigastrium, but may occur elsewhere as well. It starts immediately after eating in contrast to ulcer pain which is not aggravated but relieved by food. Details are given elsewhere (p. 183).

'Chronic appendicitis'
Pain in the right iliac fossa is a common manifestation of anxiety in young women and may have replaced the swooning of the Victorian era. More than half of these patients are dissatisfied after appendicectomy; their pain recurs or they develop other psychosomatic symptoms. For further details see p. 14.

'Chronic cholecystitis'
Complaints of vague discomfort together with belching and dyspepsia after eating fats are not due to gallbladder disease and cholecystectomy seldom relieves symptoms. Fat intolerance may occur in a few patients with any form of dyspepsia, especially duodenal ulcer, and is not a symptom of gallbladder disease. Most patients with gallstones enjoy eating fat and the intolerance usually develops only after medical advice to avoid eating fats.

Deliberate disability
The clandestine taking of purgatives can mimic colonic disease and is easily overlooked. Faeces or urine can be tested for cascara and phenolphthalein.

Munchausen's syndrome
The patients travel from hospital to hospital seeking medical attention and operation by inventing symptoms.

Pain of unknown origin
Occasionally pain is the only symptom and cannot be fitted into any category. New methods of investigation may, in the future, provide some physiological explanation.

Guidelines for handling these patients
Many are easily cured by reassurance; the doctor may arrange a follow-up visit so as to be certain that symptoms have improved or gone. Some, especially those with

long-standing pain, provide a challenge. Handling the patient is bedevilled by lack of confidence in doctors, anxiety created by unnecessary investigations and operations, worry caused by the use of obsolete labels (Table 8.4), and bitterness that no one is able to produce a cure. Aggression may conceal anxiety or a desire to escape the detection of a real emotional problem. Pains are ascribed to some disease or dysfunction of their bodies and never to an emotional cause, in contrast to those with organic disease who may even suggest that the trouble is nervous. Self-opinionated theories abound and the patient may try to 'out-talk' the doctor. Doctor–patient relationships can be strained to the utmost from mutual frustration and antagonism, so that only a sense of detachment by the doctor will save the situation.

A sympathetic and confident approach is essential. These patients are not impostors and the pain, whether organic or psychogenic, to the patient is the same. Any idea that it is imagined is naturally resented. Unfortunately, when no other organic trouble is found, the doctor may just make the frustrating statement 'there is nothing wrong with you' which is bound to create hostility. Whereas the alternative 'there is nothing *seriously* wrong with you', can have a very beneficial effect especially if the mechanism of pain is discussed.

Correction of faulty physiological ideas

This takes time, and a suitable booklet written for the lay person can be helpful. Many have wrong ideas about digestion: they blame acid and fear bile if they see it in a vomit not realizing that this is an essential physiological substance. The same applies to mucus which may be seen in stools.

Providing an explanation

This satisfies the patient's ego and provides an alibi for the reality of the pain. The term 'spasm' is easily accepted without causing anxiety; and antispasmodic tablets can be prescribed to 'relax the bowel' though often any drug, whether placebo or not, will help if dispensed by a sympathetic doctor. Discussion about nerves (neurosis) must be approached cautiously as many wrongly associate this suggestion with lack of courage and take offence, not realizing that the bravest person is sometimes neurotic. The problem of nervous tension and its effect upon the body can be explained. Headache can be given as an example of pain caused by worry or diarrhoea before school examinations as the effect of stress, for this idea is easily accepted by lay people.

Counteracting any iatrogenic component

Doctors feel compelled to tell the patient something. It is a pity if this is dogmatic and frightening. For example, one surgeon proudly stated that 'the abdomen was in a mess', meaning that he found many adhesions—though these were in fact symptomless. Doctors may remark that they are sure that the pain is organic or a psychiatrist may state that the patient is as normal a person as he is. Diplomacy is needed to counteract these statements without letting a colleague down.

Conflicting information commonly confuses. Different explanations and diagnoses may be given by doctors even working in the same department. What the patient is told should be written in the case notes for all to see, and must be reported to the general practitioner.

Searching for an emotional cause
This may be simple as in a child developing a stomach ache to avoid going to school. In adults it is usually more complex and difficult to extract. Time and privacy are needed for talking and listening.

The cause may be domestic upset, business strain, difficulties with sex, or merely the need to attract sympathy and attention. The help of a psychiatrist may be needed, but patients whose complaints are almost entirely somatic are often best dealt with by a sympathetic physician who can speak authoritatively. However, a psychiatrist can give great help to certain patients, especially those who may have delusions about their bodily function or suffer from serious depression. Treatment of depression may cure the pain.

Drugs and other treatment of pain
The effect of drugs is difficult to assess as any new ones may be effective, at any rate temporarily. Analgesics and antispasmodics may be tried but addiction-forming drugs like pethidine must be avoided. Pain may be affected by any form of suggestion, whether by hypnotism (though no controlled trials are available) or by the magic of fringe medicine like acupuncture. One patient underwent laparotomy; nothing abnormal was found but the explanation that one coil of bowel was longer than the other produced a cure.

Importance of a combined approach
Needless to say, the spouse must be kept fully in the picture with emphasis that the symptoms are genuine. All those who come into contact with the patient—other doctors, nurses, and relatives—must also be told what has been said so as to take the same hopeful approach. For example, the endoscopist and radiologist can be told of the presumptive diagnosis and act as psychotherapists reassuring the patient at the time of the investigation. Once the decision has been taken that organic disease is absent, the same supportive and reassuring attitude should be taken by all.

Malnutrition
Malnutrition may present blatantly with the picture of an emaciated patient, but diagnosis is often less easy. Causes are anorexia with inadequate calorie intake, vomiting, fever, malabsorption and diarrhoea.

The reasons given for improving nutrition are that it makes the patient feel better, helps the healing of wounds, and improves immunocompetence, though

Table 8.5. Criteria for diagnosing protein-calorie malnutrition.

Weight loss	Greater than 10% of ideal weight
Mid-triceps skinfold thickness	Less than 10 mm (men); 13 mm (women)
Mid-triceps arm muscle circumference	Less than 23 cm (men); 22 cm (women)
Serum albumin	Less than 35 g/l
Serum transferrin	Less than 2 g/l
Lymphocyte count	Less than 1500/μl
Impaired cell-mediated immunity (delayed hypersensitivity)	Skin anergy for candida, PPD (tuberculin), mumps, streptodornase and streptokinase

objective proof is still lacking because of the reluctance to perform clinical trials where malnourished patients are randomized to a controlled group.

Diagnosis

The diagnosis of protein-calorie malnutrition is based upon certain clinical, biochemical and immunological parameters (Table 8.5). Weight loss is often unreliable and it depends upon the patient's memory; there may be oedema due to hypoalbuminaemia. Also, its importance may be greater in thin than in obese patients. Anthropometric data concerning triceps skin fold and upper arm muscle size norms are available. A reliable indicator is a serum albumin of less than 35 g/l in the absence of renal or liver disease. Skin anergy occurs due to immunological changes and may be reversible.

Nutritional requirements

A normal man has only limited nutritional reserves (Table 8.6). When the carbohydrate is metabolized, and this may occur in 8–12 h, proteins and fats are used. Protein catabolism takes place in order to provide carbohydrate metabolic intermediates, as fat is unable to provide these, and indeed fat metabolism needs a steady supply of carbohydrates in order to avoid ketoacidosis. During acute starvation, catabolism occurs at a rate of 10–15 g nitrogen daily, but this may be

Table 8.6. Approximate nutritional reserves in normal man.

	Quantity (kg)	Duration
Carbohydrate	0.15–0.20	8–12 h
Fat	10–15	20–25 days
Protein	4–6	10–15 days

reduced to 3–4 g/day by giving only 100 g glucose; during these states energy supplies are derived from body fat stores which may contribute up to 50% of the calories required. An obese patient shows an identical protein catabolism so that significant nutritional deficiency can occur in the fat patient who develops, for example, ulcerative colitis, or needs an operation. Adequate feeding can reduce or even abolish the catabolic response in severely ill patients. The amount of protein needed is 1 g/kg daily, plus the loss in faeces and urine together with some extra to counteract the catabolic effect of fever if present. Hence it is wise to give about 50% more, such as 1.5 g/kg daily. The calorie content of the diet needs to be high in order to enable full utilization of the protein, and calories are needed to utilize protein at the rate of 33 kilocalories/1 g protein.

The high protein, high calorie diet
A diet is prescribed with 150 g of protein daily with a total of 2500–3500 calories and served as attractively as possible. The patient is encouraged to eat as much of this as his condition allows. However, most are unable to eat the large amounts of meat, fish and milk that are needed and many are financially unable to afford the cost. So, high protein supplements are generally required. Extra carbohydrate is supplied in the form of glucose polymers (e.g. Caloreen, Hycal, etc.) for these are less sweet than sucrose or glucose and therefore provide energy in a more palatable form—also, because of a very high molecular weight, the osmotic pressure is low and diarrhoea avoided. The market abounds with commercial preparations but a high protein, high calorie food supplement can easily be made as follows: 340 ml (12 oz) of each of the following: full cream milk powder, egg, dried skimmed milk, glucose polymer, fat emulsion (e.g. Calogen). It is made up to 2 litres to be taken daily; it tastes like a milk shake but can be flavoured as needed. It allows greater flexibility and can be tailored to the patient's needs and is cheaper than proprietary preparations.

It can either be drunk or given through a gastric tube. It only contains about 3 mg Fe per feed, so iron such as ferrous fumarate is added: 1 ml (9 mg Fe) per feed. Additional vitamins, both water- and fat-soluble are needed, but vitamin preparations may give a flavour like that of yeast to the mixture, so when given orally vitamins are often best prescribed separately. Two litres provides 90 g protein, 106 g fat, 230 g carbohydrate and so adds 2210 kilocalories daily to the intake.

Enteral and parenteral nutrition
If the patient cannot drink, or has no desire to do so, enteral nutrition through a nasogastric tube may be needed. A soft, fine-bored silicon rubber tube such as the 6-gauge paediatric tube is passed; there is no place for the long-term use of Ryle's tubes designed for gastric aspiration. A refillable plastic container like the Viomedex nutrition bag can be used to hold the feed which is attached to a delivery tube, with a drop chamber and regulating tip. Sometimes a pump is necessary. Intravenous feeding (parenteral nutrition) is only indicated in patients with a

shortened small intestine, postoperative ileus or fistula, or temporarily for intractable diarrhoea, as it is dangerous; the main hazards are blood-borne infections (septicaemia), biochemical disturbances (hyperosmolar hyperglycaemic non-ketotic dehydration and coma), hypophosphataemia (neuromuscular problems including dysarthria and paraesthesiae with weakness), hypokalaemia, metabolic acidosis, jaundice, and deficiency states due to the absence of vitamins, trace elements or other essential nutrients in the infused fluids.

Acute upper gastrointestinal bleeding

The patient with haematemesis and melaena provides one of the most worrying problems for any doctor. The course is unpredictable, and even today up to 10% of patients may die. There are certain rules for guidance but each patient must be considered individually and procrastination avoided in advising operation. The causes of bleeding are seen in Table 8.7.

Table 8.7. Causes of acute upper gastrointestinal bleeding.

---

1 Acute or chronic ulcers: (i) Chronic duodenal ulcer; (ii) chronic gastric ulcer; (iii) acute erosions; (iv) oesophagitis with ulcer; (v) stomal ulcer.
2 Mallory–Weiss Syndrome (A split in the mucosa at the gastro-oesophageal junction due to vomiting)
3 Portal hypertension with oesophageal varices (usually from cirrhosis of liver).
4 Carcinoma of stomach.
5 Rare causes: disease of the blood, hereditary telangiectasia and other vascular malformations, aortic aneurysm, pancreatic tumours, and anticoagulant therapy.

Diagnosis

The drama of haemorrhage and need for action must not deter the doctor from getting a good history either from the patient or from relatives. Enquiry must be made about drugs such as aspirin, alcohol, or antirheumatic drugs. A story of long-standing dyspepsia indicates duodenal ulcer or a short history may suggest acute erosions. Vomiting may have occurred from a cause such as migraine and the bleeding may be due to the Mallory–Weiss syndrome; then the patient initially vomits clear fluid and blood only appears in a second or later vomit. Evidence of cirrhosis may be found or general ill-health such as loss of weight and strength may point to advanced carcinoma of the stomach though this is more likely to cause melaena than haematemesis. The abdomen should be felt gently and an epigastric mass or enlarged spleen—the guide to portal hypertension—excluded.

Endoscopy

Endoscopy soon after admission has supplanted the barium meal in searching for the site of the bleeding. If done within 48 h the cause can be found in nearly 80% of patients. Earlier endoscopy is indicated if bleeding is continuous or recurrent and when operation is under consideration for it provides the surgeon with data that he could not get from laparotomy. Endoscopy also shows that erosions are not as common as previously diagnosed from a history of aspirin ingestion and negative barium meal; these patients are more likely to have bled from a peptic ulcer than from erosions. It has also shown the importance of oesophageal lesions such as oesophagitis and the Mallory–Weiss tear, and duodenal ulcers are less important than previously thought because patients with a deformed cap or duodenal ulcer may be bleeding from another site. The incidence of two potential bleeding lesions found at endoscopy is high, and may be 10% or more; this is especially relevant in those with oesophageal varices as they may be bleeding from a peptic ulcer.

Unfortunately it cannot be shown that endoscopy alters the outcome though it no doubt relieves strain on the surgeon when he knows the diagnosis before some nocturnal operation. It is slightly less safe than barium meal, mainly because of the risk of inhalation of gastric contents, and should be done by a trained endoscopist. It is more difficult because the stomach is often filled with blood clots, which obscures the view; these clots are very difficult to aspirate even with a wide-bore tube and some use intravenous metoclopramide to empty the stomach of blood beforehand. The inhalation of acid gastric contents is more likely to damage the lungs than alkali, so patients can be treated with cimetidine before endoscopy, though any beneficial effect is unproven. The forward-viewing endoscope is used first, but if no bleeding point is found, a side-viewing instrument may make the diagnosis. Sedation is a problem as it may increase risk of inhalation; so endoscopy can sometimes be done without sedation as in Japan or with smaller doses of diazepam so that the cough reflex remains intact. Spraying the throat with local anaesthetic should also be avoided. Active bleeding, a blood clot, or black slough in the base of an ulcer may be seen in over 70% of patients by an expert. The diagnostic yield declines rapidly after 48 h mainly owing to the healing of mucosal lesions.

Radiology

Plain films of the abdomen are seldom indicated. Occasionally an indirect pointer to the source of bleeding may be shown, e.g. an enlarged spleen in portal hypertension.

Barium studies in active bleeding are often disappointing because blood clot obscures all except gross lesions; so the source of bleeding may be missed in up to 30% of patients. However, if endoscopy is not available, barium studies are worth attempting as they may show oesophageal varices, a peptic ulcer or duodenal deformity, or a tumour of the stomach or pancreas. Waiting until the bleeding has stopped is better for the radiologist who, by double contrast methods, may detect unhealed mucosal lesions or chronic conditions like ulcers.

Angiography is used to locate the source of bleeding, providing it is done during bleeding when the leakage of contrast medium can be seen. Once bleeding has stopped the angiogram can only show the vascular abnormality itself and this can easily be missed.

Treatment

Anxiety must be relieved by an explanation and reassurance and a sedative injected; morphine or pethidine are seldom required and they sometimes cause vomiting. An hourly pulse and blood pressure chart is essential until bleeding is controlled—as changes will give early warning of further haemorrhage. Two-hourly milk feeds with other fluid as well, if necessary or wished, are begun. An exsanguinated patient requires fluid to replace blood volume and to prevent uraemia. Blood is taken for measurement of haemoglobin, haematocrit and blood group.

A small haemorrhage may hardly affect the patient, but loss of a litre or more of blood may cause severe shock. Estimation of blood loss in the laboratory or elsewhere is unreliable. The Hb and haematocrit may be normal on admission, for blood dilution only occurs during the next few hours or days. A simple bedside technique for estimating the blood volume is seldom available and the effect of haemorrhage must be assessed indirectly by the presence of shock and changes in the pulse and blood pressure. The criteria which indicate the need for blood transfusion are listed in Table 8.8. Initial shock must be combated by an

Table 8.8. Criteria for advising blood transfusion.

Shock
A pulse persistently above 100/min
A systolic blood pressure of 110 mmHg or less
Hb 9 g/100 ml (60%) or less

---

intravenous drip of plasma or a substitute plasma expander such as dextran until blood is available. No patients die immediately from anaemia; they die from circulatory failure due to decreased circulatory volume. Blood transfusion is not only life-saving but prevents the ill-effects of shock: uraemia from hypotension, cerebral ischaemia in the elderly and rare ocular sequelae such as blindness. However, blood transfusion keeps the bleeding patient in good condition and encourages dangerous delay in advising surgery; hence it should not be continued after 48 h unless a definite decision has been taken that operation is contraindicated. Occasionally bleeding may be torrential, as from rupture of an artery crossing an ulcer; then a drip in each arm or pump-assisted infusion is required. Central venous pressure monitoring during blood replacement is useful to judge the amount and rate of infusion if this has to be continued for any length of time; then blood filters and blood warmers may reduce some of the complications of major transfusions including shock lung and a bleeding diathesis—the latter probably being due to a disseminated intravascular coagulation; haemorrhagic problems secondary to blood transfusion are now more easily dealt with by the availability of fresh frozen plasma and platelet concentrates. With massive transfusions calcium gluconate should be given to counteract the anticoagulant effect of citrate.

The effect of drugs is disappointing. H_2 antagonists, whether given intravenously or orally, are of doubtful use except possibly when gastric erosions or duodenal ulcers have bled and in expediting the healing of chronic ulcers to prevent further bleeding later. Antifibrinolytic agents like tranexamic acid have been claimed to reduce blood loss but no controlled trials have been done; the reason for using it is to counteract the fibrinolytic activity of the stomach which dissolves newly formed clots. Vasopressin controls bleeding in only a few patients, and then often only temporarily.

Therapeutic endoscopy may help. Oesophageal varices can be injected with a sclerosant through the endoscope or compression therapy may be applied with the Sengstaken–Blakemore tube (Fig. 14.4); the major problem with this tube is aspiration pneumonia but this has been reduced by making additional suction holes above the oesophageal balloon and by nursing patients in an ITU with, if necessary, a nasal endotracheal tube in place to prevent aspiration. Reports have shown a good initial control of bleeding in the stomach and duodenum by electrocautery, with a low incidence of rebleeding, but it may damage the tissues around the ulcer and even worsen haemorrhage. In contrast the blue-green light of the Argon laser beam is selectively absorbed by blood and can produce local coagulation with minimal damage to the tissues around, but the value of this is doubtful and special expensive equipment is needed. If a bleeding point can be seen by angiography, it may be possible to introduce a catheter into the vessel feeding that point and to attempt haemostasis by infusing vasopressin or by injecting embolic material such as sterile absorbable gelatin, steel coils, acrylic polymers, or detachable balloons. However, the chance that bleeding from a peptic ulcer will stop spontaneously is so high that no method for stopping the haemorrhage can be judged clinically useful unless validated by controlled trials which include large numbers of patients.

Surgery

Operation is the surest means of stopping bleeding but as many as a third of patients operated upon because of bleeding may die after surgery. The two main reasons for the high surgical mortality are that firstly many of the patients are old and unfit before they bleed and secondly their prospects are often further impaired by inadequate treatment of blood loss and its complications. Procrastination often causes surgery to be undertaken at the eleventh hour.

Operation is most successful when performed within 48 h after admission and is advisable in the circumstances listed in Table 8.9.

Prognosis

Bleeding from acute erosions in the stomach, oesophagitis due to hiatus hernia or from the Mallory–Weiss syndrome is more likely to respond to medical treatment. The outlook in those over 60 is worse, and this may be due to associated disease such

Table 8.9. Reasons for advising operation.

---

1 For most patients with gastric ulcers, especially those over 60 years. (Mortality rate with medical treatment is higher than from other causes and operation is easier than for duodenal ulcer).
2 For patients with both gastric and duodenal ulcers.
3 For patients with duodenal ulcer which bleeds again after admision, particularly in those over 50 years.
4 For patients who bleed continuously during the first 48 h in spite of medical treatment.
5 For patient with peptic ulcer with complication like pyloric stenosis or if a coexisting perforation is suspected.
6 For patient with any suspicion of carcinoma.

---

as atheroma or heart disease. There is no evidence that routine endoscopy or the routine use of emergency surgery improves the overall prognosis, and each patient must be considered individually. Overall mortality remains between 5 and 10%.

Jaundice

Modern technology has much improved the management of the patient with jaundice. Previously diagnosis depended upon symptoms and signs supported by biochemical tests of liver 'function'. Many clinicians were unable to distinguish medical from surgical jaundice so that doubtful cases lingered in bed for weeks, with consequent cost to patient and hospital. Those that failed to recover were subjected to laparotomy, with an increased risk in ill patients. Now advances made in diagnostic techniques usually enable a correct diagnosis to be made early in the illness.

Cholestasis is the current term for the clinical syndrome that used to be known as obstructive jaundice. Whereas obstructive jaundice implies a surgical cause such as gallstones, cholestasis includes other conditions such as drug-induced jaundice which may produce a similar clinical picture. The causes of jaundice are shown in Table 8.10.

Bilirubin metabolism

Bilirubin is a waste product of haem catabolism, to which haemoglobin is the major contributor. It is highly insoluble in water and therefore does not occur in urine in its natural form and bilirubin is transported from its site of origin (spleen or bone marrow) to the liver, tightly bound by serum albumin. It is conjugated within the hepatocyte, mainly with glucuronide which renders it water soluble.

Bilirubin conjugates are normally excreted efficiently in bile; if for some reason they reflux into the blood, they will appear in the urine—being water soluble. Within the intestine bilirubin is partly metabolized by bacteria to produce urobilinogen which is water soluble and readily absorbed by the intestine. Most

Table 8.10. Causes of jaundice.

Common
    Gallstones
    Hepatitis
    Carcinoma of head of pancreas
    Secondary deposits of carcinoma in liver
Occasional
    Drugs
    Cirrhosis
    Cholangitis
    Haemolytic anaemia
    Gilbert's syndrome (usually just hyperbilirubinaemia)
Rare
    Malaria (in UK)
    Lymphomas
    Contraceptive pill
    Pregnancy
    Carcinoma of gallbladder or bile ducts

absorbed urobilinogen is efficiently extracted from portal venous blood on its first pass through the liver, but a small proportion escapes and appears later in the urine.

History-taking
Enquire regarding any previous episodes of jaundice and the duration of the current one. Is the depth of jaundice constant, fluctuating or progressively rising or falling; was the onset preceded by pain, if so what were its characteristics—severe, epigastric, radiating to the shoulder or back and so on? Dark urine, pale stools and pruritus in someone who otherwise feels well is typical of cholestatic jaundice.

    Progressive painless jaundice is characteristic of carcinoma of the head of the pancreas. A sudden severe epigastric or hypochondrial pain before the onset of jaundice suggests obstruction due to gallstones.

    Fluctuating jaundice is more typical of gallstones or carcinoma of the papilla of Vater (Fig. 8.1) than of a pancreatic neoplasm. Cholestatic jaundice and anaemia due to blood loss or iron deficiency suggests a sloughing carcinoma of the papilla of Vater.

    A prodromal illness like influenza or gastroenteritis for a week or so before the appearance of jaundice indicates hepatitis. Patients with hepatitis B, or non-A, non-B often have a history of parenteral spread from injections or transfusions. Any breach of the integument by a contaminated object may be the source, including tattoos and ear piercing. Homosexual practice may be relevant to its spread and

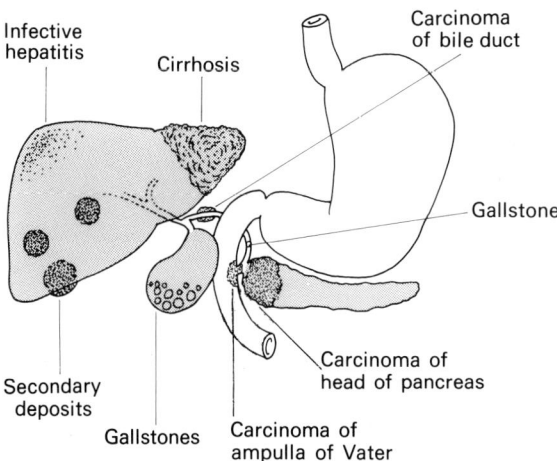

Fig. 8.1. Common causes of jaundice.

heterosexual transmission of hepatitis B also occurs during sexual intercourse. A history of foreign travel may suggest a vector-borne infection like yellow fever, though this is very rare or, more likely, hepatitis A.

Previous attacks of jaundice will indicate a possible cirrhosis, especially if there is a history of alcoholism.

A history of *rigor with jaundice* points to cholangitis or liver abscess. Testing the urine for bilirubin and microscopy for pus cells help to distinguish between cholangitis and pyelonephritis (the two common causes of illness presenting as a rigor in non-malarial zones).

Physical examination
Involvement of the sclerae distinguishes jaundice from other causes of pigmentation such as increased melanin, hypercarotinaemia, (excessive vitamin A as from overindulgence in carrots) and therapy with mepacrine or busulphan. There may be detectable differences in the tint produced by haemolytic (lemon yellow), hepato-cellular (orange-yellow) and obstructive or cholestatic (greenish yellow) causes of jaundice, though no diagnostic reliance should be based on such impressions alone. The eyes are best examined in natural light. Inspection of the palate with a torch also is a good way of detecting mild jaundice.

The body should first be searched for any signs of chronic liver disease. The most useful one is the spider naevus (Fig. 8.2) in which a central arteriole divides into a spray of tiny vessels in the skin; pinpoint pressure on the central arteriole causes blanching of the entire naevus. They occur predominantly in the distribution of the superior vena cava and more than seven are said to be

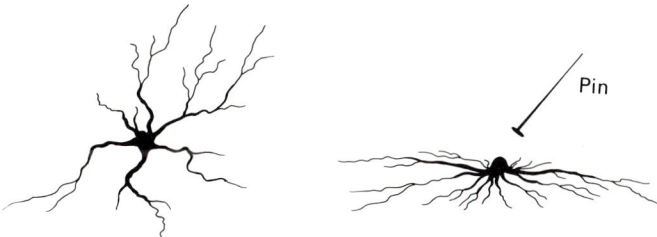

Pin

Fig. 8.2. The spider naevus.

pathological; they occur physiologically in pregnancy and are thought to indicate excess oestrogenic activity. Other less specific signs are:

1 Palmar erythema: a blotchy red discolouration of the thenar and hypothenar eminences.

2 Dupuytren's contracture (in alcoholics), gynaecomastia (especially in alcoholics or as a side-effect of spironolactone therapy), and finger clubbing.

3 Leuconychia (white nails suggestive of hypoalbuminaemia).

4 Pigmentation (e.g. primary biliary cirrhosis or the slate grey colour of haemochromatosis).

There may be no abnormal signs in the abdomen. Occasionally a lump is found indicating a carcinoma with secondary deposits in the liver. A palpable spleen points to portal hypertension from cirrhosis of the liver, a palpable distended gallbladder (Courvoisier's sign) (Fig. 2.6) indicates a carcinoma of the head of the pancreas; if due to gallstones, the gallbladder is usually small and fibrosed and cannot enlarge. Ascites suggests either malignant disease or cirrhosis.

Diagnosis

Sometimes there is doubt about the type of jaundice and this is investigated as follows:

1 Serum bilirubin may be measured by the van den Bergh reaction. Conjugated bilirubin forms a violet colour immediately on addition of sulfanilic acid (direct reacting bilirubin); unconjugated bilirubin adds to the colour subsequently, following addition of alcohol (indirect reacting bilirubin). Useful patterns seen in clinical practice are shown in Table 8.11.

2 Testing the urine can provide a valuable guide in the differential diagnosis of jaundice (Table 8.12). Urinary urobilinogen may be detected by adding Ehrlich's aldehyde reagent which produces a red colour; both urobilinogen and porphobilinogen produce a red colour, but only that due to urobilinogen may be extracted by chloroform.

It cannot be assumed that darkness of the urine is due to bilirubin without testing it. It may also be discoloured due to drugs such as sulphasalazine, rifampicin, and metronidazole. It becomes dark in the dehydrated patient and it

Table 8.11. Useful patterns of bilirubin metabolism for diagnosing jaundice.

1 Haemolysis:
  Excessive production of bilirubin
  Unconjugated hyperbilirubinaemia
  Excessive indirect reacting bilirubin in serum
  Absence of bilirubin from urine
  Excessive urobilinogen in urine (from excessive production)
2 Jaundice due to impaired hepatic removal and conjugation of bilirubin (as seen in the congenital Gilbert and Crigler–Najjar syndromes):
  Normal bilirubin production
  Unconjugated hyperbilirubinaemia
  Excess indirect reacting bilirubin in serum
  Absence of bilirubin from urine
  Normal (or reduced) levels of urobilinogen in urine
3 Jaundice from biliary obstruction (e.g. by carcinoma of pancreas or gallstones):
  Conjugated hyperbilirubinaemia
  Excess direct reacting bilirubin in serum
  Bilirubin in urine
  Reduced amounts of urobilinogen in urine (if biliary obstruction is complete, urobilinogen will be completely absent from the urine)

darkens on standing in acute intermittent porphyria and alkaptonuria. Note that making the urine alkaline may produce a pink colour due to the presence of phenolphthalein and thus provides the diagnosis in a purgative abuser who is being investigated for abdominal pain and diarrhoea.

The investigative techniques for deciding the cause of the jaundice are described in Part II and include ultrasound, ERCP and other methods.

Hyperbilirubinaemia
In a healthy person with no signs of disease, Gilbert's syndrome is a likely cause of mild hyperbilirubinaemia. This is most important to diagnose swiftly so as to

Table 8.12. Urine testing in the differential diagnosis of jaundice.

Condition	Normal	Haemolysis	Gilbert's syndrome	Obstructive Cholestatic
Derangement		Excess production of bilirubin	Impaired hepatic clearance of bilirubin	Biliary obstruction
Bilirubin	o	o	o	++++
Urobilinogen	+	+++	+/±	+/o

reassure the patient that all is well lest he become an iatrogenic wreck, unnecessarily confined to bed and warned off fat, alcohol, work and other delights! Gilbert's syndrome is one of several causes of hyperbilirubinaemia (Table 8.13), in which conventional liver function tests, AST, alkaline phosphatase, γGT show no abnormality other than a raised total serum bilirubin. The causes are classified as to

Table 8.13. Classification of the hyperbilirubinaemias.

Unconjugated
    Decreased hepatic removal and conjugation
    Common
        Gilbert's syndrome
        Physiological jaundice of the newborn
    Rare
        Crigler–Najjar type I
        Crigler–Najjar type II
        Transient familial neonatal hyperbilirubinaemia
        Breast mild jaundice
    Excess production
    Common
        Haemolysis
    Rare
        'Shunt' hyperbilirubinaemia (ineffective erythropoiesis)
Conjugated
    Rare
        Dubin–Johnson syndrome
        Rotor syndrome

Table 8.14. Differentiation of conjugated hyperbilirubinaemia.

	Dubin–Johnson	Rotor	Cholestasis
	Black liver biopsy		
Serum bile acids	Normal	Normal	Increased
BSP test			
Early clearance	Normal	Delayed	Delayed
45 min retention	($<5\%$)	($20-40\%$)	
Later increase	Yes	No	No
Urine coproporphyrin			
Total	Normal	Increased	Increased
Isomer I	$>80\%$	$<80\%$	$<80\%$
	(mean 89%)	(mean 65%)	
Isomer III ($>70\%$ in normals)			

Table 8.15. Differentiation of the hereditary unconjugated hyperbilirubinaemias.

| | Gilbert's syndrome | Crigler–Najjar syndrome | |
		Type I	Type II
Incidence	Common (>1% of the population)	Very rare	Very rare
Presentation	Occasional mild jaundice at time of stress, e.g. fasting	Deep jaundice in neonates	Variable moderately deep jaundice
Kernicterus	Never	Usual	Seldom
Bilirubin reduction in response to phenobarbital	Yes	No	Yes
Defect in bilirubin metabolism	↓Hepatic uptake ↓UDPGT activity	Absent UDPGT activity	Markedly decreased UDPGT activity

(UDPGT = uridine diphosphate glucuronyl transferase)

whether the bilirubin is conjugated (Table 8.14) or unconjugated (direct or indirect reading on van den Bergh testing) (Table 8.15).

These conditions are generally benign except in newborn infants when severe hyperbilirubinaemia can cause brain damage and kernicterus. Bilirubin that is not firmly bound by albumin may diffuse into the brain in neonates but not in later life when deep jaundice causes pigmentation of all tissue other than the brain. It is vital therefore to monitor serum bilirubin levels in jaundiced newborn infants and to prevent rises to dangerous levels by exchange transfusion or phototherapy. Kernicterus is likely if levels reach 340 μmol/l, but impaired psychomotor development may result from levels below this. Infants at risk must not be prescribed drugs which displace bilirubin from albumin, e.g. salicylates, sulfonamides, diazepam and fat-soluble vitamin K analogues. In jaundice of the newborn, reabsorption of unconjugated bilirubin formed in the intestine by action of the B-glucuronidase may be prevented by the oral administration of a non-absorbable agent which binds bilirubin. The much rarer familial causes of conjugated hyperbilirubinaemias can be differentiated by the tests listed in Table 8.14.

The medical acute abdomen

A possible medical cause must be considered in every patient admitted as an acute abdominal emergency especially if the surgical diagnosis is not typical. A detailed history and examination together with the testing of urine for sugar and protein in every surgical patient should prevent these cases being missed. Severe abdominal pain may be referred from neighbouring organs, especially from the heart, either due to coronary infarction or pericarditis. Pleurisy and renal colic may sometimes cause confusion. Early herpes zoster—before the rash appears—may cause embarrassment for the doctor who sends the patient into hospital as an emergency. Rarely involvement of a nerve route in the spine (T6–L1) from disease of the vertebra or involvement of a nerve route by poliomyelitis may mimic the 'acute abdomen'.

Two systemic disorders that must always be excluded are diabetes mellitus and uraemia and these and other general causes are listed in Table 8.16. A disorder of motility, especially irritable colon, may cause pain so severe as to require diagnostic laparotomy and young women, not uncommonly, have a normal appendix removed because of this (p. 14). Episodes of acute pain can occur in inflammatory bowel disease such as Crohn's disease of the terminal ileum. Vascular lesions can be responsible: ischaemia may cause gangrene; embolus may occur after coronary infarction, in atrial fibrillation or endocarditis; arteritis may involve the gut in connective tissue disorders (all these have a raised ESR). Finally do not forget that drugs cause abdominal side-effects which cause patients to be admitted to hospital urgently (e.g. digoxin), as well as toxins like lead poisoning (rare). The tests for diagnosing the medical acute abdomen are listed in Table 8.17.

Table 8.16. Systemic disorders mimicking the 'acute abdomen'.

1 Diabetes mellitus: diabetic ketosis causes epigastric pain sometimes with vomiting from gastric dilatation, (but abdominal catastrophe in a diabetic may precipitate ketosis so both may be present. Give emergency treatment for the diabetes: abdominal symptoms due to diabetes improve as ketosis is controlled).

2 Uraemia: vomiting or haemorrhage may also occur.

3 Diaphragmatic pleurisy.

Occasional causes

4 Herpes zoster.

5 Sickle-cell anaemia: always consider in Negroes; haemoglobin S (sickle-cell haemoglobin) gels when in reduced form. Crises occur causing pain in abdomen, limbs and jaundice (probably due to ischaemia due to stagnation of sickle cells in capillaries in abdominal viscera).

6 Coronary infarction.

7 Haemorrhage into the gut wall: this may be due to thrombocytopenia from leukaemia or other blood disorders, or from anticoagulant therapy or a leaking abdominal aneurysm (haemorrhage in peritoneum).

Rare causes

8 Lead colic.

9 Porphyria: attacks of abdominal pain occur alone or with neurological or mental changes. Passage of urine like port wine may suggest haematuria, though the urine may look normal. Consider this diagnosis in a neurotic patient with multiple abdominal scars.

10 Bornholm disease (epidemic dry pleurisy): pain is due to involvement of intercostal muscles or diaphragm. Usually in epidemics (due to virus of coxsackie B group).

11 Tabes: nerve root pain or gastric crises with vomiting can occur. Check pupils and reflexes. Treponema serology usually positive.

12 Type I hyperlipoproteinaemia: commonly familial and in children. Milky plasma after a meal, abdominal pain like pancreatitis.

13 Spinal disease (e.g. acute osteomyelitis).

14 Hereditary angio-oedema (plasma C_1 esterase inhibitor levels are low).

15 SLE serositis.

Table 8.17. Tests for diagnosing the medical 'acute abdomen'.

1 Routine examination of urine for sugar and protein.

2 Chest X-ray and ECG if a cause above the diaphragm is suspected.

3 Haemoglobin, white blood cell count and ESR to exclude a systemic disorder.

4 Plain film of abdomen: to detect calculi, dilated loops of bowel from ileus or obstruction, calcification from aneurysm or pancreatitis.

5 Tests for sickle-cell disease: sickle cells may be seen in the blood film and the plasma bilirubin is mildly increased.

6 To exclude porphyria test for porphobilinogen by adding equal quantity (2 ml) Erlich's aldehyde reagent (a pink colour is also caused by urobilinogen but can be excluded by solubility in added chloroform).

Chapter 9
Disorders of the Oesophagus

The oesophagus presents fewer difficult clinical problems than elsewhere in the alimentary tract. This is due to its relative simplicity—a hollow muscular tube about 23–25 cm long, stretching from the pharynx to the stomach. It is readily accessible to investigation by barium swallow X-ray and endoscopy.

The oesophagus conveys the bolus of food to the stomach by active peristalsis rather than by gravity, proof of which is obtained by eating or drinking while standing on the head, a skill soon lost in conditions where abnormalities of the neuromuscular mechanism occurs. The radiologist may test this by watching the patient swallow barium against gravity in the Trendelenberg position.

Sensations from the oesophagus readily reach consciousness. The warm feeling behind the sternum after swallowing hot liquid is a common example. More intense stimuli are described as heartburn, a symptom which occurs especially in oesophagitis, though also in the absence of structural disease. Other stimuli result in severe substernal pain identical to that of coronary artery disease; this has been proved by distending the lower oesophagus by a balloon in patients with angina—many are then unable to distinguish this pain from their customary angina.

The upper end is closed by the so-called pharyngo-oesophageal sphincter which prevents its contents regurgitating into the pharynx and prevents aspiration of air into the oesophagus at inspiration. The lower end is also closed—by the lower oesophageal sphincter (LOS). This is not obvious to the naked eye, but manometric studies show a high pressure zone of about 4 cm long, situated partly in the abdominal and partly in the thoracic cavity. Various agents (Table 9.1) exert some control on this, which helps to prevent reflux of gastric juice into the oesophagus. The squamous cell lining of the gullet does not share the same resistance to hydrochloric acid as shown by the columnar cells of the stomach. Hence the problem of reflux causing oesophagitis. The oesophago-gastric junction can be seen at endoscopy (38–40 cm from the incisor teeth in adults) as an irregular line where the pale pink mucosa meets the darker red gastric mucosa. The site of the cardia can be measured by the change in electrical mucosal potential as well as by manometry.

Mechanisms preventing reflux at the gastro-oesophageal junction
The efficiency of the valvular mechanism which prevents gastric contents from regurgitating into the oesophagus either at rest or when swallowing a bolus of food is proved by the exploits of the trapeze artists, in whom it remains effective in spite of the action of physical exertion and gravity. Two main mechanisms contribute to this anti-reflux barrier: the intrinsic sphincter (LOS) and the anatomy at the hiatus.

Table 9.1. Factors controlling lower oesophageal sphincter (LOS) pressure.

Increase	Decrease
Hormones	
Gastrin	Secretin
Prostaglandin F 2	Cholecystokinin
	Glucagon
	Prostaglandin E
Food	
Protein	Chocolate
	Coffee (? methylxanthines)
	Fat (cholecystokinin release)
	Smoking
	Alcohol
Drugs	
Cholinergics (acetylcholine, urecholine, etc.)	Anticholinergics
Cholinesterase inhibitors (tensilon, physostigmine)	Beta-adrenergic stimulators
Metoclopamide (direct action)	Theophylline
Antacids (gastrin release?, local reflex)	Gastric acidification
Adrenergic alpha stimulators	

The LOS
This is closed except when opened by the peristaltic wave of swallowing. Its action in preventing reflux is only partial as reflux still occurs in hiatus hernia where the LOS is the only factor in preventing reflux.

Mechanical factors
The anatomy of the hiatal orifice consists of fibres of the right crus of the diaphragm which bifurcate around the oesophagus and are attached to the vertebral column. This forms an elliptical tunnel about 3 cm long through which the oesophagus passes. Factors which are probably of importance are:
1   The oblique entry of the oesophagus into the stomach (Fig. 9.1). This method of valvular construction by the insertion of a narrow tube into a large hollow organ at an oblique angle is employed elsewhere in the body; an example is the entry of the parotid duct into the mouth—without which the trumpet player would inflate his parotid glands.
2   The flap valve effect of the positive intra-abdominal pressure upon the flaccid intra-abdominal end of the oesophagus (Fig. 9.2).
3   The mucosal rosette formed by the gastric mucosal folds; the bat which spends so much of its life upside down has a lax cardiac mucosa which blocks the entrance

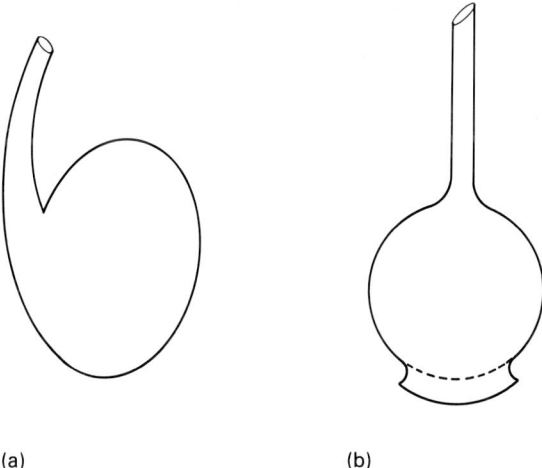

(a)   (b)

Fig. 9.1. (a) The normal oblique entry of the oesophagus resembles a retort; (b) this is lost in sliding hiatus hernia when it resembles an inverted thistle funnel.

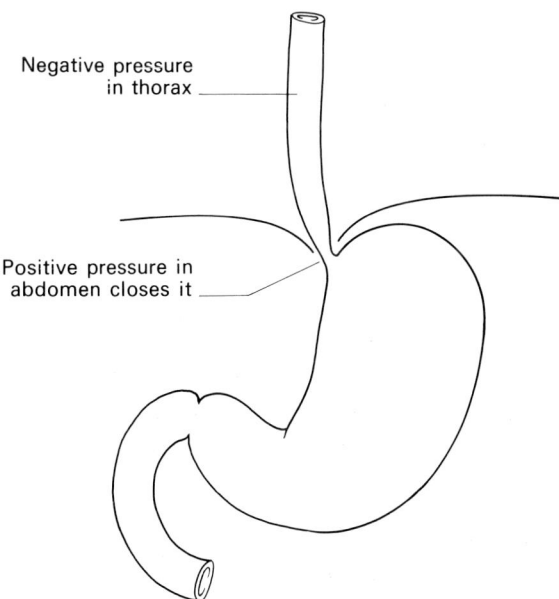

Negative pressure in thorax

Positive pressure in abdomen closes it

Fig. 9.2. The flap-valve effect at the gastro–oesophageal junction.

to the oesophagus like a cork and is as important as its ring-sphincter in preventing the stomach emptying by gravity.

Oesophagitis

Acute oesophagitis
This is the natural result of swallowing injurious substances such as boiling water, strong acids or alkalis, and corrosives like iron—for example when children mistake ferrous sulphate tablets for sweets. Inflammatory changes with necrosis of the mucous membrane occur in severe cases and strictures may result. Oesophagitis may also follow the acute pharyngitis of virus and other infections.

Various tablets and capsules may stick in the oesophagus and cause acute oesophagitis and strictures: potassium compounds, aspirin-containing analgesics, indomethacin, antibiotics and so on. The hold-up of tablets taken without water and when lying down has been shown radiologically; the mid-oesophagus is more vulnerable because of its anatomy, being indented by the aortic arch and left main bronchus. Those patients with some abnormality such as a stricture are most vulnerable and ulceration from potassium compounds has occurred where an enlarged left atrium due to mitral valve disease has caused delayed passage. Elderly patients are at increased risk.

Chronic oesophagitis
This, the commoner problem, may result from the excessive drinking of an irritant like alcohol; the 'morning vomiting' of the alcoholic is usually a regurgitation of mucous fluid collected in the oesophagus overnight—a chemical oesophagitis. Antibiotics may irritate the oesophagus or precipitate moniliasis (thrush) especially in those weakened by prolonged illness and receiving corticosteroids; this is usually, though not always, visible in the mouth or pharynx—barium swallow may be normal but sometimes shows an appearance resembling varices. Prolonged intubation of the stomach causes oesophagitis and even a stricture, for this keeps the cardia open and allows acid reflux when the patient is nursed supine; it may also follow reflux of bile and pancreatic juice after gastric operations.

However, by far the commonest cause of chronic oesophagitis is acid reflux and this is nearly always due to a hiatus hernia (see below).

Symptoms. Heartburn and dysphagia are the usual complaints; the latter may be caused either by spasm or by a fibrous stricture.

Diagnosis. Endoscopy is essential and shows a reddened oedematous mucus membrane perhaps with superficial ulceration, and biopsy may be necessary. A barium swallow is usually ordered to demonstrate reflux but its absence on X-ray does not completely exclude it. If access to an oesophageal laboratory is available, pH measurements with a tube in the lower oesophagus and recorded during the night are diagnostic, as episodes of reflux may be associated with heartburn (Fig. 9.3). The acid perfusion test (p. 61) may be helpful in patients with atypical heartburn or to distinguish oesophageal from cardiac pain.

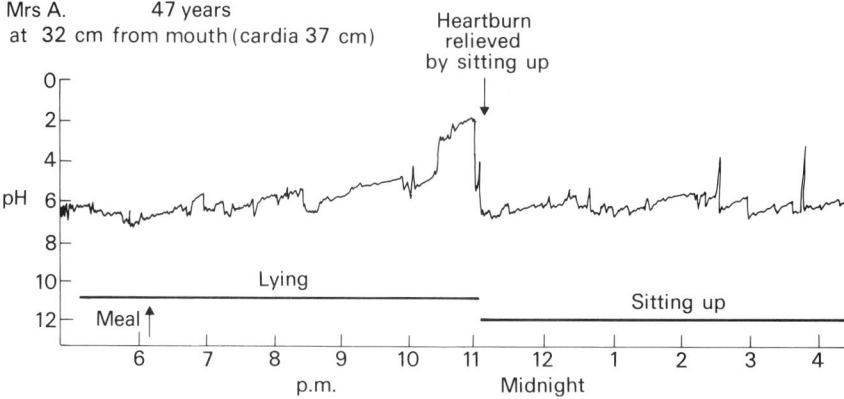

Fig. 9.3. Continuous pH record by electrode in oesophagus to show the association of pH 2 and heartburn—relieved by sitting up.

Hiatus hernia

Aetiology. Age is important, for adult hiatus hernia is commoner in middle and later life, being probably due to laxity of the hiatus occurring as part of the ageing process. There may be a developmental factor in some, though there is no proven connection between the congenital hiatus hernia of infants and that of adults. Increased intra-abdominal pressure causes it, as in pregnancy and obesity. Chest deformities such as kyphosis may predispose to it.

Hernia is traditionally linked with trauma, and injury or strain is often wrongly invoked as the cause. Hiatus hernia is possibly caused occasionally by sudden severe physical exertion, but diagnosis must be based upon an immediate relation between the exertion and the pain, this being severe and resembling that of coronary infarction.

Symptoms (Table 9.2). Hiatus hernia in infants may cause effortless vomiting or gastrointestinal haemorrhage. Many adults, about a third, go through life without symptoms. This especially applies to those with the para-oesophageal type (Fig. 9.4), for the cardia may remain in its correct position and prevent reflux of gastric juice. The sliding type typically gives rise to reflux oesophagitis. Then the heartburn is provoked by posture; it comes on at night when the patient lies down to

Table 9.2. Clinical pictures caused by hiatus hernia with reflux.

Postural heartburn
Regurgitation
'Wind' (aerophagy)
Dysphagia (from spasm or stricture)
Pain like coronary ischaemia
Haematemesis (or melaena)
Aspiration (spillover) pneumonia
Nocturnal asthma (from reflux of gastric contents into lung)
Strangulation (causing severe pain)
Gastric ulcer
Anaemia

---

sleep or bends down during the day to do housework or gardening—special long-handled tools may be used to avoid this. Other factors are large meals or tight garments around the abdomen. Heartburn may spoil the sex life of women for the combined effects of posture and raised intra-abdominal pressure disturbs sexual intercourse: heartburn or regurgitation of the evening meal occurs at the moment of bliss.

Regurgitation of food is frequent, the mouth unexpectedly fills with partially digested food, especially during exercise just after a meal. This can be confused with vomiting which, however, is preceded by nausea. Dysphagia, consisting of a temporary sticking of food, or a feeling of a lump in the chest after swallowing is also common, usually being due to spasm rather than stricture. Aerophagy is often due to the patient's belief that discomfort from oesophagitis is due to 'wind'.

Pain after eating situated over the lower sternum or high in the epigastrium can be due to oesophagitis or to a peptic ulcer, either in the oesophagus or in the pouch of the stomach lying above the diaphragm; haematemesis or melaena may occur. Strangulation and obstruction of the thoracic stomach in a para-oesophageal hernia is fortunately rare though may arise as an emergency. It mimics an upper abdominal catastrophe; vomiting is severe and the signs are those of a left-sided pneumothorax or perforated oesophagus and bowel sounds may be heard over the left chest. Immediate operation to prevent gangrene is necessary.

Iron deficiency anaemia due to oozing of blood from oesophagitis may be the only symptom of hiatus hernia.

Diagnosis. The hernia can nearly always be seen by barium meal. The patient is examined in the head–down Trendelenberg position; failure to do this explains why hiatus hernia was previously thought to be rare. Manual compression and special measures such as a deep breath, swallow or belch, may be necessary to prove reflux.

Endoscopy is usually necessary to see whether oesophagitis is present; if the

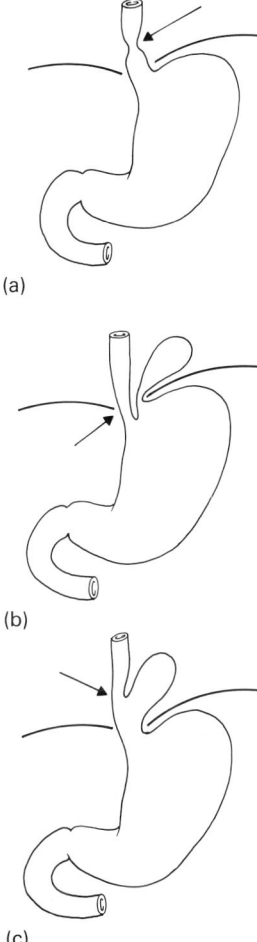

(a)

(b)

(c)

Fig. 9.4. Types of hiatus hernia. (a) Sliding; (b) para-oesophageal; (c) mixed (the arrow shows position of gastro-oesophageal junction).

oesophagus is normal, the hiatus hernia is probably irrelevant and symptomless. Strictures must be examined to exclude malignant change, a rare complication in long-standing oesophagitis.

Differential diagnosis. Occasionally pain caused by hiatus hernia may closely resemble that arising from coronary ischaemia, but a careful history is usually diagnostic. If the patient can describe the pain clearly, it will be noted that the constricting sensation of coronary disease is absent in oesophageal conditions and a history of dyspepsia may be present. Sometimes the chest physician sees the patient first; for coughing may be prominent, either reflexly or from regurgitation of food into the lungs, an event often followed by pneumonitis or lung abscess. Alternatively, the hernia itself may resemble a lung abscess when a routine chest X-ray shows a fluid level in the pouch of stomach above the diaphragm.

Treatment. Hiatus hernia in infants and children usually responds to simple medical measures: an upright position is maintained by blocking the head of the bed or by a special harness. Thickened feeds with solid foods should be started as soon as possible.

Adults with symptomless hiatus hernia require no treatment. Otherwise, simple measures after explanation and reassurance—without drugs—often suffice.

1   Reduction of weight in an obese patient may cure the hernia both clinically and radiologically. Tight garments or belts should be abandoned. Prevention of reflux at night is obtained by raising the head of the bed and not by propping up with pillows. Heartburn or regurgitation during sexual intercourse can be avoided by adopting those positions which avoid a rise in abdominal pressure.

2   Large meals should be avoided in the evening as well as any substances like chocolate (which reduces LOS pressure) last thing at night.

3   Alkali tablets containing magnesium carbonate or such like (e.g. Rennie tablets) are useful to take immediately heartburn occurs and are a helpful standby for patients.

4   Control of gastric acidity by regular medication can be considered. H_2 antagonists may be tried, though some controlled trials have cast doubt on their benefit.

5   Cholinergics and metoclopramide can be helpful by improving oesophageal emptying and increasing the LOS pressure.

6   Alginates, widely used in the food industry, increase viscosity and have suspending properties like those of a mucilage. These are used in tablets or liquid containing alkali (e.g. Gaviscon) in the hope of preventing reflux. Also some studies show that carbenoxolone is effective given by this method as it does allow some contact with the oesophageal mucosa (e.g. Pyrogastrone).

7   Occasional patients will need operation. Then it is most important to make sure that the symptoms are due to reflux oesophagitis and not due to nervous dyspepsia. Results of operation in well-chosen cases are good, but as with hernias elsewhere some recur. Strictures present a challenge to the surgeon. Some will try the effect of repair of the hernia alone, as sometimes the oedema and spasm associated with the stricture will then subside; more experienced surgeons may attempt a more radical and risky operation such as removal of the stricture and plastic repair of the oesophagus.

Other types of diaphragmatic hernia. Congenital types are rare: there may be a postero-lateral defect of the diaphragm, absence of part of the diaphragm, or a hole surrounded by the relics of the pleuroperitoneal canal (foramen of Bochdalek), when most or all of the viscera are inside the chest; borborygmi are then heard instead of breath sounds, as may occur after an accident which has caused rupture of the diaphragm—often simulating a pneumothorax. A hernia through the retro-sternal gap, the foramen of Morgani, usually contains omentum and is unlikely to present as a gastrointestinal problem.

Achalasia of the cardia

Achalasia, which is Greek for 'without relaxation', is the name given by Hurst to the condition formerly called cardiospasm, for he showed that no spasm existed and that it was due to degeneration of Auerbach's plexus. The cardia fails to relax before the oncoming bolus of food and this causes intermittent or chronic obstruction. No age is exempt, the youngest being a female infant of 6 months and the oldest over 80 years, but patients are usually between 20 and 40 years—females slightly more commonly affected.

Pathogenesis. Achalasia is a neuromuscular disorder involving the entire oesophagus and is caused by degenerative changes in the ganglion cells. Abnormal motility patterns or a complete absence of peristalsis can be shown. Failure of the cardia to open is due to the lack of the necessary stimulus of a peristaltic wave. There is hypertrophy of the muscular wall and dilatation above the obstruction. Oesopha-gitis from stasis of food is frequent and it is sometimes followed by fibrous contraction, or even malignant change, though rarely so.

Symptoms. Early diagnosis before obstruction has developed may be difficult. Discomfort from abnormal oesophageal motility may be attributed to 'indigestion' and regurgitation may be mistaken for vomiting, so peptic ulcer may be wrongly diagnosed—the dysphagia being overlooked. Barium swallow may then be normal, except for signs of disordered motility, or persistent failure of the cardia to open. Usually the patient complains of food sticking when he swallows, and points towards the lower sternum to indicate the site of obstruction; there may be discomfort though no pain. Food suddenly passes the cardia when adequate pressure has been built up by accumulation above the obstruction. The patient may notice this and find trick movements such as increasing the thoracic pressure by trying to breath out through a closed glottis useful in starting it off. Eating is slow and embarrassment may be caused by regurgitation of food. Later, the oesophagus may become enormously dilated (Fig. 9.5) and mimic a mediastinal tumour or empyema when seen on a plain film of the chest. Spill-over of food into the lungs may cause pneumonia, and starvation occurs, though patients seldom die from achalasia.

Diagnosis. Achalasia can usually be distinguished from carcinoma because of its long history. Barium swallow shows a cucumber-shaped oesophagus with a tapering

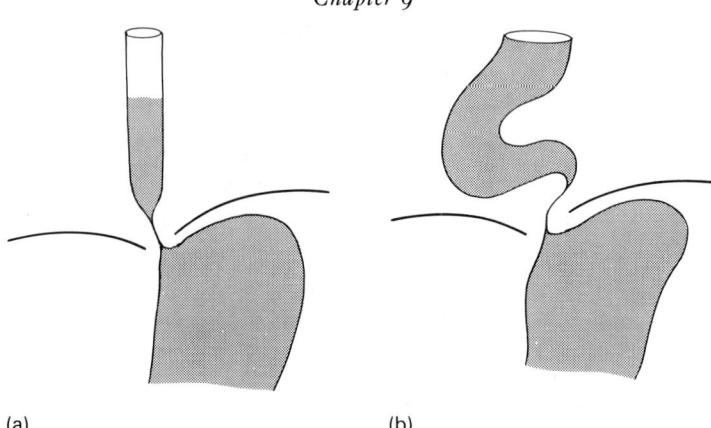

(a)   (b)

Fig. 9.5. Stages in achalasia. (a) Early; (b) late—the dilated 'sigmoid' oesophagus (note lack of air bubble in stomach).

lower end (Fig. 9.6). There is complete loss of the peristaltic wave, which is replaced by irregular segmental and tertiary contractions. The cardia is eventually forced open by the column of food when it is about 20 cm high. This column also acts as a trap so that no gastric air bubble is seen. Sometimes an enormous tortuous oesophagus called a sigmoid (shaped like the letter S) oesophagus flops into the right chest; because of its shape, the direct effect of gravity upon the sphincter is lost (Fig. 9.5).

Sometimes carcinoma looks like achalasia because of a smooth appearance at the site of obstruction instead of a ragged irregular outline (Fig. 9.6), so endoscopy is essential. Inhalation of octyl nitrite relaxes smooth muscle transiently and the oesophagus will empty in achalasia though not in other conditions. Injection of

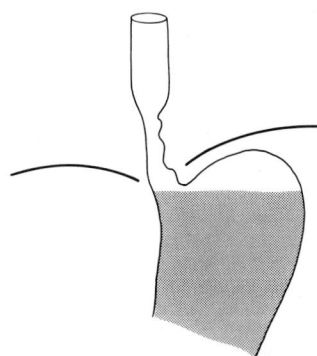

Fig. 9.6. Irregular outline from carcinoma of oesophagus.

20 mg hyoscine-N-butyl bromide (Buscopan) will, in early cases, contract the lower oesophagus and obliterate the lumen when seen by X-ray.

Treatment. The disturbance of motility cannot be corrected and drugs are seldom helpful in the treatment. The latest is nifedipine. The approach has to be an attack on the LOS which is causing the obstruction. This can be done as follows:

1   Dilatation of the sphincter is performed either by the Stark metal dilator or the Negus hydrostatic dilator which is inflated with air or water; sufficient force is used to tear the muscle fibres and cause enough damage to prevent the sphincter from resuming its state of perpetual non-relaxation. Rupture occasionally occurs and several dilatations may be necessary, but these can be done as an out-patient. The patient must be kept under observation because dilatation may provide only temporary relief and complications like oesophagitis or carcinoma may develop insidiously.

2   Heller's operation (extra-mucosal oesophago-cardiomyotomy) consists of a single long myotomy incision being made with complete division of muscle coats down to the mucosa for several centimetres at the sphincter.

Chagas' disease (South American trypanosomiasis)

Trypansoma cruzi is the causal agent of an endemic form of mega-oesophagus and megacolon met with in certain zones of Brazil. Many mammals, such as dogs and cats, act as reservoirs of the parasite and infection is conveyed through man via a bed bug. Destruction of the nerve cells in the gastrointestinal tract probably occurs during the acute phase of invasion by the parasite. Most patients have a positive complement fixation reaction. The oesophagus, and indeed most of the alimentary tract, shows a great decrease in ganglion cells. Motility studies are similar to those in achalasia and the treatment is the same.

Other disorders of oesophageal motility

Diffuse oesophageal spasm can cause intermittent retrosternal pain which mimics that of cardiac origin and sometimes causes dysphagia. Manometry shows high pressures and some develop hypertrophy of the oesophageal muscle. A corkscrew appearance is sometimes seen on barium swallow (Fig. 9.7) due to pockets of lesser pressure into which the barium is forced and this sometimes gives an outline like diverticula—indeed some develop permanent diverticula. This is regarded as separate from early achalasia, because of the motility pattern and a normal LOS. The pain may sometimes be relieved by nitroglycerine, which relaxes smooth muscle and occasionally operation—a long myotomy incision over the lower oesophagus—may be necessary. However, diagnosis must be cautious as the X-ray changes may be seen in patients without symptoms. It is a harmless condition and seldom distresses patients once the diagnosis is made. The elderly may suffer from

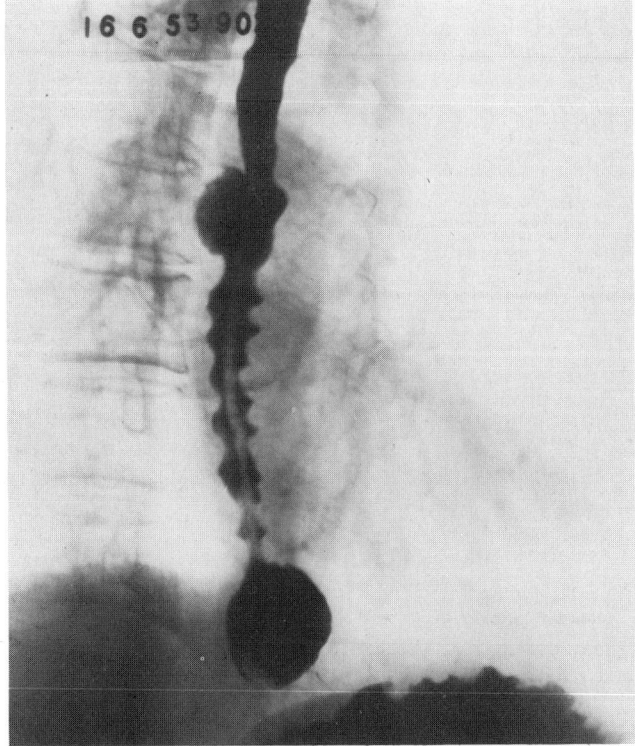

Fig. 9.7. Corkscrew oesophagus.

this and marked tertiary contractions are seen on barium swallow and cause dysphagia—the presbyoesophagus.

The oesophagus bears the main brunt when the alimentary tract is attacked in *scleroderma*. It is dilated and the transit is slow because of the absence of contractile waves; at first motility is disturbed from incoordination but later smooth muscle is destroyed, and eventually the LOS may be affected and reflux oesophagitis with possible stricture formation results. *Dermatomyositis* causes dysphagia because of weak pharyngeal muscles; the diagnosis is suggested by the dermatitis and some are due to malignant disease, either in the alimentary tract or elsewhere. *Diabetes mellitus* causes damage to the autonomic system and may affect the oesophagus causing delay in its emptying. *Myotonia dystrophica* may be associated with reduction in motility and similar motility disorders have been recorded in *myasthenia gravis* and *multiple sclerosis*.

Strictures of the oesophagus
These may be caused by the accidental or suicidal ingestion of irritants, by tablets which stick in the oesophagus or by prolonged intubation of the stomach. Rarely

rings occur in the lower oesophagus and consist of a core of connective tissue covering a bundle of smooth muscle fibres; and these may be symptomless and cause dysphagia if large pieces of meat are eaten hastily (Schatzki ring).

Treatment. Oesophageal strictures can be dilated by endoscopy. A barium swallow must be available and a forward-viewing endoscope is introduced and if possible passed through the stricture into the stomach. Biopsies for histology and brushings for cytology are taken to differentiate benign from malignant strictures. If the stricture is too narrow to permit passage of the endoscope, a narrow guide wire is threaded through the endoscope and is guided through the lumen under endoscopic control. The endoscope can be removed and the stricture dilated with successively large 'olives' by the Eder–Puerstow technique (Fig. 9.8) or by tapered bougies.

Perforation of the oesophagus is always a risk. The patient should not be allowed to resume oral feeding until subsequent examination and chest X-ray have ruled out mediastinal gas or surgical emphysema of the neck. Some patients can be taught to do their own dilatation at home with a mercury-filled tapered bougie.

Palliation of dysphagia caused by carcinoma in patients unsuitable for other forms of therapy can be done by the endoscopist. The stricture is dilated as described and then a flanged tube is introduced over the guide wire, and its final position checked by endoscopy and X-ray. This will allow swallowing. Endoscopic methods are now generally regarded as preferable to operation which requires laparotomy for placement of the tube.

Plummer–Vinson syndrome (Kelly–Patterson syndrome)

The eponymous title of Plummer–Vinson syndrome is hardly deserved as these authors regarded it as due to hysteria. Kelly and Patterson in 1919 originally described it as the long period of anaemia preceding symptoms, the presence of a pale smooth tongue and fissures at the angle of the mouth, and with the patients referring their dysphagia to the level of the larynx. Endoscopy then showed a thin atrophied mucosa in the pharynx and sometimes a pin-hole entrance to the oesophagus due to a web (Fig. 9.9) passing backwards from the larynx; there might be other changes in the hypopharynx such as superficial ulceration and leucoplakia. These authors showed the dramatic improvement from dilatation by bougies and reported that postcricoid cancer was a complication. It is seldom seen nowadays because of earlier diagnosis and treatment of iron-deficient anaemia.

Cancer of the oesophagus

This is one of the most deadly cancers, the reason being not the type of neoplastic cell (usually squamous) but the surrounding anatomy of the oesophagus. As soon as the growth trespasses beyond its walls, vital structures like the lung, bronchi, or the aorta are invaded, either directly or by lymphatic spread.

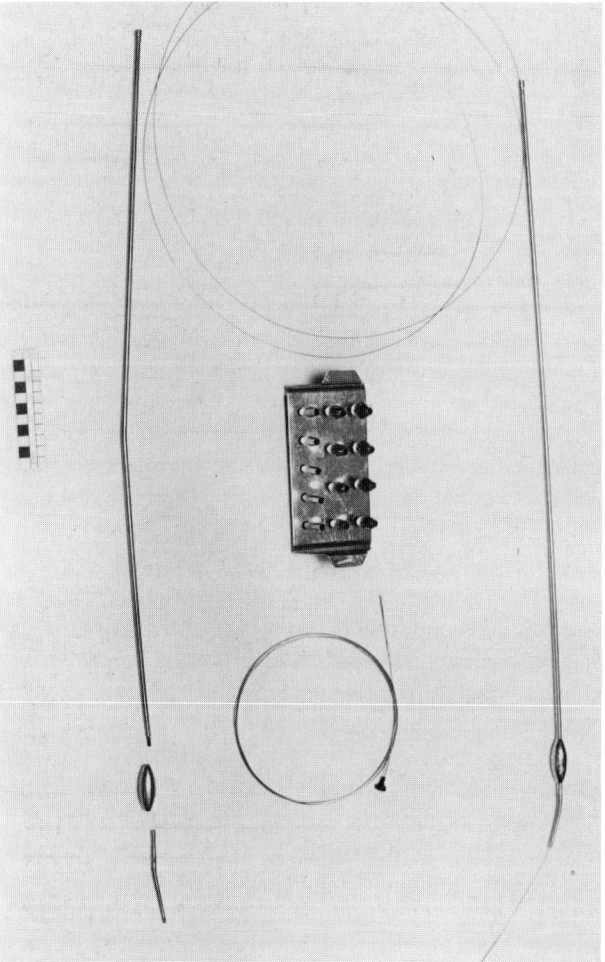

Fig. 9.8. 'Olives' for dilating oesophageal stricture.

Aetiology. It mainly affects the elderly, especially men, and occurs more in alcoholics and cigarette smokers. It may complicate achalasia of the cardia and occurs in families with tylosis (palmar plantar hyperkeratosis), though this is rare.

Its incidence varies widely throughout the world and suggests that environmental factors cause it; and because food and drink come into direct contact with the oesophageal mucosa it is tempting to assume that the environmental factors are dietary. It is very common in certain areas of Russia, Northern China and the borders of the Caspian Sea, in Iran and South Africa. In the area of China affected (Lin country), the inhabitants drink very little alcohol and there is no opium smoking; the striking fact is that the incidence is closely paralleled by that of

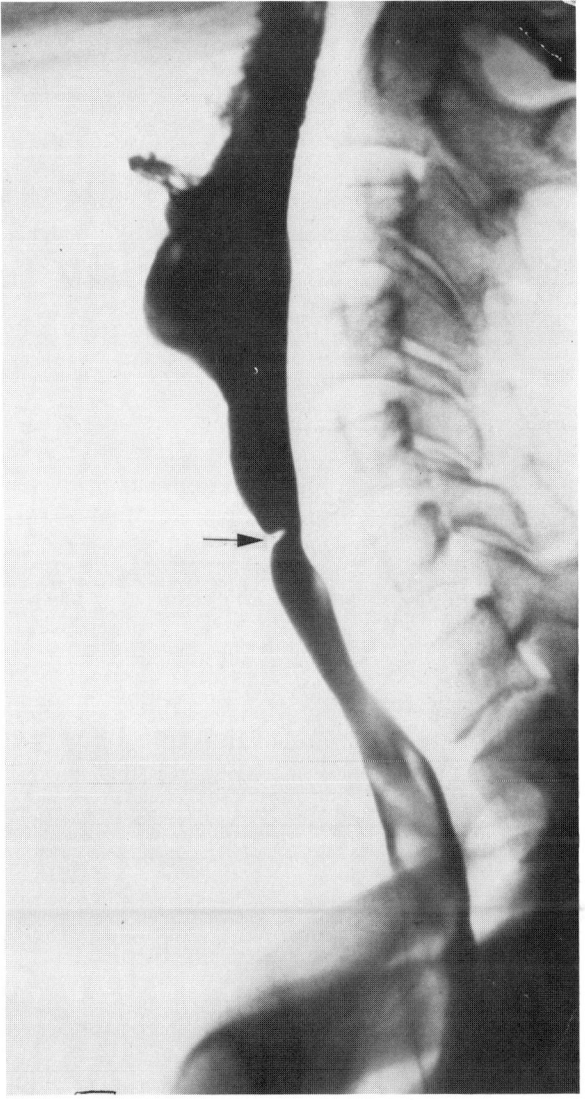

Fig. 9.9. Oesophageal web in Plummer–Vinson syndrome.

hypopharyngeal carcinoma in chickens which live largely on domestic scraps, and some evidence suggests the link between the scraps and the disease. Elsewhere in China, near Canton, cancer of the nasopharynx is commonest and there is a link between this and the Epstein–Barr virus. The barefoot doctors warn the patients of the symptoms and send to hospital any suspect.

Symptoms. Dysphagia is the commonest symptom and about half have pain in the chest or upper abdomen; regurgitation, hoarseness or respiratory difficulties are rare. Dyspepsia for several months followed by dysphagia is an ominous sequence of events and usually means an adenocarcinoma arising from the upper stomach and spreading to the oesophagus.

Diagnosis. The barium swallow appearance is usually characteristic: there is a very short narrow segment and its irregular outline, usually, though not invariably distinguishes this from achalasia (Fig. 9.6). Occasionally a longer area of minimal narrowing occurs and this is easily missed; it is caused by an extensive flat ulcerating carcinoma in which the mucosal pattern is lost. Endoscopy and biopsy confirm the diagnosis.

Treatment. This aims at both increasing survival time (quantity of the remaining life) and relieving distressing symptoms (quality). Radiotherapy is preferred for mid-oesophageal cancers, since the mortality is lower than with surgery and patients will be given symptomatic relief for 1 year. Results from operation are poor and the mortality lies between 10 and 20%. If the tumour can be removed the 5-year survival is 10%; if it is less than 4 cm it increases to 20% and if there are no local lymph nodes involved the 5-year survival is 40%. The insertion of various hollow tubes through the growth relieves the dysphagia and now can be done by endoscopy (see above).

Spontaneous rupture of the oesophagus

This dramatic condition may resemble coronary infarction or catastrophes in the upper abdomen, like perforated ulcer or acute pancreatitis. It is often not considered until shown at autopsy. The onset occurs during a large meal or vomiting, and the contents of the meal usually go into the pleural cavity; an astute house officer may recognize the presence of beer in an apparent pleural effusion. The likely explanation of the rupture is that the cricopharyngeal muscle fails to relax during vomiting and the sudden rise in intraluminal pressure splits the oesophagus at its point of least support—that is the left side of the lower third. This region has been confirmed to be the weakest point by contrast medium being injected under high pressure into the oesophagus in cadavers.

Historically Baron Wassenaer, the grand Admiral of Holland, achieved immortality as the first described case. He was a gourmet with an immense appetite. Ironically, at the time of the rupture he was atoning for over-eating by a starvation diet. He suddenly gave forth a horrifying cry at which call the servants ran to him and they heard him complain that something near the upper part of the stomach was ruptured, torn or displaced! His diagnosis was proved correct at post-mortem. The striking feature was the presence of roast duck and Danish beer in the pleural cavity and floating on this was the sweet almond oil which his doctor had given him for treatment.

Diagnosis is by a specific triad of symptoms: blood-stained vomit, followed by violent pain over the sternum, and then surgical emphysema over the upper chest and shoulders. The patient will be shocked and may have an altered voice with a nasal character. A loud clicking sound may be heard over the lower sternum synchronous with the heart beat and due to mediastinal emphysema. A plain X-ray of the chest may show air in the mediastinum, with slight separation of the mediastinal pleural leaves, and a hydropneumothorax usually on the left side.

Surgical repair must be done as soon as possible. In rare cases, where operation is impossible or where rupture has not taken place into the pleural cavity, conservative treatment by an indwelling duodenal tube can be advised. Antibiotic therapy is necessary as death often takes place from fatal mediastinitis or empyema.

Mallory–Weiss syndrome

This is a fairly common cause of haematemesis, and the mechanism is similar to that of ruptured oesophagus which is rare. The mucosa is only split deep enough to cause bleeding. The history is often diagnostic: a bloodless vomit is followed either shortly or within a few hours by haematemesis. It may follow vomiting from any cause including alcohol and pregnancy, and the fissures are painless. It is probably more common in patients with hiatus hernia.

Diagnosis is by endoscopy which should be done as soon as possible otherwise the tear heals and cannot be seen. Bleeding usually stops but occasionally an operation is needed to suture the tear.

Chapter 10
Peptic Ulcer

The marvel of the stomach is that it can secrete gastric juice which digests food though not the stomach itself. Remarkable also is its capacity to digest so many bizarre foods and to tolerate insults such as alcohol or biopsy; and gastric juice digests meat and even living tissue without digesting its own mucosal lining. Little is known about the mechanisms which protect the mucosa from injury and autodigestion; these protective mechanisms stop immediately after death so that fixation with formalin is necessary if histological studies are to be done.

The gastric mucosa

The mucosa of the stomach is orange-red and glistens from its surface covering of mucus when seen through the endoscope; it is thicker at the pyloric and thinner at the cardiac end and the numerous rugae or folds flatten out when the stomach is distended with air. The superficial lining is made up of columnar or cylindric cells which extend into the gastric glands. In the glands, peptic (zymogen) cells secrete pepsinogen which is converted by acid to the enzyme pepsin which has its optimal activity at pH 2. Parietal (oxyntic) cells secrete hydrochloric acid; the number of these correlate with the acid output and the highest number occurs in some with duodenal ulcer but especially in the rare Zollinger–Ellison syndrome (p. 180). Normal secretion of gastric juice varies between 10–250 ml/h.

Mucous (goblet) cells secrete mucus and alkaline gel which is a lubricant and also forms an adhesive protective layer preventing damage by acid or trauma. Its exact chemical composition is uncertain but it is a glycoprotein in which the terminal sugar residues have characteristic blood group specificity. It is normally resistant to the action of pepsin but degradation is brought about by bile acids, alcohol and salicylates so that the mucus ceases to perform its protective function.

The gastric mucosa also secretes a heat-labile mucoprotein (intrinsic factor) which binds vitamin B_{12} and this has the specific property of promoting the absorption of B_{12} from the ileum. Electrolytes such as sodium and potassium are also secreted; the fact that chloride has to be secreted against high concentrations in gastric juice and against electrical gradient accounts for the term 'the chloride pump'. There is a specific tributyrinase in the stomach; the smell of vomit is largely due to butyric acid set free from milk products.

Motility and emptying of the stomach

The stomach is a reservoir to store food while it is mixed, diluted with gastric juice and liquefied into chyme. Small samples are then propelled into the intestine at regular intervals to allow mixing with pancreatic juice. It is only possible for certain fat-soluble substances like alcohol to be absorbed from the stomach. The stomach can be regarded as having two components: the distensible fundus and body with the reservoir function and the more muscular antrum where mixing occurs; liquification is generally complete when contents reach the duodenum. There are two types of motor activity: tonus which holds the walls of the fasting stomach together and determines its shape, and peristalsis which starts especially after meals, waves of contractions beginning in the body of the stomach and passing towards the pylorus at the rate of three per minute. Emptying of the stomach is exponential so that a fixed fraction of 2–5% of gastric contents is delivered to the duodenum each minute, a fundic pacemaker starts the electrical activity of peristalsis. Hormones, except possibly motilin, play no part in gastric-emptying though they may inhibit motility. The driving force behind the emptying process is the pressure difference between the antrum and duodenum; the stomach therefore acts like a pump, periodically increasing its pressure above that of the duodenum.

Various factors influence emptying: the type of food, carbohydrates leaving rapidly and fat delaying emptying; the consistency of food, fluid leaving more rapidly than solids; the osmolarity of the meal as the stomach by its secretions makes its contents nearly isotonic; emotion—sadness delaying, and anger increasing emptying; and mechanisms initiated in the duodenum and small intestine. The speed of emptying in patients with duodenal ulcer is more rapid than normal though may be delayed with antral ulceration, but is usually normal with gastric ulcers. It can be measured radiologically (the stomach being empty 4–6 h after the start of a barium meal) by intubation, by isotopic methods and more recently using ultrasonography.

Mechanism of secretion

The secretion of gastric juice is carefully controlled and synchronized so that a quantity sufficient to digest food is secreted and production of excessive amounts which would injure the mucosa is prevented. The flow depends upon three mechanisms:

1   The psychic stimulation from the sight and smell of food which acts reflexly through the vagus and lasts for about 15–20 min.

2   Food comes into contact with the antrum and releases the hormone gastrin (p. 67) which continues to stimulate the secretion of hydrochloric acid throughout the meal.

3   An intestinal phase occurs when various products of digestion reach the duodenum and jejunum; this probably contributes about 10% or more of the total acid response to a meal.

There must be a mechanism to check further secretion of acid, otherwise the gastric contents would become sufficiently corrosive to damage the mucous membrane; this inhibitory mechanism, the antral 'cut-off' mechanism, involves both the antrum and duodenum and occurs when the gastric contents become too acid. In the duodenum, receptors which respond to fats and high concentrations of sugar (as well as to acid) also inhibit secretion of acid. Furthermore acid in contact with the duodenal mucosa stimulates the flow of the hormone secretin which stimulates the flow of alkaline pancreatic juice. Glucagon also inhibits acid and lowers serum gastrin. There may be some disorder of inhibition in patients with duodenal ulcer, where highly acid juice not only flows after eating but continues throughout the night. Recently the importance of the small intestine in controlling gastric secretion has been shown. Surgical resection causes acid to increase and there are probably receptors which respond to fat and decrease acid secretion by the hormone enterogastrone.

Peptic ulcer

The term peptic ulcer refers to any ulcer in an area where the mucosa is bathed by the hydrochloric acid and pepsin of gastric juice: gastric and duodenal ulcer as well as oesophageal and stomal ulcers (which follow gastric operations)—and the rare ulcer in Meckel's diverticulum where aberrant gastric mucosa sometimes occurs.

Aetiology of gastric and duodenal ulcer
The cause is not known but the following factors could be relevant.

Environment. Accurate knowledge of the geographical incidence of peptic ulcer is difficult to obtain compared with a disease like malaria where precision in diagnosis is easier. It is widely distributed and not a prerogative of Western society, for it occurs in African subjects of varying tribal origins, and duodenal ulcer is common in southern India where it is often large and causes stenosis rather than haemorrhage or perforation. The ratio of duodenal to gastric ulcer varies greatly in different countries and sometimes gastric rather than duodenal predominates.

Genetics. Gastric and duodenal ulcer often affect more than one member of a family; this could be due to coincidence, a similar response to the same environment, or a shared genetic predisposition. The last is supported by the fact that peptic ulcer is common in those of blood group O, these being 40% more liable to develop ulcer than those of groups A, B or AB. The risk of gastric ulcer developing in persons of group O is less than that of duodenal ulcer but 20% greater than in others. Complications of ulcers, especially bleeding and stomal ulcer, are also particularly liable to occur. However, the association between group O and peptic ulcer is not strong and it is unlikely that blood group substances have any direct role either in causing or protecting against disease, though the blood group genes may also control the type of gastric mucosa or mucus which one inherits. Twin studies suggest that genetic and environmental factors are about equal in importance in duodenal ulcer.

Food. Irregular meals, different foods, inadequate teeth, tobacco and alcohol are no longer regarded as causes.

The modern consumption of refined carbohydrates unaccompanied by roughage has been blamed by Cleave (1974) for causing ulcers. The idea is that these stimulate acid without any substance in the stomach to buffer it; this perhaps could apply to those who take frequent nibbles of biscuits and sweets on an empty stomach.

That the presence of a noxious substance in food or drink could cause peptic ulcer cannot be dismissed; perhaps a chemical or one of the many additives or preservatives used in preparation, or something concerned with tinning or cooking utensils. It is only in this century that there has been a transfer of the manufacture of food from the home to the factory, a change which has coincided with increased duodenal ulcers.

Psychosomatic. Worry is often regarded as the cause and duodenal ulcer is widely regarded by the layman as the penalty of pressure and the prerogative of the successful businessman. It is flattering to think of our civilization as causing a greater strain than in the World's previous history. Perhaps different types of stress have different types of psychosomatic significance, and the perpetual frustrations of everyday life may be more important than single calamities such as famine or plague. Emotions certainly have a remarkable effect upon the alimentary tract, as shown by the studies of Wolf & Wolff (1947) on their subject Tom with the gastric fistula whose gastric mucosa could be observed directly: hostility and resentment profoundly altered gastric secretion and caused congestion with easy bleeding. However, there is surprisingly little evidence otherwise to support the idea that the ulcer is caused by the worry and stress of modern life. Surveys show it to be widely distributed throughout the population; there is a slight increase in those in responsible positions and also in doctors, though the increased accuracy of diagnosis may here be a factor. Whether or not an 'ulcer personality' exists is very doubtful. Emotional disturbance may be important as a factor in precipitating organic disease, but is unlikely to be the cause of peptic ulcer.

Sex. The influence of sex is notable. Peptic ulcer, especially duodenal ulcer, is a hazard for the adult male. This sex difference is not seen in children until puberty. Women are protected against developing peptic ulcer and when it does occur, it runs a milder course though after the menopause these advantages are lost. No significant difference in acid secretion exists between males and females. Pregnancy has a beneficial effect and generally relieves symptoms, possibly due to an agent acting directly on mucosal repair. Neither oestrogen nor progesterone affect hydrochloric acid secretion, but female sex hormones have been shown to benefit men with duodenal ulcer, though at the unacceptable price of feminizing side-effects. Both sexes do just as well after operation.

Association with other diseases. The fact that it is so common makes it difficult to be certain of true links with other diseases. Peptic ulcer, mainly duodenal, was thought to be more common in patients with chronic obstructive lung disease; if this be true there is no obvious explanation, for anoxia tends to depress gastric secretion. Ulcers are said to be more common in hepatic cirrhosis (especially after portacaval shunt) and a secretagogue, perhaps arising in intestinal mucosa acting directly upon the stomach without modification by the liver, is blamed. Gastric ulcer may be more common in patients suffering from rheumatoid arthritis though this could be due to the drugs used in treatment. Peptic ulcer is definitely more common after renal transplantation (see later); the serum gastrin is high probably owing to failure of the kidneys to degrade gastrin.

Pathophysiology

Gastric acid secretion. The capacity to secrete acid is determined mainly by the number of parietal cells in the gastric mucosa, and this is mainly genetically determined. Acid secretion is estimated by measuring the response to a high dose of a stimulant such as pentagastrin. The secretory capacity is less in women than in men, partly due to the difference in body size; it decreases with age probably because increasing gastritis destroys the acid-secreting cells. These sex and age differences are the same in patients with ulcer as in controls.

An increased capacity to secrete acid is certainly involved in duodenal ulcer, for it is more common in those with acid output, such as 40 mmol/h or more, though secretion in some is normal. Also the flow of acid gastric juice continues unabated throughout the night—hence the occurrence of pain at about 2.00 a.m. Hypersecretion of acid stays relatively constant during relapses and remissions of an ulcer. Possibly an increased sensitivity to stimulation may be present, or perhaps defective inhibitory mechanisms may contribute to this.

Mucosal resistance. The special protective mechanism against hydrochloric acid is lost at death and the stomach digests itself. Possibly this loss of resistance occurs in states of severe illness, sometimes when the patient is almost moribund, so that multiple erosions form in the stomach and duodenum—the so-called stress ulcers. Since most gastric and some duodenal ulcers occur in patients without any increased gastric secretion, a decreased resistance of the mucosa to acid-peptic injury is probably important. Possible factors include blood flow, regeneration of epithelium, the secretion of mucus and the resistance to back diffusion of hydrogen ions. The idea that mucus protects the mucosa against damage is probably correct but so far present methods have not shown any defects in the secretion or quality of mucus of patients with peptic ulcer.

Back diffusion. Acid secreted into the stomach diffuses back into the mucosa only very slowly when the mucosa is normal. Various chemical agents, for example drugs, can break this barrier to back diffusion and allow a leak-back of acid. To break the barrier the chemical must enter the mucosa, and if ionizable, it must be in its un-ionized lipid soluble form to enter the mucosa; for example aspirin must be in an acid solution. Bile acids and alcohol both break the barrier. Signs of a broken barrier include decrease in the electrical potential difference across the gastric mucosa and increased bi-directional permeability to sodium with increased accumulation of sodium in the gastric lumen. As acid diffuses through the broken barrier, it causes further damage and this is shown by leakage of interstitial fluid and plasma into the gastric lumen as well as by bleeding.

Other possible factors. Pepsin may be as important as hydrochloric acid in causing ulcers. The increase in gastric secretion in patients with duodenal ulcer and decrease in those with gastric ulcer involve both acid and pepsin. Reflux of bile from the duodenum into the stomach may be important and those with gastric ulcer reflux more than controlled groups; this could lead to breaking of the gastric barrier through back diffusion of hydrogen ion and make the mucosa less resistant to ulceration. Patients with duodenal ulcer have a considerable increase of the parietal cells of the stomach; this appears to be a work hyperplasia, analogous to the thyroid gland in thyrotoxicosis, and it is not known whether this excess of gastric secretory tissue is present from birth or is induced by nervous or hormonal factors like gastrin, and it is assumed to be a cause rather than effect of an ulcer.

In the stomach, prostaglandins regulate blood flow and exert a protective effect upon the gastric mucosa; inhibition of their action may start a series of events which lead to mucosal damage and probable ulcer formation. Aspirin and all non-steroidal anti-inflammatory drugs inhibit prostaglandin synthetase and their anti-inflammatory action partly depends upon this; hence they may all have an adverse effect upon the stomach.

Incidence of peptic ulcer. Duodenal ulcer, according to necropsies, was unusual during the nineteenth century. Then it was gastric ulcer, probably acute, which was more common and caused the deaths of young ladies under 25 years; haemorrhage or perforation swept off beautiful and healthy creatures within a few hours. Deaths in young women are now rare, and ulcers for some environmental or other reason have changed their sites. Duodenal ulcer has emerged as a major disease afflicting the young and middle aged of the twentieth century. Fortunately, the incidence has probably begun to decline. Duodenal ulcer is several times more common in men and the incidence of gastric ulcer increases with age. Probably a high proportion of the population have an ulcer at some time in their life.

Symptoms

Pain is the cardinal symptom, described as discomfort by some and severe by others, and is felt in the epigastrium. Pain is referred elsewhere when the ulcer penetrates surrounding structures such as pancreas, and backache may then be present; occasionally low abdominal pain may follow involvement of mesentery.

Many describe their pain as gnawing or burning, though few could have experienced these happenings in life. A highly discriminating symptom is spontaneous night pain: the patient is awoken by pain at about 2.00 a.m. and relieves it by taking milk or alkali. Pain occurs 2 or 3 h after a meal when the stomach is empty and relief by eating or drinking is typical, especially for duodenal ulcer; patients tell of immediate relief by neutralizing the acid with antacids, or by diluting it even with a glass of beer. Relief is also obtained by vomiting, the vomit usually being small and bile-stained, in contrast to the large amounts from pyloric stenosis. Food rarely causes pain, except in patients with nervous dyspepsia and occasionally with gastric ulcer; when pain starts immediately after food, it supports the old adage that patients with gastric ulcer are afraid to eat but those with duodenal ulcer are afraid not to eat.

Periodicity has a high discriminating value. Although one attack of peptic ulcer only may occur, the usual pattern is for attacks to appear intermittently throughout the patient's life coming and going for no apparent reason; this picture is only blurred at a later stage when complications such as penetration of the ulcer or pyloric stenosis develop. Then relief by alkalis is less distinct and the pain is more severe or continuous and likely to be referred to the back or elsewhere.

Clinical impression has suggested that gastric and duodenal ulcer can sometimes be separated by symptoms. Pain may come on just after food and the story is often atypical in gastric ulcer; it is felt more to the left, whereas in duodenal ulcer it is more central or to the right, and hunger pain with relief by food is typical. Waterbrash, the sudden filling of the mouth by saliva from some reflex mechanism, and heartburn is complained of by many, though there is no oesophagitis from hiatus hernia nor reflux to explain the latter.

Signs
Generally none. The pointing test (Fig. 10.1) where the patient points to the site is often helpful: an ulcer is probable if the patient points with one finger to a localized area in the epigastrium, possible if he indicates the upper abdomen but improbable when areas in both upper and lower abdomen are indicated. Tenderness is not usually a sign of peptic ulcer unless penetrating or perforated; it more often indicates an apprehensive patient perhaps with nervous dyspepsia. A succussion splash, if the patient has neither eaten nor drunk for 4 h, points to pyloric stenosis.

Diagnosis

Barium meal. This is usually necessary to confirm the diagnosis, but should not always be done in women of child-bearing age with a typical history. False negative reports may occur up to 20% of duodenal ulcers. A specific sign is an ulcer crater, easily seen in the stomach, though less often in the duodenum; duodenal deformity

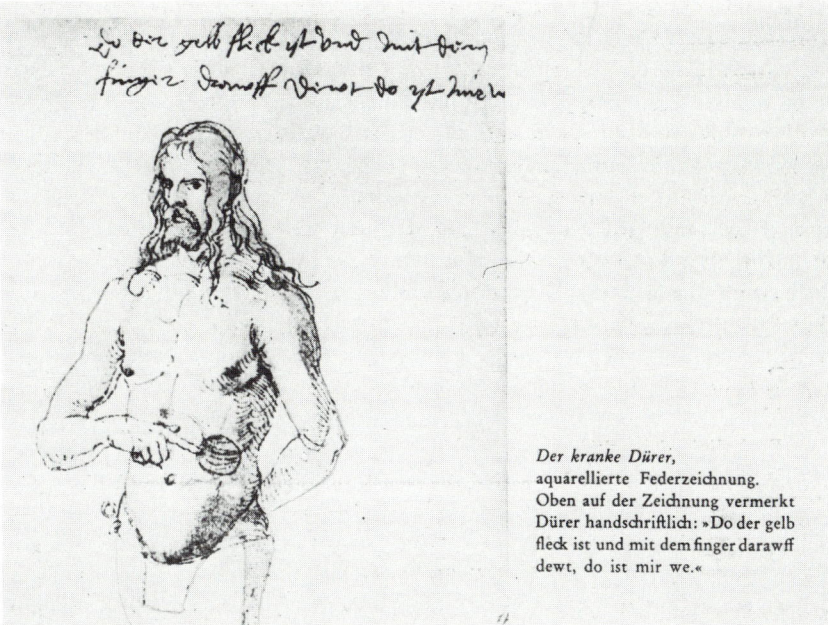

Der kranke Dürer,
aquarellierte Federzeichnung.
Oben auf der Zeichnung vermerkt
Dürer handschriftlich: »Do der gelb
fleck ist und mit dem finger darawff
dewt, do ist mir we.«

Fig. 10.1. Pointing test. The idea originated from the engraver and painter Dürer who drew this picture of himself to show where he had pain and sent it to his doctor. (Eine Bildbiographie Dürer Max steck München: Kindler. 1957.)

may result from scarring from an ulcer, pylorospasm, or from distortion by an adjacent structure. Once a duodenal ulcer is diagnosed, no further X-ray is needed unless outlet obstruction of the stomach is suspected. A postbulbar duodenal ulcer is easily missed.

Endoscopy. This is more accurate and biopsies can be taken; also the discomfort is hardly more than from a barium meal. Indications are:
1 Symptoms suggestive of peptic ulcer, when the barium meal is normal or shows doubtful changes.
2 To prove the diagnosis of duodenal ulcer by seeing the crater.
3 All patients with duodenal ulcer for operation (in the past no ulcer has been found in some at operations and these, where the true diagnosis may be nervous dyspepsia, continue with their symptoms).
4 To exclude malignancy in a gastric ulcer and, sometimes, to confirm healing.
5 In haematemesis and melaena.

Medical treatment
The aim of treatment is to aid the healing of an ulcer and to keep it healed, but the

latter is seldom possible; generally, all that can be done is to relieve pain and allow a normal life to be lived despite the ulcer. Operation is only required in a minority, perhaps 10%. Ulcers come and go for no apparent reason, so assessing the effect of drugs is difficult and large numbers of patients are needed for controlled trials.

Additional hardships and restrictions from well-meaning doctors should be avoided. Emotional problems probably increase acid, and a traditional piece of advice has been to instruct patients to avoid all worry and stress. This, to be effective, ought to be accompanied by a gift of a suitable income, a carefree occupation and provision of a different spouse if necessary! Much, however, can be done to modify a patient's reaction to the usual and inevitable stresses of life. Variety, with interests and hobbies, creates a more tranquil mind than is usually possible in one obsessively devoted to his job alone. Most are treated as ambulant cases, but bed rest does hasten healing and relieves pain, so may be used if there is failure to respond to other measures. Stopping smoking cigarettes allows the ulcer to heal more quickly. There is no hard evidence about the effect of alcohol but this, like coffee, is a stimulant of acid so should only be taken on a full stomach.

Proper communication is important to reassure and to relieve worry about cancer, for relief of anxiety lowers the pain threshold. Patients are liberated from the dietetic regimes of the past as controlled trials have shown that diet has no effect on the course of an ulcer. The patient should be told to eat properly, especially those with gastric ulcer where nutritional deficiency may be important. Food relieves pain by neutralizing acid, so some people benefit by eating frequently but must avoid obesity. Milk is no better than other foods in neutralizing acid and in excess may raise the serum cholesterol.

Evidence provided by endoscopy indicates that any of the following remedies approximately doubles the proportion of ulcers healed during short-term treatment though none has been proved to prevent relapse: intensive antacid treatment, H_2 receptor antagonists, carbenoxolone, and chelated bismuth.

Alkalis. An alkali relieves pain by reducing acidity temporarily, but it is impossible to neutralize acid effectively during the day let alone at night unless taken in large amounts; 60 g sodium bicarbonate daily would be needed by intragastric drip to keep the pH of the stomach contents above 4 in patients with a gastric ulcer, the amount needed being much greater in those with a duodenal ulcer. Some workers have shown that antacids given in such doses by mouth will induce ulcer healing, but many develop diarrhoea. Only an obsessional patient could keep to the regime.

Many, however, find antacids very helpful and carry tablets with them. They then live normally while the ulcer heals spontaneously—as usually occurs.

A satisfactory antacid is cheap, harmless, palatable, and should not interfere with bowel action. Popular and suitable preparations contain either aluminium hydroxide or magnesium trisilicate; these are not readily soluble, so they are not absorbed and do not produce alkalosis. Magnesium salts have the advantage of a slight laxative effect in those who are constipated whereas aluminium preparations are slightly constipating. Soluble preparations like sodium bicarbonate probably relieve pain most quickly but this can cause alkalosis particularly if renal damage is present.

Antacids can alter drug kinetics by affecting their absorption or excretion though this is probably rare. Mechanisms may be delayed gastric emptying, the binding of the drug in the intestine, or excretion in urine affected by alkalosis if sodium bicarbonate is used. Antacids with a high sodium content must be avoided in patients whose dietary sodium intake needs to be restricted as in hepatic or heart failure, or pregnancy.

H_2 receptor antagonists. These, cimetidine and ranitidine, work by blocking the effect of histamine on the acid-producing cells of the gastric mucosa. This blockade prevents the stimulation of the cells by acetyl choline via the vagus nerve and by the hormone gastrin from the antral mucosa, histamine probably being the final common pathway of both routes of stimulation. They therefore reduce gastric acid but within 24 h of stopping the drug—even after taking it for a year—acid secretion returns to pre-treatment levels, neither more nor less. Recurrences are therefore expected as the factors which cause ulceration are still operating.

Using 1 g daily of cimetidine or 300 mg daily of ranitidine, most trials report ulcer healing in 70% of patients after 4 weeks, and up to 80% after 6 weeks; figures in control patients taking placebo tablets vary, the average being 40%. After 6 weeks, a night-time dose of cimetidine 400 mg or ranitidine 150 mg only is given and this can be continued for 6 months or longer. The recurrence rate with a maintenance night-time dose is about 25% and this is reduced to 10% if given twice daily, both these figures being lower than the control group. This protection only lasts as long as the drug is being taken and reluctance has been felt about continuing it for longer than 1 year owing to possible side-effects (Table 10.1). Endoscopy is the only way of proving healing, but healed ulcers can recur even if the patient is asymptomatic, so clinical remission and ulcer healing are not synonymous. If there is a previous history of bleeding, confirmation of healing by endoscopy is important and failure to heal is an indication for operation. If symptoms do not disappear after a week or two after starting treatment, an alternative cause for the pain should be suspected such as gallbladder, pancreatic, or colonic disorder.

Trials have also shown that cimetidine and ranitidine in the doses stated above are effective in healing about three-quarters of gastric ulcers, which is rather better than with other treatment.

H_2 antagonists should only be used when an ulcer has been confirmed and should not be prescribed for non-specific dyspepsia. Also malignancy must be excluded before starting treatment as the drug may mask the symptoms.

Carbenoxolone. Observations in Holland indicated that liquorice helped patients with gastric ulcers. Hence came carbenoxolone which has no effect upon the secretion of acid or pepsin but probably acts by changing the nature and volume of

Table 10.1. Side effects of H$_2$-receptor antagonists.

Common (about 2%)
    Diarrhoea
    Dizziness
    Rashes (transient)
    Muscle pains
Occasional
    Mental confusion
Rare
    Gynaecomastia
    Increase in serum transaminase and plasma creatinine values

---

(The idea that sudden withdrawal causes a 'rebound' perforation or haemorrhage is only anecdotal. Nor is there any evidence that cancer of the stomach is a risk though bacterial colonization associated with prolonged hypochlorhydria could cause an excessive production of carcinogenic nitrosamines.)

the protective mucus and aids the enzyme processes involved in cellular regeneration. It has a local anti-inflammatory effect; 50 or 100 mg three times daily after meals is given for about 6 weeks or until the ulcer is healed.

Because of its local effect, treatment of duodenal ulcer is more difficult for gastric contents pass through the duodenum so rapidly that close contact of the drug with the mucosa is unlikely. So gelatin capsules intended to rupture in the duodenum (duogastrone) are used, the dose being the same but given 15–20 min before meals for about 6–12 weeks.

Carbenoxolone is more effective in gastric than duodenal ulcer and better suited for younger rather than older patients because of its side-effects which include sodium retention and hypokalaemia; these may aggravate oedema, hypertension and cardiac failure, and cause muscle weakness. These adverse effects can be managed by concurrent administration of a thiazide diuretic with a potassium supplement.

Deglycyrrhizinized liquorice (Caved S) has been developed to retain the healing effect of the active principle of liquorice without the adverse effects and may have a slight healing effect. It is certainly a good placebo both for doctor and patient for it has the taste of liquorice yet is harmless; it also contains other substances such as alkali and fangula bark.

Sucralfate. This is an aluminium salt of sucrose octasulphate. It forms a viscous paste in the acid environment of the stomach which adheres better to an ulcer base than to normal mucosa. This is probably because the anion of sucralfate binds to the positively charged protein molecules exposed in an ulcer base. It does not alter the acidity but may inhibit pepsin and prevent hydrogen ion diffusion locally. It also binds bile acids, and possibly reduces their damaging effect upon the gastric mucosa. It therefore seems to exert a protective effect. Controlled trials have indicated that it hastens the healing of both gastric and duodenal ulcer.

One gram four times daily, 1 h before meals is prescribed; this, together with the large size of the tablets, may be a problem for some patients. So far, it does not appear to cause serious side-effects. Constipation is most common and occasional nausea and discomfort. There is appreciable aluminium absorption.

Other drugs. Anticholinergic drugs have been used widely in attempts to control acid but results have been unsatisfactory. A maximum effective dose, sufficient to cause blurred vision and a dry mouth, will reduce basal, postprandial and peak acid output but this does not affect intragastric acidity throughout 24 h. Controlled trials failed to produce consistent evidence that anticholinergics either encourage healing or prevent relapses; so the term 'medical vagotomy' is a euphemism and these drugs are no more than 'logical placebos'. The tricyclic antidepressant trimipramine has been claimed to be effective in both duodenal and gastric ulcers and with antacids was almost as effective as cimetidine; if proved, it could be either due to a weak antisecretory action, or to the sedative effect. Prostaglandin E_2 is a normal constituent of human gastric mucosa and gastric secretion, and may have a protective effect on the mucosal cells as well as reducing acid output. Prostaglandin E deficiency could be a factor in human peptic ulcer. Synthetic analogues of prostaglandin E have been used for treating duodenal ulcer but proof is not yet available. Irradiation therapy to the gastric mucosa only temporarily reduces acid output. Placebo treatment using injections of saline reduces the number of days of pain compared with no treatment at all.

Surgical treatment

The indications for operation are given in Table 10.2. Medical treatment is not usually regarded as failed until a full course of cimetidine or ranitidine together with a maintenance evening dose for 6 months or longer has been given. Some patients who have had an obvious duodenal ulcer with much scarring for many years and who are unlikely to respond could be referred for operation without it. How soon

Table 10.2. Indications for advising an operation for a peptic ulcer.

1	Failure of medical treatment.
2	Complications such as perforation, stenosis and haemorrhage.
3	Gastric ulcer where there is any suspicion of malignancy.
4	Stomal ulcer if uncontrolled by H_2 antagonists.

operation is considered depends upon the degree of disability as assessed by loss of time from work or inability of the housewife to cope with the family.

No patient should have an operation unless an obvious ulcer crater is seen in the stomach by X-ray or in the duodenum at endoscopy. Caution is necessary in advising neurotic patients to undergo surgery especially where dyspepsia occurs on a background of psychosomatic symptoms; for they may become gastric cripples from exaggeration of minor postoperative sensations. Nevertheless neurosis may be the result of prolonged dyspepsia and cured by operation.

Purpose and choice of operation. The choice of operation should be based on known facts about operative mortality, side-effects and incidence of recurrent ulceration. The aim of operation is to reduce the capacity of the stomach to secrete acid and pepsin, so allowing healing of the ulcer and protection against further ulceration. The fact that various operations (Fig. 10.2) are available indicates that none is perfect. Most surgeons now regard some form of selective vagotomy as the first choice. Vagotomy was used to treat duodenal ulcer about 30 years ago; the acid output falls by 50–70%, allowing duodenal ulcers to heal in most patients. Gastric stasis usually occurs as well as diarrhoea, perhaps due to contamination of the small intestine by bacteria from a stagnant stomach. Incidence of recurrent ulcers was high. *Selective vagotomy* cuts only branches of vagus supplying the stomach so that autonomic nerves supplying the rest of abdominal viscera are left intact. *Proximal gastric vagotomy* (PGV) is highly selective: the fibres of the vagus supplying the acid-secreting gastric mucosa are dissected and divided, the extra-gastric nerves and innervation of gastric antrum and pylorus being preserved—so a drainage procedure to counteract stasis is not needed. PGV has a high recurrent ulcer rate (5–15%) but a very low mortality and no side-effects compared with gastric resection. Results depend upon the experience of the surgeon in achieving complete denervation. The incidence of recurrent ulcers increases with time, probably due to a slow increase in acid secretory response, reflected in a positive insulin (Hollander) test one year after operation though a positive response is associated with a recurrent ulcer in only a few patients. It is difficult to do in a fat person and necrosis of the lesser curve has been reported. PGV, performed by an experienced surgeon, is now the procedure of choice for uncomplicated duodenal ulcer. Mortality rate is 0.5% or less.

Other operations are PGV with drainage, either pyloroplasty or gastroenterostomy. If partial gastrectomy is preferred, the Billroth I operation (Fig. 10.2) is preferable, for it preserves the normal channel through the duodenum; so troublesome steatorrhoea is less likely as pancreatic juice can mix properly with food and no blind afferent loop is left; but this may be impossible, especially if much scar tissue is present and where there is an unnecessary risk of trying to join the two ends together, so a Polya partial gastrectomy or Billroth II (Fig. 10.2) is carried out instead and the remaining stump is anastomosed to jejunum. The mortality rate may be as high as 2%, and the occurrence of stomal ulcer perhaps 10%.

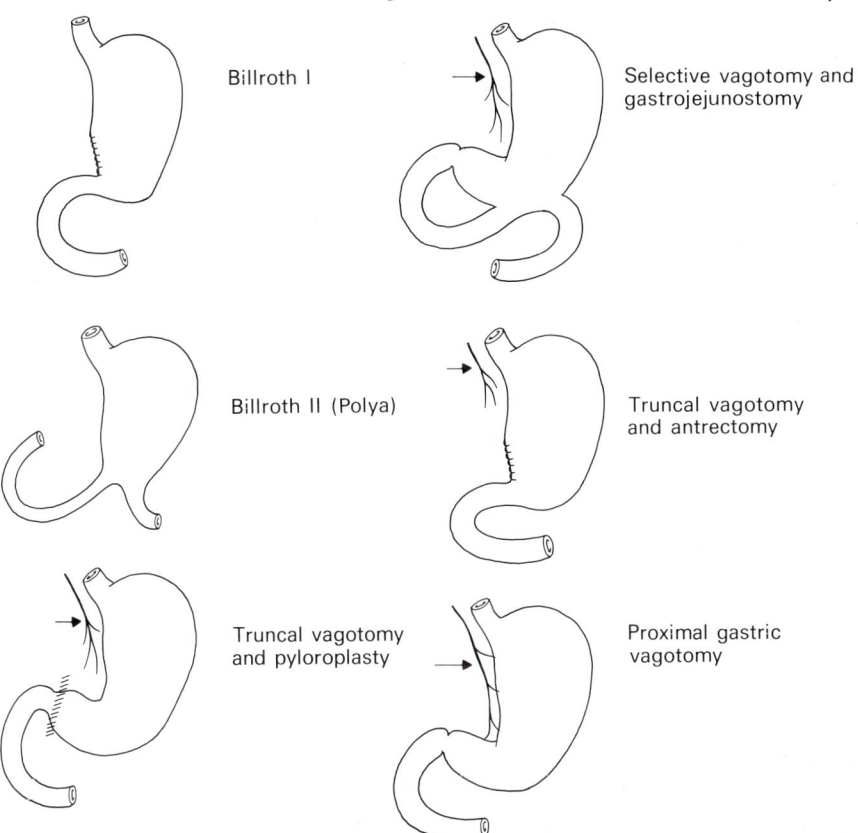

Fig. 10.2. Types of operation for duodenal ulcer.

Most after gastric resection enjoy the luxury of an unprotesting alimentary tract but a few, possibly 15%, do suffer from various symptoms:

1 Small stomach syndrome. When much stomach has been removed, discomfort or distension may be felt towards the end of a meal. The patient should eat little and often, and be reassured that it usually subsides.

2 The dumping syndrome. The typical complaint is of epigastric fullness with a sudden profound weakness and feeling of faintness when eating. It starts soon after the operation and has a tendency to get better. It is probably due to sudden distension of the jejunum, for it usually occurs only in the upright position. Patients are reassured and advised to eat dry meals with the minimum of fluid. If necessary, they should lie down during or after a meal.

3 Hypoglycaemia. This occurs (rarely) about 2 h after eating, and has been wrongly called 'late dumping'. The low blood sugar follows an excessive insulin release, probably due to the sudden absorption of carbohydrates. Dizziness, light-

Table 10.3. Causes of dyspepsia after gastric surgery.

Common
    Stomal ulcer
    Recurrence of original ulcer (if not removed)
Occasional
    Nervous dyspepsia
    Oesophageal reflux
    'Bile vomiting'
    Drugs, e.g. analgesics
Rare
    Carcinoma in gastric remnant
    Zollinger–Ellison syndrome

---

headedness, sweating, palpitations and even confusion may occur. It is treated by frequent small meals low in sugar and ingestion of sugar once symptoms have developed.

4 **Bilious vomiting.** Vomiting small amounts of bile may occur for a while after operation and is likely to disappear. Vomiting of bile collecting in the afferent loop (after partial gastrectomy) follows a period of good health and is more troublesome. Adhesions may be causing partial obstruction to its entry into the gastric remnant and operation may be required. Symptoms may subside or be relieved by the patient lying on his left side to drain the loop.

5 **Recurrence of dyspepsia.** Dyspepsia after gastric operations (Table 10.3) is most commonly caused by a stomal ulcer, though it can be due to the original ulcer if it was not removed, or to some other condition. Stomal ulcer may occur after any anastomotic gastric operation and begins either at the suture line or a short distance down the efferent loop of the jejunum. The risk is as much as 10–20% in some series and it is most frequent after duodenal ulcer because of the high acidity. Stomal ulcer may perforate or penetrate surrounding structures giving a gastro-jejuno-colic fistula.

Diagnosis is by endoscopy as radiography is difficult due to the effects of the operation. The first line of treatment should be with H_2 antagonists for 6 months or 1 year. If this fails, further operation is needed.

When no cause is found for postoperative symptoms, nervous dyspepsia should be considered. Some patients are operated upon for non-existing ulcers and the findings of the original operation should be reviewed. A routine use of endoscopy to prove the presence of an ulcer in doubtful cases should prevent this happening in the future.

6 **Diarrhoea.** Any gastric operation may have a laxative effect upon the bowel. Indeed, some patients are pleased when they receive the unexpected bonus from an operation to cure their ulcers that their life-long constipation is cured. Others are

less happy because of diarrhoea; vagotomy may cause it due to a disturbance in intestinal motility. This tends to improve with time and may respond to drugs such as dihydrocodeine or cholestyramine.

7   Steatorrhoea. This may be caused by rapid passage of food through the absorptive area of the small intestine. After a Polya operation (Fig. 10.2), bile and pancreatic secretions follow the food instead of being mixed with it; or adhesions may cause narrowing of the exit of the afferent loop, so that trapped secretions become stagnant, allowing bacterial growth which affects the small intestine. A mild degree of steatorrhoea is expected after any gastric surgery and is usually symptomless and can be ignored.

8   Weight loss. Failure to gain weight is common and of no significance except that it causes unnecessary worry to the patients. Even if associated with steatorrhoea, there is no contraindication to increasing fat in the diet and it may be better to give it at frequent intervals. Otherwise it is usually only necessary to explain and reassure the patient. Pulmonary tuberculosis must be excluded.

9   Anaemia. Iron deficiency anaemia particularly affects women of child-bearing age, as loss of iron through menstruation places them in a precarious state of iron balance. Defective absorption of the iron in food may be due to achlorhydria after surgery or to the rapid passage of food through the gut. In either case, release of the ionic iron will occur lower down in the intestine and a smaller area is available for absorption. Absorption of inorganic iron occurs normally and these patients respond to ferrous sulphate. Serum B_{12} levels fall after gastric operations but megaloblastic anaemia is rare.

10   Metabolic bone disease. Osteomalacia with bone pains and pseudo-fractures occasionally occurs after partial gastrectomy. The serum calcium and alkaline phosphatase should be checked whenever this is expected.

11   Carcinoma. Gastric cancer is a slight risk after any stomach operation, especially resection. It occurs in about 3%, increasing with time—those who had the operation 10 years or more ago being especially at risk.

Complications of peptic ulcer

Uncomplicated peptic ulcer is a benign disease and not a cause of death. Mortality rate is accounted for by perforation, haemorrhage, obstruction, and by operation. Perforation, potentially the most lethal, occurs in about 5% and haemorrhage in up to 15% of patients.

Haemorrhage. A branch of one gastric artery may open into the floor of a gastric ulcer, or a branch of the pancreatico-duodenal artery may cross the duodenal ulcer and be liable to bleed. The risk of death from bleeding increases with age, partly because atheroma may prevent the closure and retraction of vessels, so clotting and arrest of haemorrhage is less likely—and partly because other diseases often coexist. Bleeding is also likely to be worse in old and chronic ulcers where vessels are fixed and rigid.

Perforation. Rapidly penetrating acute or subacute ulcers are more likely to perforate than chronic ones as fibrous tissue has not formed on the outer surface of the stomach or duodenum. For example, two ulcers may be present on opposite sides of the duodenal cap. The posterior may be old and chronic while the acute anterior one perforates; then free gastric juice leaks into the peritoneal cavity whereas this is less likely with posterior ulcers. The incidence of perforation appears to be declining from its highest peak at the end of the Second World War, though it is still a common surgical emergency.

Symptoms start so suddenly that most know the exact time of onset—in few other acute abdominal conditions does this happen. There is immediate prostration with severe pain. Board-like rigidity, which may prevent deep palpation, is expected except in the debilitated, in those receiving corticosteroids, and the aged. Shoulder-tip pain may occur from irritation of the diaphragm; when gastric juice flows downwards, it may occur in the right iliac fossa, perhaps simulating appendicitis, and may cause a pelvic abscess. Bowel sounds disappear because of ileus. Resonance over the liver because of free gas is a valuable sign though it sometimes can occur from a distended colon. A plain X-ray of the abdomen taken upright to show gas under the diaphragm often confirms the diagnosis. Pain is treated by pethidine or other analgesics intravenously; gastric suction to prevent further leakage is started and immediate operation arranged.

Simple oversewing is the simplest life-saving procedure and is carried out in the desperately ill or elderly patient or if perforation has been present for 24 h or more, when there will be peritoneal sepsis. Once life is saved, the patient should be reviewed and definitive surgery advised only if he has an undoubted chronic duodenal ulcer or if symptoms indicate it; about 20% of patients having repair of an acute perforation with a history of less than 3 months need later operation, compared with over 40% of those with chronic ulcers. However, under good conditions an experienced surgeon can perform gastrectomy or vagotomy and

Table 10.4. Causes of pyloric stenosis.

Common
    Duodenal ulcer
Occasional
    Carcinoma of pyloric antrum
Rare
    Gastric ulcer
    Benign tumour of stomach
    Congenital hypertrophic pyloric stenosis (in adult)
    Prolapsed gastric mucosa
    Bezoar

drainage in the presence of a perforation, but few would perform PGV under these conditions as it requires a meticulous and rather tedious technique.

Pyloric stenosis. The commonest cause of pyloric or, more correctly, duodenal stenosis, is scarring from a duodenal ulcer. Gastric ulcers rarely produce obstruction of the pylorus, but it occurs with carcinoma of the pyloric antrum. Other causes are given in Table 10.4. Vomiting, especially towards the end of the day, is the cardinal symptom; the quantity of vomit is large in contrast to the small bile-stained vomit of simple ulcer and it may contain food remnants such as tomato skins hours or days after being eaten; offensive eructations due to fermentation from gastric stasis may be noticed. Pain is not troublesome unless obstruction is due to a growth. Inanition together with electrolyte disturbances such as alkalosis, uraemia and potassium deficiency is a sequel to vomiting.

There may be no abnormal signs. Peristaltic waves travelling to the right across the upper abdomen usually indicate a benign origin as the slow development of obstruction will have allowed time for hypertrophy of the stomach wall to develop. The stomach should be empty 4–6 h after eating and gastric stasis is diagnosed by succussion splash, aspiration of more than 250 ml, or the presence of barium still in the stomach at this time.

Occasionally the clinical picture may be confused by mental changes, uraemia, tetany, or even coma from alkalosis. Although constipation is the expected companion to obstruction, some have diarrhoea; a possible explanation is that stale food in the stomach leads to the production of a compound irritating to the intestine or that bacterial contamination of the small bowel occurs.

Operation is performed as soon as abnormalities of electrolytes and blood urea have been treated. Some respond temporarily to aspiration and hydration, probably because obstruction of the pylorus is partly due to spasm and oedema; indeed complete stenosis from scarring alone is uncommon. Most surgeons prefer a drainage operation, usually gastroenterostomy with some form of vagotomy.

Special problems

Gastric ulcer benign or malignant? An ulcer lying on the lesser curve between the angulus and cardia as a button-like projection, the surrounding mucosa appearing normal and pliable, with folds radiating out from the crater as healing takes place, is almost certainly benign (Fig. 10.4). An ulcer on the greater curvature or in the pre-pyloric region is often neoplastic and may protrude as a shallow plateau *into* the lumen of the stomach, and a filling defect may be seen (Fig. 10.3).

Endoscopy with multiple biopsies and aimed brushings to obtain cytological material is always necessary for gastric ulcers but not with duoenal ulcers. The endoscopic suspicion of malignancy is strong if the surrounding mucosa is irregular or heaped up, or if the ulcer has an unusually irregular appearance or seems to be on

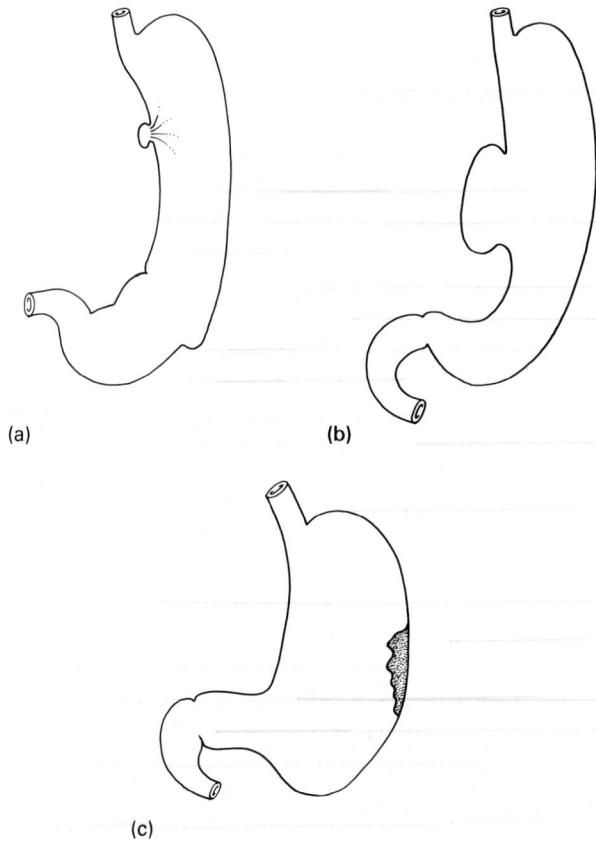

(a)   (b)

(c)

Fig. 10.3. Benign gastric ulcer (a and b) lie outside extended line of the stomach but malignant ulcers (c) project inside.

a mass. Biopsies should be repeated if the ulcer does not heal with medical treatment; always advise operation if there is the slightest indication of malignancy.

Do benign gastric ulcers become malignant? A benign ulcer seldom, if ever, becomes malignant. Confusion has arisen in the past probably because of a wrong diagnosis at the start. Also atrophy due to gastritis is associated with a gastric ulcer especially in the vicinity around it, so carcinoma may occur nearby.

Giant lesser curve ulcer. Giant ulcers with a 'punched out' crater (Fig. 10.5) are usually benign. They occur at any age, though especially in mid-life, and have the usual sex incidence, so probably are of similar aetiology to small ulcers. Situated on the lesser curve, they may spread to the posterior wall of the stomach and must be

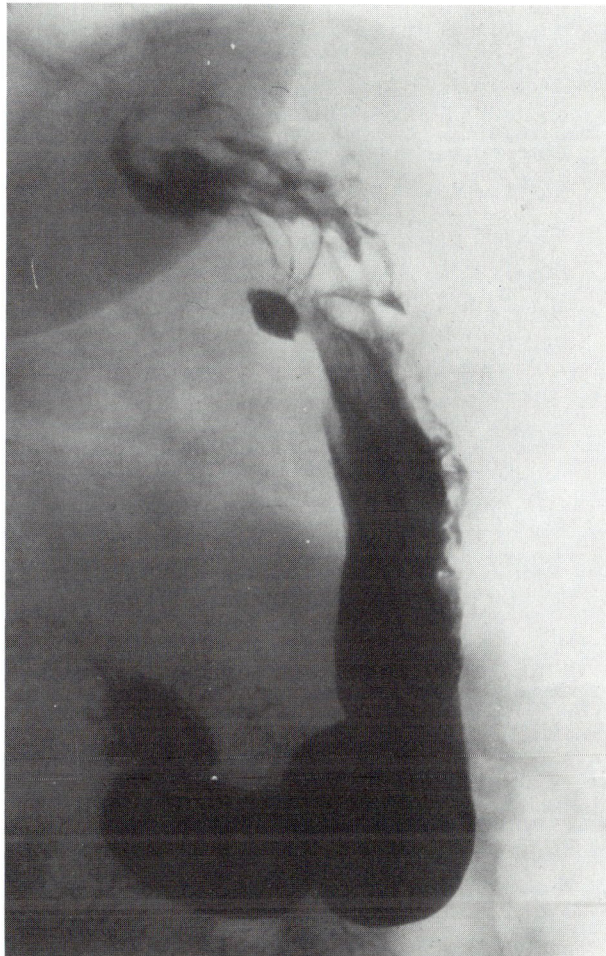

Fig. 10.4. X-ray of benign gastric ulcer.

distinguished from giant carcinomatous ulcers, but the latter are more likely to be beyond the angulus, and in the pyloric canal.

Symptoms are often atypical; vomiting may be severe and haematemesis fatal. If proved benign by endoscopy and biopsy, treat medically for 6 weeks as many heal; if not, advise operation.

Stress ulcers. Multiple small erosions occur in the fundus and body of the stomach and are usually symptomless apart from haematemesis or melaena. Diagnosis is by

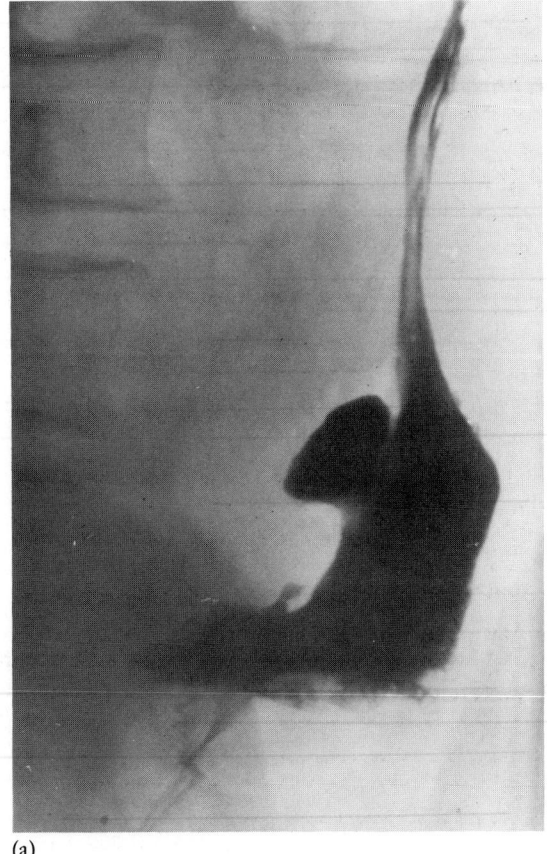

(a)

Fig. 10.5. (a) X-ray of large benign gastric ulcer; (b) (*opposite*) ulcer almost healed after 6 weeks.

endoscopy as, being so superficial, they are not seen by routine barium meal except by the double contrast method.

They occur in patients who are seriously ill from some other cause, such as those in an intensive care unit. They have been traditionally associated with burns (Curling's ulcer) and lesions of the brain, especially after neurosurgical operations (Cushing's ulcer). Why they occur is unknown and factors suggested include reduced gastric mucosal blood flow (many patients are collapsed with shock), bile salts, and 'malnutrition'. Hydrochloric acid is usually present but hypersecretion is absent. The erosions heal in a few days.

Peptic ulcer after renal transplantation. Patients with renal transplants are liable to many gastrointestinal complications including fungal oesophagitis, pancreatitis,

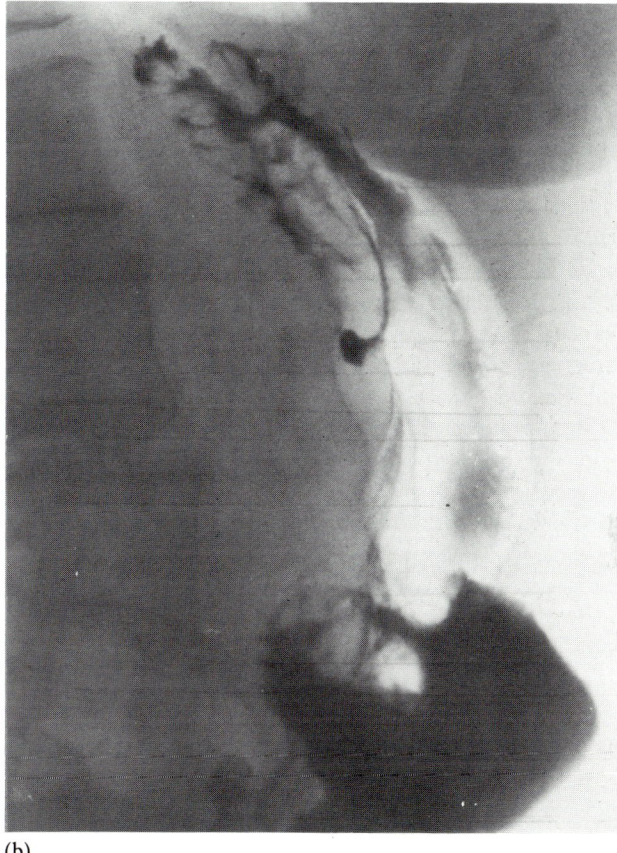

(b)

small bowel obstruction or infarction, ischaemic colitis, and colonic perforation. The commonest is peptic ulcer with the frequency as high as 18%. It is complicated by perforation or haemorrhage, carrying an overall mortality of over 40%.

The ulcers may have developed before transplantation, for peptic ulceration is not uncommon in renal failure. Then the serum gastrin can be high owing to failure of kidneys to degrade gastrin. Both the basal acid output and peak response to pentagastrin can be raised, especially in patients on haemodialysis; after transplantation, serum gastrin falls rapidly, but curiously acid secretion can increase further.

Corticosteroids in large doses probably increase the risk but azathioprine is not guilty. A possible factor is virus infection since cytomegalovirus (CMV) is often present in the mucosa of the stomach and duodenum after transplantation, but evidence for this is not strong. Immunosuppression does not prevent these peptic ulcers from healing and H_2 antagonists may prevent them. If haemorrhage or other symptoms recur, surgery still seems the safest treatment. Prophylactic ulcer surgery before transplantation would not reduce complications since most ulcers arise in those with no previous ulcer symptoms. Cimetidine has been used for prophylaxis and for treatment. At present it is impossible to identify patients at risk by acid or other studies.

Drug-induced ulcers. Aspirin undoubtedly causes acute erosions though this may be rare. The epidemiological evidence that aspirin causes chronic peptic ulcer is controversial. In Australia, analgesic abuse is probably important in causing gastric ulcer, but in the USA the risk of ulcer in habitual consumers has been compared to that of venous thrombosis in women taking oral contraceptives.

Antirheumatic drugs receive much blame though this may sometimes be unfair as peptic ulcer may be more common in patients with rheumatoid arthritis. However, both phenylbutazone and indomethacin are a cause of bleeding from acute ulcers and should be avoided in patients with chronic peptic ulcers. Indomethacin when originally introduced as a tablet did cause large gastric ulcers and so it was made as a capsule. Corticosteroids in large doses (above 15 mg daily) probably cause chronic peptic ulcers though the risk of this in doses of less than 15 mg daily is probably negligible.

Recent research has revealed that most of these drugs exert their beneficial effects partially by inhibiting prostaglandin synthetase activity in the joints. This enzyme is also found within the gastric mucosa where it seems to be involved in maintaining the mucosal barrier to back diffusion of acid. Drugs inhibiting prostaglandin synthesis may interfere with mucus production, so permitting acid peptic damage to the mucosa, resulting in erosion or ulceration. This theory is supported by some animal and human studies which show that simultaneous administration of prostaglandin E_2 can prevent mucosal damage.

Peptic ulcer in children

Peptic ulcers are somewhat rare in children, but may cause melaena in a newborn infant or abdominal pain and wake the child at night in early childhood; vomiting is more common than in adults probably because of the small duodenum which easily becomes obstructed by oedema and spasm.

In late childhood, the typical history of duodenal ulcer emerges and it is interesting to note that many adults with duodenal ulcer date the onset of symptoms to their 'teens. Diagnosis depends upon the awareness of the doctor that chronic peptic ulcer occurs in children. Their cause invites speculation: the acute ulcers in infants may have a separate aetiology, since, however precocious the child, financial worries and alcoholism, or excessive cigarette smoking are unlikely to be factors, particularly in those under 10 years.

Zollinger–Ellison syndrome (ulcerogenic tumour of the pancreas)

In this rare syndrome an islet-cell tumour of the pancreas secretes gastrin which stimulates the parietal cells of the stomach to produce large quantities of highly acid gastric juice, causing ulcers in the stomach, duodenum, or upper jejunum (Fig. 10.6). Repeated gastric operations may fail to stem the flow of acid or to cure the ulcers.

Symptoms and complications of peptic ulcer generally dominate the picture. Diarrhoea is an early symptom, sometimes before peptic ulceration. This is probably due to irritation of the jejunum by gastric juice, too copious to be neutralized by the alkaline pancreatic secretion. The pH in the upper jejunun is acid. Alkali or aspiration of gastric juice may correct this and temporarily improve the diarrhoea.

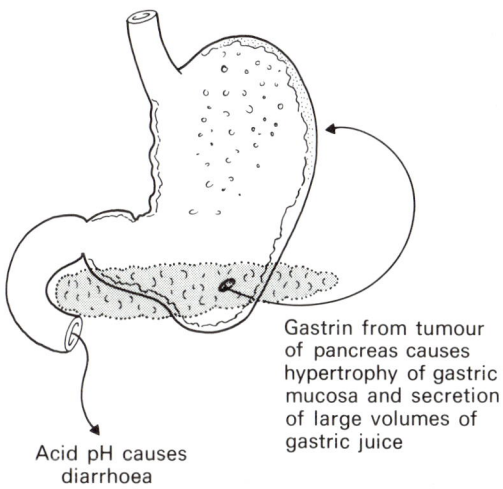

Gastrin from tumour of pancreas causes hypertrophy of gastric mucosa and secretion of large volumes of gastric juice

Acid pH causes diarrhoea

Fig. 10.6. Zollinger–Ellison syndrome.

Diagnosis. This can be made by measuring fasting plasma gastrin (p. 68). A barium meal shows large folds or even polyposis from hypertrophy of gastric mucosa due to the perpetual stimulus to secretion. Aspiration of the stomach provides vast quantities of gastric juice including basal specimens; all have a high acid output so that the basal and maximal stimulus by pentagastrin is usually the same.

A CT body scan may show a tumour of the pancreas, providing this is larger than 1 cm in diameter. An even rarer condition is over-production of gastrin due to antral-gastrin cell (G-cell) hyperplasia (plasma gastrin levels are normal in patients with duodenal ulcer).

Treatment. This is often best carried out by total gastrectomy, for partial gastrectomy is followed by stomal ulcers, haemorrhage and perforation. Operations directed at the pancreas can be unsatisfactory, for the tumour may be multifocal, malignant, or never found. An adenoma is likely to be in the body or tail of the pancreas in two-thirds of the patients and multiple adenomas may occur in one-third. Microscopic malignancy is present in two-thirds and there are metastases, usually in the liver, in one-third of the patients when first seen. However, the metastases are often slow growing and some patients have lived for some years with them; they may or may not influence gastric secretion. Acid levels fall to normal if the syndrome is due to a single lesion when this is removed. Lesions are found within the pancreas in 90% but in the rest appear in aberrant pancreatic tissue, either in the hilum of the spleen, along the superior border of the pancreas or buried in the gastric or duodenal walls; sometimes they look like a lymph node adjacent to the pancreas.

Chapter 11

Dyspepsia, Gastritis and Tumours of the Stomach

Nervous dyspepsia

Dyspepsia often arises from disturbances in the psyche rather than in the alimentary tract and is due, like tension headache, to stress or to an unfounded fear of having cancer. Symptoms may so resemble organic disease that operations upon normal organs are performed, events that may cure by the power of suggestion, or prolong a neurosis. The stomach, according to studies by Wolf & Wolff (1947) on their technician Tom with the gastric fistula, undergoes changes in secretion, motility and blood flow which reflect the attitude of mind of its owner. So, in certain patients, symptoms such as anorexia, nausea, vomiting and diarrhoea merely symbolize emotions such as sadness, disgust and anxiety and do not indicate disease. The symptoms of other patients in this group may be due to the irritable bowel syndrome and indeed often occur with irritable colon, or possibly due to some hitherto unknown effect of an upper gut hormone.

Symptoms. Pain or discomfort may be localized to the epigastrium though more often it occurs elsewhere as well. It starts immediately after eating, in contrast to ulcer pain which is not aggravated but relieved by food. Alkalis may have little effect and victims are not awakened from sleep because of pain as in peptic ulcer; more often they are unable to sleep because of a disturbed mind.

Other symptoms (Table 11.1) distinguish these patients. The appetite may be good, yet a feeling of satiety develops soon after a few mouthfuls so that the meal has to be discontinued. Sensitivity to food occurs and patients become introspective about eating, finding that various, and in some cases every type of food and drink causes symptoms. Even the smell of food may start trouble. One patient stated that she knew by telepathy whether food was about even if she could not see or smell it. Another was able to enjoy New Zealand lamb but English lamb made her ill for several days afterwards. No-one's stomach has this remarkable power of discrimination and any 'allergy' usually lies in the psyche and not in the gastric mucosa. Vomiting may be prominent and even continue for years without loss of weight; indeed the patient may appear remarkably robust in spite of it.

Other symptoms which support the diagnosis are nausea, burning feelings, dislike of anything tight around the waist and so on. 'Heartburn' may be a complaint but this is not true heartburn, which lasts for 2 or 3 min; it may continue for 24 h and is a typical nervous symptom. In contrast to the peptic ulcer patient who is usually fit apart from the dyspepsia, they are often unwell otherwise due to complaints of nervous origin (Table 11.2).

Table 11.1. Differential diagnosis between dyspepsia due to peptic ulcer and nervous dyspepsia.

	Ulcer	Nervous dyspepsia
Complaint	Pain	Various symptoms: wind, discomfort, burning, acidity, dislike of clothes touching abdomen or tight garments around waist.
Reaction to foods	Eats anything (except perhaps fat)	'Sensitivity' to various foods
Effect of alkali	Immediate relief	Variable
Pointing test	+	—
Health otherwise	Fit	Tiredness, headaches, insomnia, etc.

Diagnosis and treatment. Reassurance after thorough examination and investigation often cures. Unfortunately, this may not happen: instead of immediate reassurance when the barium meal is normal, the patient may be told that this does not exclude an ulcer and and that he is to be put on the list for endoscopy; this puts doubt in the mind and there may be a waiting list of 2 or 3 months. If endoscopy is normal, reassurance may be ineffective because of amnesia from diazepam. Next the patient may fail to contact the general practitioner or communication from the hospital may be defective. Worst of all is the doubt cast by reporting a mucosal variation such as gastritis, for neither the doctor nor one's colleagues in other specialities may know its significance. It is always more rewarding to 'find something', especially by junior staff whose clinical acumen may lag behind their technical competence. However, both gastritis and duodenitis are often incidental. If given an organic label, neurosis may be perpetuated and patients condemned to dieting or tablets instead of being cured by reassurance. Correct diagnosis must be made before treatment. Prescribing an H_2 receptor antagonist may cure by a placebo effect but can do harm;

Table 11.2. Complaints that are more likely to originate from the psyche than soma— especially if several are present.

1	Tiredness	5	Dyspareunia
2	Headache	6	Sexual difficulties
3	Dizziness	7	Insomnia
4	Depression		

instead of instant reassurance, it fixes the idea of the trouble being organic and due to acid.

Fear of cancer, so often present, must be dispelled. Faulty ideas concerning digestion must be corrected. The idea that some foods cannot be digested is imaginary, as could be proved by sampling through a stomach tube. Similarly worry is caused by so-called wind which is sometimes thought to be a form of marsh gas due to unnatural fermentation; most is swallowed air (aerophagy) and explaining this will relieve anxiety. A normal diet should be prescribed with confidence as some will have developed food fads. A careful search for an emotional cause should be made.

Prognosis. Most with nervous dyspepsia can be cured if diagnosed early. Some spend their lives with their 'delicate stomach', their enjoyment of food curtailed and their leisure spent in consuming digestive remedies. Where the diagnosis has been missed or not accepted, the patient may have gone from doctor to doctor labelled with mythical diagnoses such as adhesions, chronic appendicitis, chronic cholecystitis, gastritis and so on. They present pathetic pictures with a battle-scarred abdomen, where numerous viscera have been tampered with. Their original symptoms remain and at this stage are often incurable.

Dyspepsia due to disease of the gallbladder or pancreas

Gallstones cause colic and acute cholecystitis, both easily recognized as clinical entities. Chronic cholecystitis as a cause for flatulent dyspepsia is a diagnosis that, like chronic appendicitis, has become obsolete, for so many of these patients have the same symptoms after cholecystectomy. Flatulence in someone with gallstones is likely to be due to other causes such as hiatus hernia, peptic ulcer, or nervous dyspepsia. Gallstones, with or without cholecystitis, may cause pain in the epigastrium or right hypochondrium after eating, and, in the absence of other disease, the gallstones should be removed.

Chronic pancreatitis may cause pain after eating and is often overlooked because it is not considered in a differential diagnosis of dyspepsia.

Gastritis

Gastritis, when used as a lay term to explain an otherwise unexplained dyspepsia, should not be confused with gastritis used in a pathological sense, for there is often no association between the two.

Acute gastritis

To this group belong types of gastritis where the cause is known, e.g. the swallowing of irritant substances and food poisoning. The gastric mucosa is protected by a thick layer of tenacious mucus so irritants may provoke no more than erythema, though they cause tissue damage when applied to the skin. The protective powers of mucus can be overwhelmed, e.g. ferrous sulphate tablets swallowed by children in mistake for sweets will cause necrosis of the mucosa. Acute gastritis used to be seen in children dying of diphtheria, or in adults succumbing to influenza; today it may account for gastric distress and vomiting seen in some acute febrile illnesses.

However, the two common causes of acute gastritis are alcohol and staphylococcal endotoxin. Symptoms of alcoholic gastritis may occur soon after a drinking bout, but are especially notable next morning when the victim experiences nausea, epigastric discomfort and vomiting. Gastric biopsies will show damage to surface epithelium, but the glandular structure remains intact so full recovery takes place—as is usual after acute gastritis. Staphylococcal gastroenteritis due to food poisoning starts about 4–6 h after eating contaminated food and causes vomiting and diarrhoea, usually self-limiting, and symptoms subside after 12–24 h.

Acute erosive gastritis

This may cause haematemesis or melaena. The gastric mucosa looks red and oedematous with multiple small erosions from the size of a pin's head to several millimetres in diameter. They are often symptomless apart from bleeding. Diagnosis is by endoscopy or by double-contrast barium meal.

Usually no cause is found and recurrent attacks may occur. Aspirin, however, is important: haemorrhage occurs with both soluble aspirin and plain tablets, but as undissolved particles probably 'burn' holes in the gastric mucosa especially taken with alcohol, patients should be advised to take soluble aspirin, dispersed by a drink of water. Haematemesis and melaena are caused by aspirin or alcohol and may require urgent blood transfusion, but bleeding generally stops spontaneously within 36 h, and complete healing of erosions occurs within a few days.

Slight oozing of blood from the stomach occurs in 70% of patients who take aspirin for rheumatoid arthritis, whether soluble, insoluble, or effervescent preparations are used; enteric-coated aspirin (Nu-seals) make this less likely as judged by occult blood tests on stools and by using chromium-labelled red blood cells. This bleeding is no reason for withholding aspirin; the daily loss of about 5 ml blood is hardly more than from repeated venesection in blood donors but the Hb must be watched as anaemia certainly occurs, especially in women before the menopause.

Chronic gastritis

The fact that most people with chronic gastritis are eupeptic, being able to enjoy their food without dyspepsia, compels caution in trying to link symptoms with histology. Chronic gastritis is a common finding at endoscopy and usually incidental; so do not use this label in a patient with symptoms of nervous dyspepsia else a permanent neurosis may be induced. Dr Beaumont (1833), who studied the gastric mucosa of his patient Alexis St Martin through the fistula produced by a gun shot wound, first noted that traumatic and intense mucosal changes could be induced without causing any symptoms whatsoever; this observation has been repeated and confirmed.

At endoscopy reddening of the mucosa is often striking, but biopsy alone confirms chronic gastritis; for erythema may be produced by circulatory changes possibly due to the psychic trauma of the endoscopy itself, for emotional upset produces changes in the stomach. Such gastritis is a normal and incidental finding after gastric drainage operations and is due to bile reflux. No treatment is needed and it is best either not to mention it to the patient, or to reassure him.

Chronic atrophic gastritis

This is common in symptomless, healthy people and increases with age. The atrophy affecting the glandular portion of the mucosa may be partial or complete; there is an inflammatory cell infiltration mainly of lymphocytes. Surface epithelial cells are commonly stunted and abnormal and in severe cases the mucosa may look like intestinal epithelium with finger-like projections similar to villi, a change termed intestinal metaplasia. This can be premalignant.

It may follow chronic gastritis or perhaps be a separate condition as in pernicious anaemia where atrophy is complete and acid-producing parietal cells are absent. It causes achlorhydria and failure of intrinsic factor secretion; so vitamin B_{12} cannot be absorbed in the ileum and pernicious anaemia will result. About 5% of patients with pernicious anaemia develop gastric carcinoma. Constitutional factors may be significant as the gastric atrophy of pernicious anaemia runs in families; the presence of gastric auto-antibodies implies an autoimmune process; whether such antibodies are a cause or merely a result of the abnormal mucosa is unknown.

Iron-deficient anaemia is more common in patients with atrophic gastritis. Achlorhydria does not affect absorption of therapeutic iron though it may depress absorption of food iron because ionic iron is split off from organic food iron lower down in the alimentary tract, hence a smaller area of gut is available for absorption. Achlorhydria may tilt the iron balance adversely in patients where dietary intake is only just sufficient to keep pace with the need, such as replacement of iron lost by women at menses or in childbirth. Treatment with iron while curing epithelial changes such as cheilosis, glossitis and koilonychia, seldom improves the gastric mucosa.

Virtually nothing is known concerning the cause of chronic gastritis. The fact that it is common in man and not seen in animals makes it tempting to blame the bizarre foods and drinks that has been one of the rewards of civilization. The stomach mucosa, like the skin, is subject to damage by trauma and distension as well as by spices, spirits, heat and cold. The wonder is that we do not all get chronic gastritis.

Rare forms of gastritis

Hypertrophic gastritis was diagnosed as a cause for prominent folds of gastric mucosa seen in the past by radiologists and endoscopists, but biopsy has shown no evidence for this. The size of folds of gastric mucosa depends upon the degree of distension of the stomach and coarse gastric folds may be normal. In the Zollinger–Ellison syndrome a great increase in the number of parietal cells, together with a high acidity, may be present together with a polypoid appearance of the mucosa.

Giant folds

These are sometimes seen by barium meal and may mimic either a tumour or gastric polyposis. They look like convolutions of the cerebrum and are especially seen along the greater curvature and fundus. This condition is called Ménétrièr's disease and is often symptomless. If dyspepsia occurs, it may be due to infection or ulceration of the folds.

If extensive, it may be a cause of protein-losing enteropathy: the loss of protein oozing from the folds causes the serum albumin to be under 35 g/l while loss of immunoglobulin may impair the immune defences. It is a rare cause of oedema of the feet and elsewhere. It is three times more common in men than in women and usually diagnosed between 30–50 years. Full thickness biopsy specimens show proliferation of all mucosal cells, but of mucus-secreting ones more than parietal pepsin cells; there may also be lymphoid hyperplasia. Acid secretion is reduced. It is not yet proved to be a premalignant condition. The cause is unknown and there is no genetic aspect. No treatment needed if it is symptomless. Irradiation gives bad results. Partial resection is slightly more risky than in peptic ulcer disease, perhaps from suturing unhealthy gastric tissue, so total gastrectomy is occasionally indicated.

Duodenitis

Endoscopy sometimes shows inflammation of the duodenal mucosa, perhaps dotted with 'pepper and salt' erosions. Barium studies are usually normal unless scarring is present from previous ulceration. Duodenitis is often asymptomatic, but it can produce the same symptoms and respond to the same treatment as duodenal ulcer and be followed by overt ulceration.

Duodenal diverticulum

Diverticula in the first part of the duodenum are either due to epithelialization of a large ulcer crater or represent the pouching of the duodenal wall opposite the ulcer which has contracted by scarring; a similar bilateral appearance may follow the myotomy of a pyloroplasty. Those in the rest of the duodenum are usually protrusions of the mucosa and submucosa through the muscular coat, as happens elsewhere in the alimentary tract or may be congenital. Careful judgement is needed before blaming duodenal diverticula for dyspeptic symptoms. Diverticula in the rest of the alimentary tract are usually symptomless unless there are complications such as inflammation, torsion, perforation, or bleeding; these can occur with duodenal diverticula but are rare.

Adult hypertrophic pyloric stenosis
This is rare and diagnosis is usually only confirmed at laparotomy. It is usually a congenital neuromuscular dysfunction of the pyloric canal similar to the condition in infants. It is doubtful whether it causes any symptoms apart from obstruction. The problem is to distinguish it from carcinoma or from a thickened fibrosed pylorus secondary to a nearby ulcer. The mucosa is normal in appearance and in flexibility.

Tumours of the stomach

Benign gastric tumours
The incidence of benign lesions varies, according to patient selection and method of detection, from 0.5% at necropsy to 3% at endoscopy. Approximately 50% are gastric polyps, which mainly cause concern because of their malignant potential. Two types of polyp occur: *hyperplastic polyps* which are regenerative lesions associated with gastritis and not true neoplasms, easily recognized as small (less than 2 cm) smooth protrusions which often occur on the tops of gastric folds and often regress spontaneously; *adenomatous polyps* which occur mostly in the antrum and are sessile, papillary or villous and are often associated with intestinal metaplasia in the adjacent mucosa. These should always be removed entirely through the endoscope as they are premalignant, an associated carcinoma either in the polyp or elsewhere in the stomach being present in about 50% of cases. Biopsy is essential in all gastric polyps whatever their size.

Leiomyomas
These are the commonest mesenchymal tumours of stomach—arising from the muscular wall. Bleeding is their main symptom, usually slow and continuous, causing iron-deficient anaemia, though occasionally profuse. If close to pylorus, they may cause obstructive symptoms. Bleeding is due to central ulceration giving the appearance of a volcanic crater at the apex of the mound and this produces a typical radiological picture by barium meal. Although most remain benign, the difficulty of being certain of the diagnosis and the possibility that about 10% are or may become malignant indicates wide local excision.

Bezoar
A bezoar, usually formed from vegetable fibres, may rarely appear as a round mass in the stomach and mimic a tumour. The trichobezoar or hair ball forms when young women chew and swallow their hair. It may extend further down the gut as a 'tail' and has been named as the Rapunzel syndrome, named after the princess in Grimm's fairy tale.

Cancer of the stomach

While the incidence of cancer of the stomach is undoubtedly decreasing in the Western world, it remains the third commonest cause of death from malignant disease in Britain, exceeded only by tumours of the lung and large bowel. Usually it is diagnosed late and the prognosis is gloomy, with a survival rate of only about 10% after 5 years.

Detecting early lesions

The Japanese, who are more liable to develop gastric cancer, have pioneered its early diagnosis. Then the lesions cause no symptoms and screening of the population is necessary; this is done by the gastrocamera (as with mass radiography of the chest in the UK), and by double-contrast barium studies.

Gastric cancer is defined as 'early' when the depth of invasion is histologically limited to the submucosal layer of the stomach. The endoscopist must have a suitably developed sense of suspicion when he sees small areas of mucosal thickening, nodulation or roughening, in addition to the more conventional lesions which show ulceration. Target biopsies and brushings for cytological analysis are then made. No screening of healthy people has taken place outside Japan and the expense hardly justifies it unless the cancer is common. Certain high-risk patients could, in the future, be subjected to regular screening: those with a family history of gastric cancer, those likely to have atrophic gastritis and hypochlorhydria, pernicious anaemia, Polya partial gastrectomy more than 10 years before, chronic atrophic gastritis, intestinal metaplasia, and gastric ulcer.

Predisposing factors

Gastric cancer is worldwide and twice as common in men as in women, usually being seen in the middle-aged or elderly. It is particularly common in Finland, Japan, Chile and Iceland. The mortality from gastric cancer in the Western world is rapidly declining (by 30% every 10 years in the USA) due to a decrease in the incidence of the disease, the reason for which is unknown but environmental factors in food or cooking may be responsible.

Certain families have had a special tendency to develop cancer of the stomach, one example being the family of Napoleon Bonaparte. The risk is slightly greater in patients of blood group A, possibly due to a lower secretion of acid which may imply a greater tendency to gastric atrophy. Dietary nitrate, which may form carcinogenic nitrosamines in the stomach, could predispose to malignant change; high dietary nitrate levels have been found in several countries with a high incidence of this cancer.

Nitrates in such common foods as cooked potatoes are easily reduced to potentially carcinogenic nitrites by incorrect food storage—without refrigeration. Some experimental evidence indicates that nitrites may be formed by bacterial overgrowth in a hypochlorhydric stomach. This has led to fears that suppression of gastric acid as by drugs or vagotomy could eventually be carcinogenic.

Achlorhydria is a known predisposing factor and 10% of patients with pernicious anaemia develop gastric cancer; the incidence is increased after most ulcer surgery, especially Polya gastrectomy. Adenomatous polyps of the stomach are premalignant.

Symptoms. Cancer of the stomach must be considered in any middle-aged or elderly person with recent dyspepsia though, curiously, 20% or more give a history of dyspepsia for many years beforehand. Early symptoms, in contrast to the late 'textbook' picture so often seen in hospital, bear no relation to site of growth and are vague: feelings of discomfort in epigastrium, inability to finish a large meal or sense of fullness, complaints also made by those with nervous dyspepsia. Others give a story similar to ulcer dyspepsia, and ocasionally ulcer dyspepsia or haematemesis is a presenting symptom. Obstructive symptoms such as dysphagia from carcinoma at the cardia or fundus (Fig. 11.1), or pyloric obstruction are usually late symptoms.

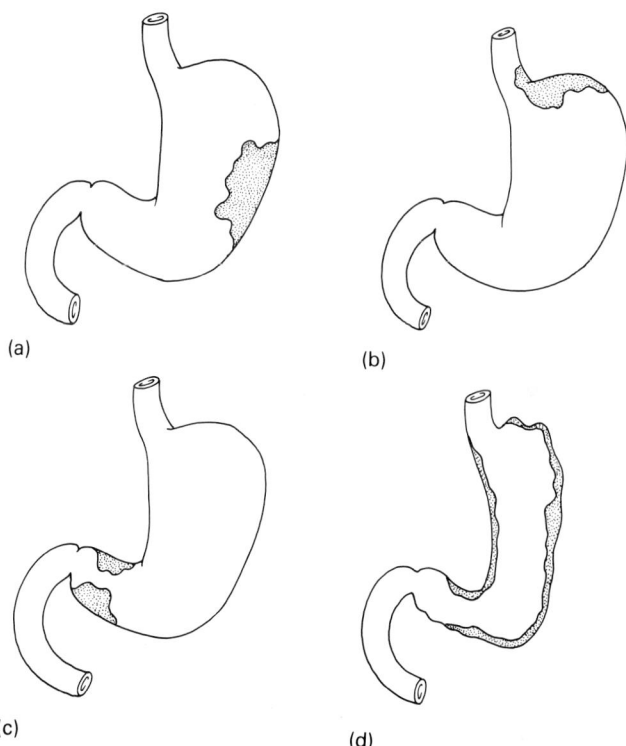

(a) (b) (c) (d)

Fig. 11.1. Carcinoma of stomach. (a) Ulcerating adenocarcinoma; (b) carcinoma of fundus causing dysphagia; (c) pyloric obstruction; (d) linitis plastica (leather-bottle stomach).

General symptoms may precede those from the stomach, such as anaemia from iron deficiency due to oozing of blood or leucoerythroblastic anaemia from deposits in the bone marrow which indicates a hopeless prognosis. Occasionally there is a disturbance of bowel action with either constipation or diarrhoea. Loss of weight is only a late symptom.

Signs. A palpable tumour may be felt in about half of the patients but this is no proof that the cancer is inoperable. Search should be made for the presence of deposits: peritoneal involvement is indicated by ascites and there may be a mass in the pelvis (or Kruckenberg's ovarian tumour) following transperitoneal invasion, and the liver may be enlarged, or a hard umbilical nodule felt; another late sign of inoperability is the enlarged lymph node in the supraclavicular fossa, Virchow's sign.

Diagnosis. The barium meal is the traditional method of diagnosis and detects about 80% of cases but it misses early lesions even when the double-contrast method is used.

Routine endoscopy on healthy people is the surest way of detecting early mucosal lesions, as has been shown in Japan where cancer of the stomach has been common; this would not be justified on a cost-benefit basis in countries elsewhere. However, endoscopy is always indicated in doubtful lesions and in many with a negative barium meal, especially if symptoms persist in spite of the reassurance of the X-ray. A combination of biopsy and brush cytology increases the diagnostic accuracy. Also, biopsy by endoscopy may be indicated with obvious malignant lesions, for example to exclude the rare but more treatable lymphoma of the stomach; but may be wasting the endoscopist's time whenever operation is going to be necessary anyway.

The three types of carcinoma of the stomach are: scirrhous growth causing either the narrow rigid aperistaltic leather-bottle stomach or pyloric stenosis, usually easily diagnosed by barium meal; the fungating (cauliflower) adenocarcinoma—poorly differentiated in young men giving a bad prognosis but well differentiated in elderly men resulting in a better outlook; or the malignant ulcer. Malignant ulcers are more likely in the pyloric antrum, or on the greater curvature and can usually be distinguished from the punched-out appearance of large benign ulcers.

Treatment. The prognosis of gastric cancer is poor, so incurable patients must be spared unnecessary surgery. The Japanese have produced a 95% survival rate after 5 years when minute early lesions of the mucosa are operated upon, as may be discovered when screening the healthy population by endoscopy. Discussion has occurred as to whether these lesions are different from early cancer in the UK but a consensus of opinion is that they are the same.

Generally, 60% may survive to 5 years if the cancer is detected early but 10–30% is a more likely figure. Prospects for cure may remain good even if lymph nodes are invaded from an intramucosal carcinoma; this could suggest that patients with early gastric cancer present immunological or other self-protective advantages, and the Japanese have noticed phases of healing in some lesions. It also seems that the intramucosal phase is likely to last very much longer in some patients than others.

Radiotherapy is not often of value for the surgically hopeless patient with gastric cancer. Hard data is lacking and difficult to obtain; further studies are needed with chemotherapy. At present the following are being used; 5-fluorouracil, mitomycin, and *bis*-chloronitrosourea either alone or in combination and may help in disseminated gastric cancers. However, there are serious difficulties in treating patients with a large solid tumour. Much of the tumour is insensitive to cytotoxic drugs and the degree of penetration into the tumour is uncertain. Hence there should be well-defined clinical indications and objectives before a patient with advanced gastric cancer is subjected to the misery and toxicity of chemotherapy. The quality of life may be a more important consideration than its prolongation.

Chapter 12
Disorders of the Gallbladder, Biliary Tree and Pancreas

Gallstones

Gallstones occur commonly in people of all races, though their prevalence varies. At least 15% of adults have formed gallstones when they die, but most of these appear to be incidental findings at necropsy and so are silent in life. The rest may cause severe pain and life-threatening diseases. It is hardly surprising, therefore, that not all doctors agree that a conservative approach is indicated if gallstones are discovered coincidentally, as often happens during radiological studies of the abdomen.

Predisposing factors

The aphorism that the typical patient with gallstones is a fat, fair, fertile, 40-year-old female should be buried. Any clinician relying on that stereotype would not only investigate many patients unnecessarily but also miss most gallstones. Firstly, fat: the evidence is circumstantial only and conclusive proof is lacking— indeed, many patients are slim and body build should not influence ideas about individuals. Next, the association with a fair complexion is nonsense. Fair-haired people are no more prone to gallstones than the rest of the community and the highest prevalence in the world occurs in American Indians. Although high parity has been linked with gallstones, nulliparous women also are commonly afflicted. The most important modern factor is the use of oestrogens in oral contraceptives; these probably double the frequency of gallstones by causing a deterioration in the cholesterol saturation of bile. Nor is the concept of a middle-aged peak in their prevalence supported by any evidence. Gallstones can occur in children and young women but generally the prevalence increases steadily with age, so that men in their eighties are more prone to the condition than women in their forties. Finally gallstones are common in men as well as in women. The sex differential changes with advancing age; under 40 years female to male ratio is 3 : 1, whereas over 80 years the ratio is 3 : 2.

Iatrogenic causes are clofibrate therapy for hyperlipidaemia and ileal resection. Patients with Crohn's disease of the ileum are also more likely to develop gallstones.

Pathogenesis

How and why gallstones are formed remains enigmatic but current research promises to provide us with efficient means of their prevention and dissolution. It is common to speak of three classes of gallstones: pigment, cholesterol and mixed stones (a mixture of pigment and cholesterol). This, however, is an over-simplification since nearly all are a mixture of many constituents.

Pigment stones
These contain various proportions of calcium bilirubinate, carbonate, phosphate and palmitate as well as some cholesterol. Bilirubin dominant pigment stones are commoner in patients with:
1   Haemolytic disease (increased bilirubin production).
2   Cirrhosis.
3   Infections of the biliary system (infection by organisms which contain β-glucuronidase, e.g. *E. coli*, results in production of insoluble bilirubin from bilirubin glucuronides).

These stones are often calcified and therefore visible on plain X-ray. Biliary colic due to pigment stones can be difficult to differentiate from an abdominal sickling crisis in HbS patients.

Cholesterol stones
Cholesterol is extremely insoluble in water. Its excretion from the body is therefore dependent on the detergent quality of bile. (Maximum cholesterol solubility in water $= 27$ nM; in bile $= 5$ M; i.e. it is 200,000 times more soluble in bile). The solubility of cholesterol in bile depends on the ratio, cholesterol : phospholipid + bile acid. When this ratio is too high, bile is supersaturated with cholesterol which then precipitates to form microcrystals with potential gallstone formation.

Clinical picture
Why some stones cause trouble and others do not is not known; large single stones are more likely to remain silent as they are too big to enter the cystic duct. Complications (Table 12.1) of gallstones are, particularly:
1   Colic. Mild to agonizing pain is caused when a stone lodges in the common bile duct. The pain is felt in the epigastrium or right hypochondrium and although called biliary or gallstone *colic*, it is usually a pain of varying intensity on a

Table 12.1. Complications due to gallstones.

1   Obstruction of the neck of the gallbladder (Hartmann's pouch).
2   Cholecystitis.
3   Biliary colic (cystic or common bile duct).
4   Cholangitis.
5   Pancreatitis.
6   Gallstone ileus.
7   Perforation of the gallbladder. ⎫ Rare
8   Carcinoma of the gallbladder. ⎭

background of constant pain, and lasts a few hours. Radiation of the pain to the lower end of the right scapula is common and is accompanied by vomiting or sweating. Characteristically the patient is restless and rolls about in agony. Obstructive jaundice usually follows. Rarely a stone can be passed painlessly, more so in the elderly.

2   Acute cholecystitis. If a stone becomes impacted in the gallbladder outlet or cystic duct, the gallbladder wall becomes inflamed due to the irritation of the concentrated bile within it producing a chemical cholecystitis. The gallbladder fills with pus which is usually sterile on culture, but infection with intestinal bacteria soon supervenes. There is fever with marked toxaemia and leucocytosis. The upper abdomen is extremely tender and often a palpable mass develops in the region of the gallbladder; this represents the distended inflamed gallbladder wrapped in inflammatory adhesions and the omentum. The stone may dislodge and the infection settles or an empyema of the gallbladder develops. Rarely, perforation takes place into the peritoneal cavity or stones may rupture through the gallbladder wall and cause a fistula into the duodenum or other neighbouring organs. If the inflammation is sterile, a mucocele of the gallbladder may form. Acute cholecystitis is usually associated with gallstones but may occur in children without them.

Treatment is often expectant, giving antibiotics and intravenous fluids as necessary. Some surgeons operate during the acute phase whereas others prefer to do an elective cholecystectomy 2 or 3 months afterwards.

3   Intestinal obstruction from gallstones. Rarely, a large gallstone, having ruptured into the duodenum, may cause obstruction of the lower ileum (gallstone ileus). A gallstone entering the colon has been known to lead to acute large bowel obstruction in the presence of diverticulitis or carcinoma of the colon.

4   Cholangitis. Partial obstruction of the common bile duct is the commonest cause of acute and suppurative forms of cholangitis, as the biliary tree is invaded by gut organisms. Then Charcot's triad or intermittent biliary fever is caused: intermittent jaundice, pain and fever. Other forms of cholangitis are dealt with later.

5   Chronic cholecystitis is not a cause of flatulent dyspepsia as symptoms remain in so many patients after cholecystectomy. Gallstones are associated with cancer of the gallbladder and with acute pancreatitis when a stone blocks the pancreatic duct.

Diagnosis
Techniques used for detecting gallstones are listed in Table 12.2.

Treatment
Symptomless gallstones should probably be left alone, though many surgeons dispute this point of view. They may disappear spontaneously. The risk of their removal surgically is at least equal to the risk of leaving them (infection and rarely, carcinoma of the gallbladder). For symptomatic gallstones the choice is between medical and surgical therapy.

Table 12.2. Techniques used for detection of gallstones.

Without jaundice
  1 Plain radiograph (for radio-opaque stones).
  2 Oral cholecystogram or ultrasound.
  3 Intravenous cholangiogram (rarely).
With jaundice present
  1 Plain radiograph.
  2 Ultrasound.
  3 (a) ERCP or PTC for suspected CBD (common bile duct) stones. ERCP preferable since in addition to diagnosis it offers opportunities for curative treatment.
     (b) HIDA scan if acute cholecystitis is the favoured diagnosis.

Medical treatment. This consists of oral medication with one of the following given on a milligram per kilogram body weight basis:
1 Chenodeoxycholic acid.
2 Ursodeoxycholic acid.

The principle of the method is that by expansion of the bile salt pool, bile becomes undersaturated with cholesterol, thus enabling cholesterol stones to dissolve. Secondly the bile acids used have an inhibitory effect on HMGCoA reductase, the rate limiting enzyme in cholesterol synthesis (Fig. 12.1).

Requirements for medical therapy
1 Radiolucent gallstones.
2 Functioning gallbladder.
3 Compliant patient.
Dissolution is favoured by a high surface area : volume ratio i.e. small stones (Fig. 12.2).

Disadvantages of medical therapy
1 Prolonged course of treatment usually required, i.e. 6 months to 2 years.
2 Success not guaranteed.
3 Patient may experience biliary colic during the time of dissolution.
4 Stones often recur after cessation of therapy.
5 A small hepatotoxic risk from chenodeoxycholate which can also cause diarrhoea.

For these reasons, and because in an otherwise healthy subject cholecystectomy is a reasonably safe procedure which rapidly resolves the situation, medical treatment should be reserved for patients who have symptomatic gallstones but are unfit for surgery, e.g. because of heart or lung disease.

Treatment of retained common bile duct stones. Sometimes a gallstone is inadvertently

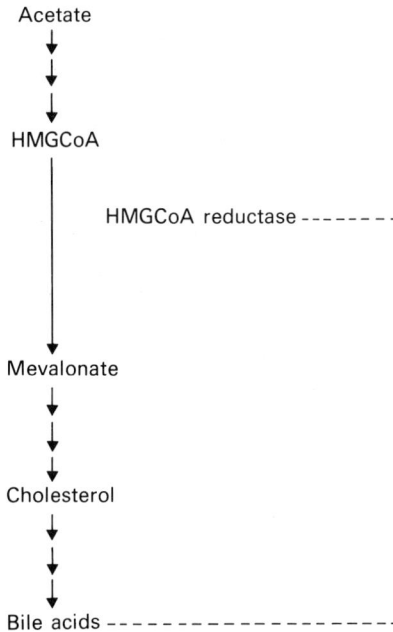

Fig. 12.1. Metabolic pathway for cholesterol and bile acid synthesis. The rate-limiting steps during cholesterol synthesis and conversion of cholesterol to bile acids are schematically drawn. Bile acids which are useful for dissolving gallstones have as one of their actions an inhibitory feedback activity on HMGCoA reductase.

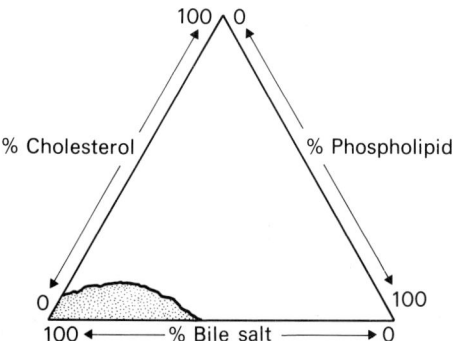

Fig. 12.2. The composition of bile shown on triangular coordinates. Any composition of bile with respect to its three main constituents cholesterol, phospholipids and bile acids can be represented as a single point within a triangular coordinate provided the quantity of each is represented as a percentage of the total. Only compositions within the shaded area maintain cholesterol in solution, and those with cholesterol gallstones usually have a higher percentage of biliary cholesterol.

left in the common bile duct after cholecystectomy. Then a second laparotomy and exploration of the common bile duct carries a high risk especially in the elderly or when the original cholecystectomy proved difficult. So other methods of removing the stone should first be tried. It all depends on whether or not a T-tube remains in position. If it does, there are the following possibilities:

1   The biliary system can be perfused with an organic solvent. The monoglyceride mono-octanoin dissolves cholesterol stones but not pigment ones. If a stone has been kept after cholecystectomy, it can be tested: rapid solubility in ethyl ether will indicate that it is likely to respond well to a mono-octanoin infusion.

2   It may be grasped by an instrument and pulled out through the T-tube track. For this, a wide T-tube needs to be left *in situ* for 6 weeks.

If no T-tube has been left in position, another operation may be necessary. However, endoscopic papillotomy is often successful for stones in the common bile duct (CBD).

The technique (Fig. 12.3), is as follows:

1   Selective cannulation of the CBD with radiological confirmation.

2   The sphincter at the opening of the CBD into the duodenum is cut by diathermy.

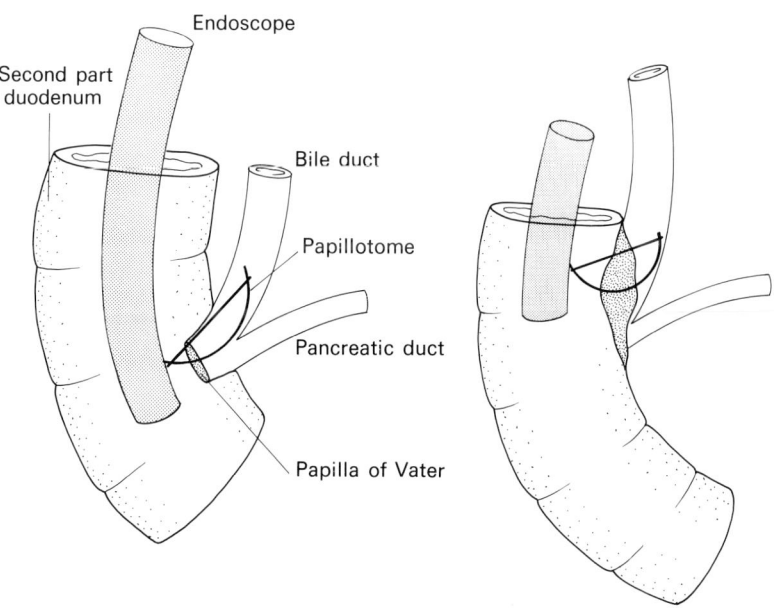

Fig. 12.3. Technique of endoscopic papillotomy. A catheter is introduced into the bile duct and its position checked radiographically by injection of contrast. A diathermy current is passed through a bowed wire which cuts through the sphincter of Oddi and up the medial wall of the duodenum, thus opening the lower end of the bile duct and facilitating the extraction of gallstones.

3   Stones may be allowed to come out spontaneously or extracted with a Dormia basket (Fig. 12.4).

If gallstones are thought to be too large to pass through in spite of the papillotomy, a tube can be introduced into the biliary system at the ERCP and left there for the subsequent infusion of mono-octanoin through the naso-biliary tube. This also allows drainage and so lessens the risk of stone impaction or cholangitis following sphincterotomy.

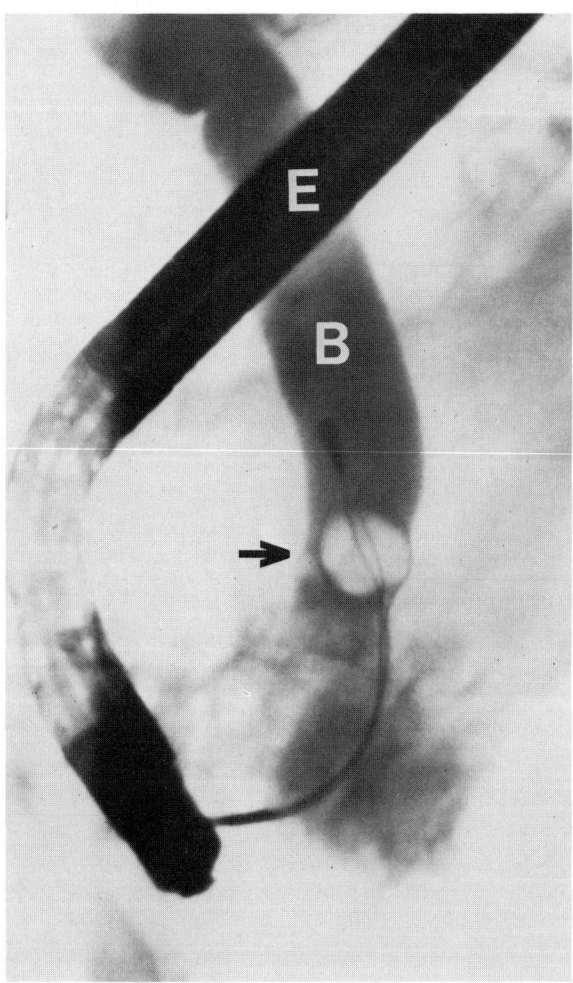

Fig. 12.4. Stone extraction with a Dormia basket. The endoscope (E) is positioned within the duodenum following endoscopic sphincterotomy. The wires of a Dormia basket can be seen to surround a lucent gallstone (arrow) within the common bile duct (B).

Cholangitis

Cholangitis means inflammation of the bile ducts. In the acute and suppurative forms the cause is nearly always bacterial infection, but the aetiology of sclerosing cholangitis is unknown.

Acute ascending cholangitis

This is a syndrome caused by bacterial infection of the biliary tree. The symptoms are fever, shivering or rigor, right upper quadrant abdominal pain and passing of dark urine. Examination usually reveals tenderness over the liver, high fever and bilirubinuria. The organisms involved can usually be grown from blood taken during an attack, the commonest by far being *E. coli*. There is always an underlying anatomical abnormality which predisposes to infection, of which the commonest is common duct gallstones. Others include:

1   Intrahepatic gallstones: these are particularly common in patients from the Far East in whom there is infestation by *Clonorchis sinensis*.

2   Acquired strictures of the bile ducts: postsurgical, sclerosing cholangitis, cholangiocarcinoma, carcinoma of the papilla of Vater.

3   Congenital deformity of the biliary tree: Caroli's syndrome (dilatation of bile ducts), choledochal cyst.

Ascending infection is extremely rare when obstruction is due to a malignant stricture, except when infection is introduced by manipulation (e.g. by ERCP).

Diagnosis is based on the findings of fever, leucocytosis, tenderness in the right hypochondrium with a positive Murphy's sign and bilirubin in the urine. A HIDA scan will help if acute cholecystitis needs to be excluded.

Treatment. Antibiotic therapy is commenced as early as possible. In mild attacks amoxycillin or co-trimoxazole may suffice. In severe attacks a combination of gentamicin and metronidazole is recommended.

The cause of biliary obstruction should be removed wherever possible.

Suppurative cholangitis

This occurs as a complication of acute cholangitis. The content of the obstructed bile duct is infected pus which must be drained with extreme urgency to relieve symptoms and prevent other complications such as septic shock. Antibiotics alone are insufficient to control the high swinging fever.

Treatment. Urgent drainage under antibiotic cover. There must be no delay and the patient may be too ill for a laparotomy. A tube is introduced to drain the infected bile either transhepatically or via an endoscopic papillotomy. Successful drainage usually gives a prompt and satisfying response.

Primary sclerosing cholangitis (Fig. 12.5)

Jaundice and pruritus are the commonest symptoms. Some patients experience mild right upper quadrant discomfort. Often the diagnosis is made before symptoms develop, usually during investigation of patients with ulcerative colitis for a raised serum alkaline phosphatase. The disease is sufficiently advanced to produce complications of portal hypertension (e.g. bleeding varices) as the first symptom in a few patients.

Associated diseases

Common. Ulcerative colitis is present in a half to two-thirds of patients.

Rare. Crohn's disease, Riedel's thyroiditis, retroperitoneal fibrosis, chronic pancreatitis.

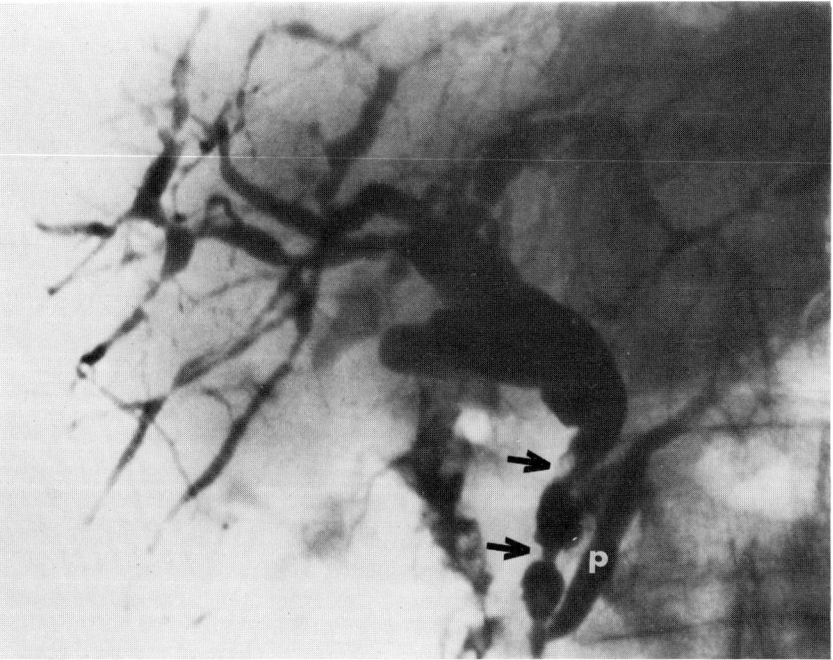

Fig. 12.5. Sclerosing cholangitis. This radiograph was taken after removal of the endoscope at ERCP. Strictures (arrows) can be seen within the common bile duct and the intrahepatic biliary system is also grossly irregular. The appearances are typical of sclerosing cholangitis and, as in this patient, are frequently associated with ulcerative colitis. The pancreatic duct (p) is also shown.

Diagnosis. The serum alkaline phosphatase is nearly always raised. ERCP is the preferred method of diagnosis since it gives the best definition of the whole intra- and extrahepatic biliary tree (Fig. 12.5). Prophylactic antibiotics are essential for ERCP in this condition.

Treatment. Is largely symptomatic, e.g. for pruritus. Acute ascending cholangitis and acute suppurative cholangitis may rarely occur as complications and are treated in the usual way. Vitamin A, D, E and K supplements may be required. Although used at times the efficacy of steroids, azathioprine or penicillamine is not proven; indeed they may be quite ineffective. In some patients sclerosing cholangitis and chronic active hepatitis appear to coexist and in those patients corticosteroids are usually of symptomatic benefit.

Prognosis. About 50% of patients are alive 7 years following diagnosis. The presence of cirrhosis and portal hypertension adversely affects the prognosis.

Cholangiocarcinoma

A cholangiocarcinoma is a primary carcinoma of bile duct origin. It is usually a slow growing and late metastasizing tumour. Its incidence is increased in patients with ulcerative colitis and in areas of the world where *Clonorchis sinensis* is found. In some patients neoplasia appears to be a late response to radiothorium present in thorotrast, a contrast medium used in radiology decades ago.

In view of the slow growing nature of the tumour, cholestasis may have an insidious onset with pruritus preceding jaundice by a year or more. It is important to bear this in mind when considering the differential diagnosis of primary biliary cirrhosis and sclerosing cholangitis. The serum alkaline phosphatase is usually raised and may be the only serological marker when only intrahepatic bile ducts are obstructed.

Cholangiocarcinoma at the hilum of the liver is commonly the cause of pitfalls. A surgeon who has waived the assistance of preoperative cholangiography (Fig. 6.2) may conclude at laparotomy that he was wrong to diagnose obstructive jaundice because the gallbladder and bile ducts are collapsed. If he then closes the abdomen without performing operative cholangiography he will have proved himself doubly foolish by completely missing the small obstructing neoplasm at the bifurcation of the common hepatic ducts.

Diagnosis should always be suspected on the basis of preoperative cholangio- graphy by PTC or ERCP. Laparoscopy may further the diagnosis and aid the assessment of operability. Histological confirmation is essential but can be extremely difficult on small samples of tissue.

Treatment is by surgical resection whenever possible. Otherwise percutaneous transhepatic, endoscopic or operative intubation or the neoplastic stricture may provide prolonged and effective palliation. Radiotherapy is also probably of value.

Adenomyomatosis of the gallbladder

In this condition there is (i) proliferation of the mucosa, (ii) hypertrophy of the muscle coat and (iii) intramural diverticular formation known as Rokitansky–Aschoff sinuses.

It may be (a) diffuse, involving the entire gallbladder or (b) focal. This form often involves the apex of the gallbladder and may be associated with a septum which gives the gallbladder an hour-glass shape (Fig. 12.6).

There is doubt regarding the relationship of this condition to symptoms, and

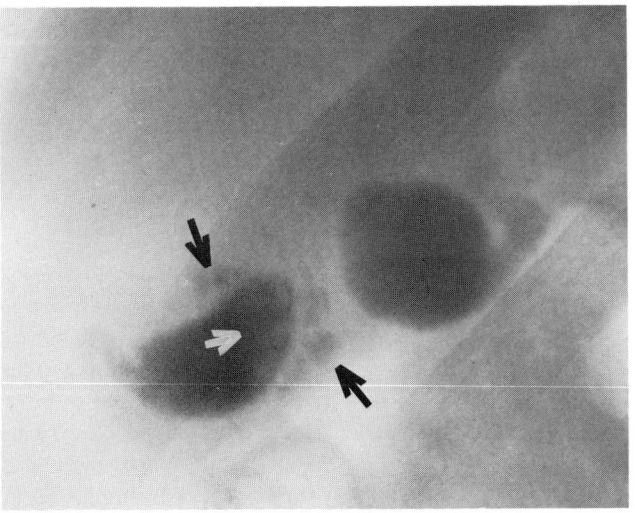

Fig. 12.6. Adenomyomatosis of the gallbladder. This oral cholecystogram shows the typical features of adenomyomatosis with a bilocular gallbladder, the lower of which has a halo of Rokitansky–Aschoff sinuses surrounding it (black arrows) and gallstones within its lumen (white arrow).

the indications of cholecystectomy are uncertain unless gallstones coexist or the septum can be seen to obstruct emptying of the gallbladder during cholecystography.

Acute pancreatitis

Acute pancreatitis produces a wide spectrum of clinical illness ranging from almost insignificant upper abdominal pain, such as that which may be associated with mumps, to an abdominal catastrophe that is rapidly fatal. In order of increasing severity, the process may be characterized pathologically as oedematous, haemorrhagic or necrotizing.

Its causes are listed in Table 12.3.

Table 12.3. Causes of acute pancreatitis.

Common
    Alcoholism
    Gallstones
Occasional
    Hypercalcaemia
    Hyperlipidaemia
    Drugs, e.g. corticosteroids, thiazides
    Virus, e.g. mumps, coxsackie
    Hypothermia

Clinical features. Pain is nearly always a prominent feature and may be severe. It is felt in the epigastrium and may penetrate through to the back. Vomiting is common. There may be a preceding history of biliary colic to suggest gallstones. In others, there is a history of heavy alcohol intake, or a particularly heavy meal preceding the attack.

There is usually epigastric tenderness with some guarding. Bowel sounds may be reduced. The patient may be shocked with tachycardia, thready pulse and hypotension. Haemorrhagic pancreatitis may lead to superficial bruising in the periumbilical region (Cullen's sign) or costovertebral angles (Grey–Turner's sign)—both rare. Anuria and cyanosis are also indicative of a relatively poor prognosis.

Diagnosis. The diagnosis is usually made by a combination of clinical, biochemical and radiological features. The serum amylase is usually markedly elevated (lipase and trypsin levels are also raised though less frequently measured), but the finding is not specific for pancreatitis since other intra-abdominal catastrophes, e.g. perforated peptic ulcer or strangulated bowel, also frequently cause a rise in serum amylase.

Other common findings include a polymorphonuclear leucocytosis, hypocalcaemia, glycosuria with hyperglycaemia, methaemalbuminaemia, and hypoxia. Because hypocalcaemia is a common feature of acute pancreatitis, hypercalcaemia can only be excluded as a possible cause of acute pancreatitis if blood has been taken following a satisfactory convalescence.

Hyperlipidaemia (Table 12.4), another possible cause of pancreatitis, should be suspected if plasma appears milky. Hyponatraemia (a spurious result due to replacement of plasma water by fat) may be a clue to the presence of hypertriglyceridaemia. Type I is seen in infants who present with abdominal pain due to pancreatitis. These children lack the enzyme lipoprotein lipase which is normally responsible for catabolism of chylomicrons. Treatment is by removal of all

Table 12.4. Types of hyperlipidaemia associated with pancreatitis.

Type I   —hyperchylomicronaemia
Type IV—raised very low density lipoproteins (VLDL)
Type V —hyperchylomicronaemia and raised VLDL
(Aide memoire. Type V=features of I plus IV)

---

triglyceride from their diet. Types IV and V may be induced by carbohydrate or fat in the diet. Alcoholism is the usual trigger in those patients who develop associated pancreatitis.

Radiology. Erect and supine plain abdominal radiographs are necessary to exclude a perforated viscus. A localized segment of adynamic bowel known as a 'sentinel loop' may be apparent in the region of the pancreas. If gallstones are visible their position should be assessed and their number and position should be compared with previous radiographs if any are available. The presence of air in the biliary tree and multiple fluid levels within the small intestine is known as 'gallstone ileus' and is indicative of recent extrusion of a large gallstone into the intestine.

Chest X-ray may show a left pleural effusion. Analysis of the amylase concentration in aspirated pleural fluid can serve to confirm the diagnosis of pancreatitis.

Treatment. Any of the following may be useful:
1   Intravenous fluid to replace plasma volume lost by exudation, vomiting, etc.
2   Analgesia: pethidine is a satisfactory choice.
3   Intravenous calcium gluconate to correct hypocalcaemia.
4   Oxygen for hypoxia.
5   Rarely hyperglycaemia may be sufficiently severe to require insulin for its control.
6   If gallstones are responsible, their removal is necessary at some stage.

The following have *not* been shown to be efficacious, and there is probably no good indication for their continued use:
1   Aprotinin. This bovine salivary antitrypsin has been given in an attempt to prevent pancreatic autodigestion by activated trypsin.
2   Glucagon.

Complications. The following have been shown to be possible complications:
1   Acute renal failure   ⎫
2   Respiratory failure   ⎬ Early
3   Pancreatic abscess   ⎫
4   Pseudocyst formation   ⎬ Late

Chronic pancreatitis

Whereas it is assumed that the pancreas reverts to normal following an attack of acute pancreatitis, the diagnosis of chronic pancreatitis implies irreversible pancreatic injury. Diagnostic criteria are given in Table 12.5.

Table 12.5. Criteria for diagnosis of chronic pancreatitis.

Morphological
    Calcification visible on plain X-ray
    Disorganized duct pattern on pancreatography
    Fibrosis and chronic inflammation seen histologically
Functional
    Impaired exocrine secretion in the absence of another cause, e.g. carcinoma

In some patients the clinical course is punctuated by a series of acute illnesses identical to that described above for acute pancreatitis; it is the presence of irreversible injury which then differentiates *chronic relapsing pancreatitis* from *acute relapsing pancreatitis* (recurrent acute pancreatitis). Chronic relapsing pancreatitis is common in alcoholism (Table 12.6). Other patients with chronic pancreatitis

Table 12.6. Causes of chronic pancreatitis.

Common
    Alcoholism; by far the commonest in 'Western society'
    Malnutrition; the commonest in deprived peoples
Occasional
    Cystic fibrosis
Rare
    Other familial disease. In some of these families there is an association with cyclical
    neutropenia

have an indolent course without any clinical crises and may be totally asymptomatic until they develop steatorrhoea or diabetes as a result of advanced disease. This pattern is common in cystic fibrosis.

Clinical features. Pain is often troublesome. Though not always typical this characteristically is felt in the back as well as in the epigastrium. It may also radiate around the left upper quadrant of the abdomen and flank.

    Steatorrhoea may be the presenting complaint. The appetite is usually well maintained; the concurrence of a voracious appetite with continuing weight loss (reminiscent of thyrotoxicosis) due to steatorrhoea is strongly suggestive of chronic pancreatitis.

Diabetes often complicates chronic pancreatitis and may on occasion be its presenting feature. Rarely, biliary obstruction is a late feature of chronic pancreatitis.

Diagnosis. Blood chemistry does not give much assistance in diagnosis. Blood amylase because it also originates from several non-pancreatic sources is usually normal, unless there is superimposed relapsing pancreatitis when it may be elevated. Serum trypsin, measurable in some centres by radioimmunoassay, is often subnormal.

Plain X-ray of the abdomen is diagnostic if it reveals calcification on both sides of the vertebral column in the region of the pancreas (Fig. 12.7).

Functional testing either by duodenal intubation, (S-CCK or test meal) or by the less sensitive tubeless pancreatic function tests (pp. 90) shows subnormal exocrine function.

Pancreatography obtained by ERCP may show a characteristic morphology (Fig. 6.11). If doubt exists, cytology or biopsy may be required to differentiate chronic pancreatitis from carcinoma.

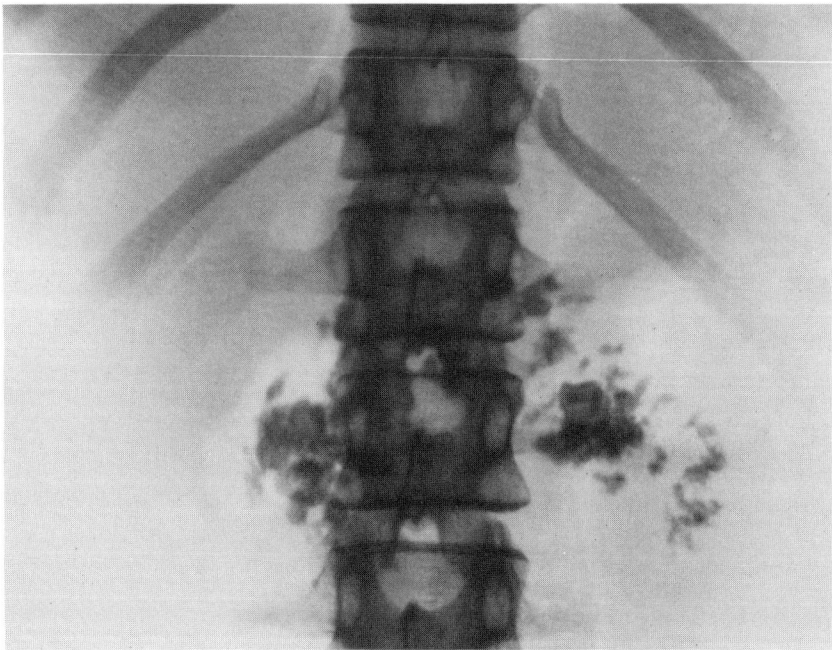

Fig. 12.7. Calcific pancreatitis. This plain abdominal radiograph shows gross changes of chronic calcific pancreatitis in an alcoholic patient with massive steatorrhoea.

Management. In alcoholic chronic pancreatitis the most important single measure is complete lifelong abstinence from alcohol; if this is achieved the pain gradually recedes in most patients.

Analgesics are often required, and many patients with the susceptibility shown by prior alcoholism are at high risk of becoming narcotic addicts. If pain is severe and persistent, surgery planned on the basis of the pancreatogram obtained by ERCP may be helpful.

Steatorrhoea is initially treated by pancreatic enzyme supplements taken at meal times. If, despite full dosage, the response is unsatisfactory, antacid preparations or H_2-antagonists may be used to prevent destruction of the pancreatic enzymes by gastric acid. These measures in combination usually suffice. If diarrhoea due to steatorrhoea is still unresolved, a low fat diet is required.

Supplements of fat-soluble vitamins are occasionally required especially when, as may occur in cystic fibrosis, there is coexistent hepatobiliary disease. Diabetes mellitus is treated routinely.

Carcinoma of the pancreas

Carcinoma of the pancreas is usually diagnosed late and, therefore, has a generally poor outlook. Initial symptoms depend on the part of the gland affected. Tumours arising in the head will often present with painless jaundice. Tumours in the body and tail are more likely to cause pain and weight loss. Only when tumours arise from the papilla of Vater (not strictly speaking pancreatic in origin) is there a reasonable prospect of surgical cure. Results of therapy are therefore generally disappointing and the prognosis poor.

Its aetiology is largely unknown. It is much commoner in smokers than in non-smokers and has an increased incidence in workers exposed to benzidene and β-naphthylamine. Diabetes mellitus may slightly increase the chances of developing pancreatic carcinoma.

Clinical features. The jaundiced patient may appear in good general health. Scratch marks may be present. The liver is usually smoothly enlarged and the gallbladder may be palpable (Courvoisier's law Fig. 2.6). When tumours arise in the body or tail, jaundice is a late feature; a mass may be palpable in the epigastrium or left hypochondrium; recent weight loss may be apparent. A bruit audible over the pancreas suggests splenic artery involvement, and the spleen may enlarge from splenic vein obstruction. Distant metastases may be palpable as a Virchow's node in the neck or an irregularly enlarged liver or visible on chest X-ray. If retroperitoneal extension is producing pain the patient may find relief from leaning forward, preferring not to sleep in bed but to lean on the side of the bed with arms outstretched making a 'crucifixion sign'.

Investigation. Ultrasound may show dilated bile ducts or a mass in the pancreas. Aspiration cytology via an ultrasonically guided probe may confirm the diagnosis rapidly.

ERCP may outline abnormalities of the duct to localize the tumour and permits biopsy of any duodenal areas involved or aspiration cytology from the pancreatic duct. The ratio of lactoferrin to trypsin in pancreatic or duodenal juice may help to differentiate cancer from chronic pancreatitis.

Treatment. Surgery is rarely necessary for diagnosis. It is also indicated occasionally for resection of potentially curable lesions and more commonly for palliation.

Preoperative assessment of the resectability of pancreatic cancer usually requires angiography and venography to demonstrate freedom from tumour-invasion of the inferior vena cava and portal vein and lack of hepatic metastases.

Palliative surgery usually includes:

1 Choledochojejunostomy with Roux-en-Y to bypass obstruction of the lower common bile duct.

2 Gastroenterostomy to avoid symptoms from later duodenal obstruction.

3 Injection-destruction of the coeliac ganglion as an attempt to interrupt pain fibres from the pancreas.

Chemotherapy and radiotherapy for pancreatic cancer have not shown any great benefit. Future advances may include:

1 Intra-operative radiotherapy: permits high dosage irradiation of the pancreas while other radiosensitive tissues, e.g. intenstine, are held aside.

2 Multiple chemotherapy. Favoured agents currently used in combination are 5-fluorouracil, adriamycin and mitomycin C (FAM) but more effective agents are required.

Carcinoma of the papilla of Vater

As noted this is usually regarded as carcinoma of the pancreas but there are several important differences—most notably, the prognosis is much better following surgical resection. Three-year survival after pancreatoduodenectomy is 50%, compared to only 10% for carcinoma of the head of the pancreas. Carcinoma of the papilla usually presents as cholestatic jaundice, which may fluctuate as central necrosis of the tumour intermittently permits improvement of bile drainage. Tumour ulceration gives the classical triad of anaemia due to blood loss, jaundice and pruritus which should always suggest the diagnosis.

Diagnosis. ERCP is the method of choice. This permits taking of diagnostic samples for histology and cytology.

Treatment. Unless tumour spread is apparent, the fit patient should be offered radical surgery with the prospect of curative resection.

Cystic fibrosis (Fibrocytic disease, mucoviscidosis)

Inheritance. This is an autosomal recessive disorder. The incidence of the carrier state in Caucasian Europeans is about 1 in 25, producing the disease in about 1 in 2,000 live births.

Pathology. Several exocrine glands produce thickened secretions. In the respiratory tract tubular obstruction by viscid mucus and superadded infection culminate in bronchiectasis, respiratory failure and cor pulmonale. The exocrine pancreas eventually becomes non-functional behind blocked secretory passages, although 10–15% of sufferers continue to have clinically insignificant pancreatic disease. In those who survive two decades, inspissated bile may lead to biliary cirrhosis.

Clinical examination reveals an increased anterio-posterior diameter of the chest in a frail child with marked finger clubbing and a productive cough whose sputum usually contains *Staphylococcus aureas* and *Pseudomonas pyocyaneos.* Pancreatic disease may be manifest as steatorrhoea and failure to thrive. Meconium ileus produces the picture of intestinal obstruction in the newborn due to inspissated bowel contents; later intussusception is also seen; the incidence of rectal prolapse in teenage patients with cystic fibrosis may be ten times that seen in their healthy peers.

Diagnosis. This is confirmed by the sweat test. Sweat is collected following stimulation, e.g. by pilocarpine iontophoresis. In cystic fibrosis (and adrenal insufficiency) the concentration of sodium and chloride ions is abnormally elevated.

Treatment of exocrine pancreatic insufficiency and fat-soluble vitamin deficiency is as described above for chronic pancreatitis. Treatment of chest infections by antibiotics has markedly increased life expectancy in these patients.

Chapter 13
Acute and Chronic Hepatitis

Acute hepatitis

Hepatitis refers to a spectrum of illnesses whose common factor is necrosis of liver cells and associated inflammation. The common causative insults are viral infections and drugs but occasionally metabolic diseases and toxins such as the poisonous Amanita mushroom or industrial solvents may be responsible.

Viral hepatitis

Several viruses cause hepatitis: hepatitis A (HAV) and B (HBV) and also the non-A and non-B where the virus has eluded discovery. A mild form of hepatitis, often a complication of infectious mononucleosis (glandular fever), is due to the Epstein–Barr (EB) or cytomegalovirus (CMV). It also occurs in yellow fever in areas where sandfly fever exists.

The spectrum of diseases due to hepatotropic viruses is wide (Fig. 13.1) and the severity is partly related to the vigour of the patient's immune response.

Acute viral hepatitis

The commonest clinical syndrome resulting from infection with one of the hepatotropic viruses is a self-limiting illness with a characteristic course.

Prodromal phase. The patient experiences anorexia, nausea, and in smokers there is usually aversion to smoking. Fever, headache and myalgia may lead to a misdiagnosis of influenza. Occasionally abdominal discomfort and diarrhoea suggest gastroenteritis. In some a rash and arthralgia or arthritis mimic serum sickness.

Jaundice. This becomes apparent. The urine is dark and stools may be pale. Fever usually settles. Fatigue is common.

Recovery phase. The appetite returns and constitutional symptoms recede. Jaundice fades with darkening of the stool and clearing of the urine. Occasionally, despite generalized symptomatic improvement in other respects, jaundice and pruritus become more severe and persist for several months—the late 'cholestatic phase' of viral hepatitis.

Post-hepatitic syndrome. Some patients complain of persistent lethargy, malaise and depression long after resolution of clinical signs of the illness. This is commoner in

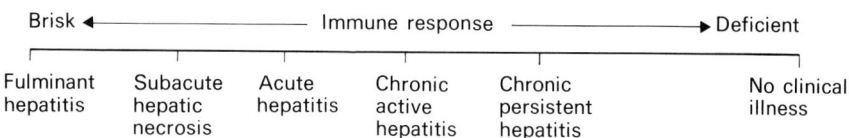

Fig. 13.1. Spectrum of diseases due to hepatotropic viruses.

well-informed, intelligent patients. Avoid suggesting to the patient that this prolonged convalescence is to be expected, since this may induce unnecessary introspection.

Management. A controlled study among reasonably fit American soldiers failed to show benefit from enforced rest during the acute illness. However, in the more severely ill patients it is usual to advise rest during the early stages and exhaustion should be avoided.

Although it is fashionable to withdraw fat, this need only be done if it relieves troublesome symptoms, e.g. diarrhoea, and a normal diet may be resumed in early convalescence. Patients often lose a lot of weight and this may be aggravated unnecessarily by forbidding fat.

Isolation of patients is usually not necessary since those with hepatitis A are first jaundiced towards the end of the period when their faeces are infectious. Gamma globulin should be administered to close contacts of hepatitis A victims who are pregnant or immunosuppressed (e.g. on steroids). Recent sexual contacts of patients with acute hepatitis B should receive anti-HBs-rich antiserum prophylactically.

Progression to chronicity. Sometimes acute hepatitis fails to resolve. If liver function tests are persistently abnormal for 6 months from the onset, the patient, by definition, has chronic hepatitis. Chronic liver disease following hepatitis A has not been reported but both hepatitis B and non-A non-B hepatitis carry this risk. Persistence of HBeAg more than 3 months after the onset of hepatitis B indicates a high probability of progression to chronic hepatitis.

Subclinical hepatitis

With hepatitis A this is common. The infection may occur as an epidemic amongst school children. Surveys in institutions show that many have raised serum transaminases, but neither symptoms nor jaundice. Thus many will acquire immunity without giving any history of the disease. There is no known chronic carrier state for hepatitis A but hepatitis B can cause this and infected individuals may have no symptoms or signs of liver disease at any stage. Histology may show little or no abnormality.

Fulminant hepatitis

This is characterized by rapid progression, usually over very few days and always within 8 weeks of prodromal symptoms, to acute liver failure with deep jaundice and disturbance of conscious level. Death is the outcome in more than 80% of the cases. In those who survive, recovery of liver function is usually complete.

Acute liver failure

Acute liver failure is the clinical syndrome which includes hepatic encephalopathy resulting from recent severe (acute) liver injury (Table 13.1).

Table 13.1. Causes of acute liver failure.

Viral hepatitis — fulminant A, B, and non-A and non-B
— subacute hepatic necrosis
Toxins, e.g. carbon tetrachloride and *Amanita phalloides*
Drugs, e.g. paracetamol
Anaesthetics, e.g. halothane
Metabolic, e.g. Wilson's disease and Reye's syndrome
Acute fatty liver of pregnancy

Management. Monitor the level of consciousness, blood glucose, liver size and prothrombin time. Treat encephalopathy with neomycin, lactulose, enemas and protein withdrawal; treat any bleeding tendency when prothrombin ratio approaches 5:1 with fresh frozen plasma. Avoid sedation (precipitates coma) and all possible sources of infection, e.g. arterial lines, bladder catheterization if possible. Maintain gastric pH above 5 (by H_2-antagonist usually). Multicentre trials of high dose corticosteroids have failed to show any benefit. Measures to counteract cerebral oedema may also be required; this may be exacerbated by infusions of fresh frozen plasma.

Subacute hepatic necrosis

The onset is usually typical of acute viral hepatitis but recovery does not commence at the expected time and the course thereafter is one of relentless progression of liver 'necrosis' over 4–8 weeks.

Persistence of very high transaminase levels, recurrence of nausea and sudden diminution in liver size after 3–8 weeks of acute hepatitis indicates a grave prognosis.

Other sequelae

Polyarteritis nodosa, acute glomerulonephritis and Henoch–Schönlein purpura are all possible manifestations of immune complex disease produced by an aberrant immune response to hepatitis B infection in some patients.

The hepatitis viruses

Hepatitis A

Hepatitis A virus is spread by the faecal–oral route. It is excreted in the faeces during the incubation phase. Poor hygiene contributes to spread, and epidemics occur in crowded institutions. Poor sewage treatment leads to transmission via shellfish in some countries.

The virus is a 27 nm RNA virus particle which, despite some atypical features, is currently classified with the enterovirus subgroup of picornaviruses.

Diagnosis. Detection of IgM class anti-HAV in the blood indicates hepatitis A infection within the past year. IgG class anti-HAV indicates an immune status due to infection in the more distant past. Passive *immunity* is conferred by all commercial immunoglobulin preparations. For a 6-month jaunt to an endemic area it is advisable to have 0.05 ml/kg body weight of immune serum globulin before leaving and a second dose 4 months later.

Clinical course. Either symptomless infection or a typical self-limiting acute hepatitis is usual. Rarely fulminant hepatitis occurs. Chronic hepatitis is unknown.

Hepatitis B

The hepatitis B virus was first recognized as 'Australia antigen'. The complete virion is a 42 nm sphere known as the Dane particle consisting of an outer surface envelope and an inner 27 nm core. The core contains double-stranded circular DNA with a short gap in one strand, and an enzyme known as DNA-polymerase (Fig. 13.2). HBsAg, HBeAg and DNA polymerase are usually detectable in blood if it is taken at the onset of hepatitis B (Fig. 13.3). Persistence of HBeAg after 2–3 months can be a harbinger of chronicity. Anti-HBc does not confer immunity; its detection is a useful indicator of infection in the 'window period' between disappearance of HBsAg and detection of anti-HBs. Immunity is conferred by anti-HBs and anti-Dane antibodies. Sequelae are shown in Fig. 13.4.

Associations. Male homosexuality; Down's syndrome; the mentally subnormal in residential care; certain racial subgroups; immunosuppressed patients, e.g. those on renal dialysis and transplantation programmes.

Transmission. Hepatitis B is transmitted in two main ways:
1 Via blood.
2 Across mucous membranes especially by sexual intercourse.

There is no evidence for excretion of the virus in faeces. Patients should be advised to dispose of anything contaminated by their blood with extreme care. They should not allow anyone to use their shaving razor or toothbrush. Unless their sexual partner has been shown to be immune to hepatitis B, the male partner should

Hepatitis B virus

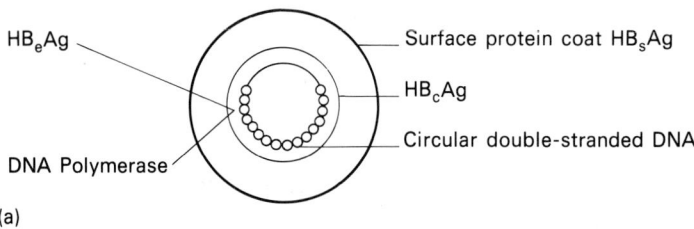

(a)

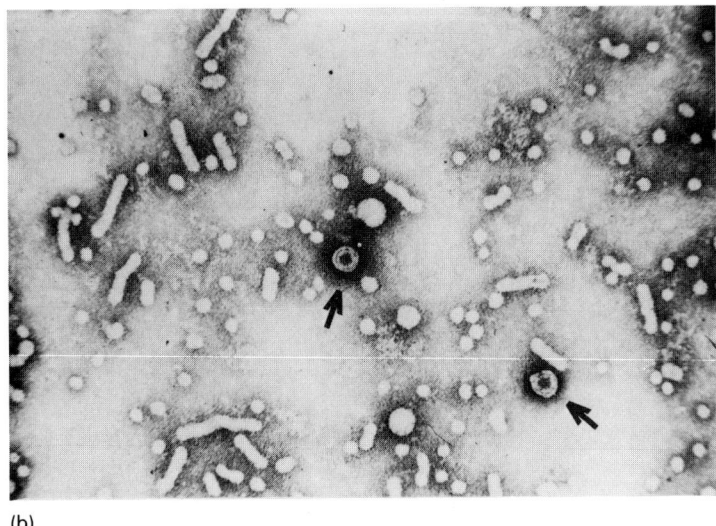

(b)

Fig. 13.2. (a) The hepatitis B virus. The diagram shows the hepatitis B virus to have an incomplete ring of circular DNA within a core particle and surrounded by surface protein. The virus also contains the replicating enzyme DNA polymerase and the 'e' antigen. (b) These are the appearances of hepatitis B material (formerly known as Australia antigen) on electronmicroscopy of a patient's blood. As well as the complete virions which have a double ring (arrowed) there are a large number of spheres and tubules which consist of excess surface antigen which is devoid of any core material.

wear a condom for sexual intercourse. All transfused blood is now screened for hepatitis B, but it is still just possible that hepatitis B may be transmitted by transfusions and in such cases the infected donor must be traced and advised accordingly.

Incubation period. Anywhere between 30–130 days.

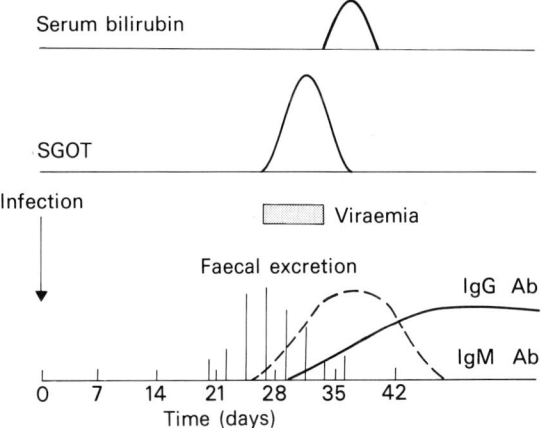

Hepatitis A

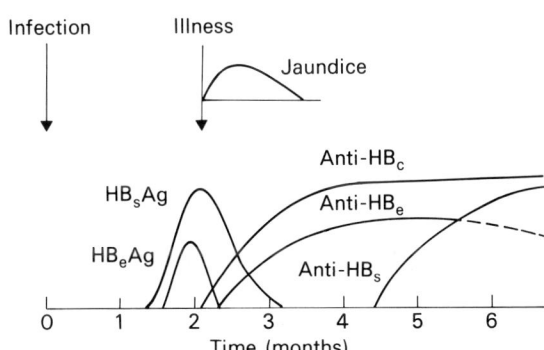

Hepatitis B

Fig. 13.3. Serological events in hepatitis A and B infection. The time course for detection of viral antigens and antibody is shown schematically during typical spontaneously resolving attacks of acute hepatitis due to virus A and virus B.

Carrier state. The prevalence varies markedly between countries, e.g. 1 : 500 in UK, 1 : 400 in USA, 1 : 10 in Senegal, 1 : 5 in Taiwan. Healthy carriers appear to be immunologically tolerant of the virus. Thus the virus is not cytopathic, it is the host's immune response which destroys the infected liver cell; some immunosuppressed patients infected with hepatitis B had minimal liver disease, but developed fulminant hepatitis on withdrawal of their immunosuppressive therapy.

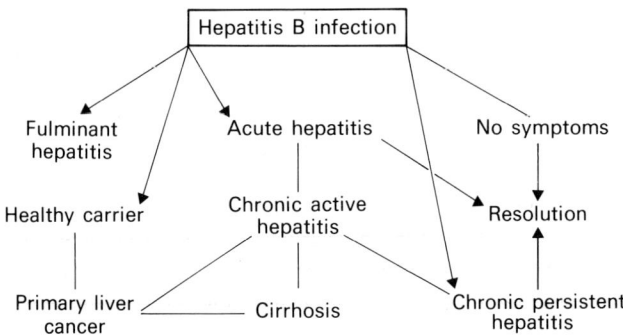

Fig. 13.4. Sequelae of hepatitis B. The diagram shows the various clinical responses and disease states which may develop as a consequence of infection with the hepatitis B virus.

Oncogenicity. The hepatitis B virus has oncogenic properties. The areas of the world where carrier status is common also have a high incidence of primary hepatocellular carcinoma. Transmission in those communities is often 'vertical', i.e. from parents to offspring, and commonly occurs near the time of birth. Evidence of past and present hepatitis B infection is much commoner in the mothers of patients with primary liver cancer than in the mothers of a control population (with cirrhosis).

Experiments have shown that viral DNA from the hepatitis B virus has been incorporated into the host's DNA in human primary hepatocellular cancer cells. Successive generations of those cells, grown in the laboratory, synthesize hepatitis B viral protein though the virus itself is not present.

Antiviral therapy. Several agents are under trial for their antiviral effect but none is generally available. Promising results were found in some of the patients treated with interferon or adenine arabinoside (Ara–A).

Immunity. Passive immunity can be conferred by serum with high titres of anti-HBs, and is effective if given early and repeatedly following exposure. This is especially relevant to health care workers who suffer needle-prick exposure and offspring of mothers infected during the third trimester of pregnancy.

Active immunity follows inoculation with HBsAg which produces an anti-HBs response in more than 90% of subjects who thus become immune. Early evidence suggests that such immunity is effective even when immunization commences early during the incubation period although after the date of exposure.

Non-A, Non-B hepatitis

This diagnosis is currently made by exclusion of the other infectious agents discussed above in an otherwise typical case of acute infectious hepatitis. Cases occur sporadically and after blood transfusion. Administration of pooled blood products, e.g. Factor VIII to haemophiliac patients, has produced a series of illnesses which suggest at least two forms, one with a short incubation period of 7–10 days and the second with a much longer incubation period. Progression to chronicity has been described. Some patients experience a prolonged acute attack with an undulating course.

Paracetamol toxicity
Paracetamol is frequently taken in overdose during attempted suicide. When hepatic reserves of reduced glutathione (GSH) are exhausted, reactive intermediate metabolites of paracetamol combine with macromolecules, resulting in cell damage and death. Hepatocellular necrosis is predominantly centrolobular.

Clinical features. The patient may have only a few symptoms or signs for 1–2 days following ingestion of a paracetamol overdose. However, prolongation of the prothrombin time, or an impaired ^{14}C-aminopyrine breath test may already indicate a grave prognosis during this interval. Severe hepatic necrosis may lead to hepatic coma and death during the following days.

Management. The stomach is washed out if there is a likelihood of recovering unabsorbed paracetamol. The concentration of paracetamol in the blood is measured. If it falls above a line connecting 200 μg/ml at 4 h with 50 μg/ml at 12 h, treatment is instituted immediately and always before 12 h post ingestion by giving an agent which substitutes for the SH groups of GSH. This agent may be methionine, N-acetyl cysteine or related compounds. If adequately treated during the early post-ingestion phase most patients recover without developing acute liver failure.

Halothane hepatitis
The widely used anaesthetic agents halothane (in UK) and methyoxyflurane (in USA) are capable of producing severe liver damage in a small proportion of exposed patients who develop a hypersensitivity reaction.

A typical case history involves unexplained fever following a first operation. Jaundice may or may not develop during the second week, and if blood is analysed an eosinophilia and raised aspartate transaminase level is observed. These features are often unheeded and may not be noted because the patient leaves hospital soon after a minor procedure. Anorexia, vomiting and jaundice indicate a relatively severe hepatitis after a single exposure. Following the second exposure fever occurs early, and jaundice develops within a few days. Acute liver failure, often fatal, not uncommonly ensues. The reaction appears to be commonest in elderly, obese females.

Prevention. Halothane's safety understandably makes it the anaesthetic of choice for most patients, but an awareness of its potential to cause severe hepatitis, albeit rarely, is essential. The previous anaesthetic history is routinely checked, and should an unexplained fever, eosinophilia or raised serum transaminase have followed a surgical procedure, repeated use of the same agent must be avoided. In view of the 'hypersensitivity' nature of the reaction, this involves the use of anaesthetic machines which have not been contaminated by that anaesthetic.

Weil's disease (Synonym: leptospirosis due to *leptospira icterohae-morrhagiae*)

The disease was first described in 1886 by Adolph Weil, Professor of Medicine at Heidelberg. The causative spiral organism *L. icterohaemorrhagiae*, is harboured in the kidneys of rats and field mice. It infects humans who are usually exposed by working in wet conditions with abrasions on their hands, especially sewer workers, farmers, slaughterers and veterinary surgeons, though organisms may also be acquired by inhalation and ingestion. Many other serotypes of leptospira are capable of infecting man but they tend to cause less severe illnesses.

Clinical features. Following an incubation period of 7–14 days, the patient develops fever, often with rigors, headaches and myalgia. Jaundice develops within a week of onset; widespread haemorrhages into the skin, mucous membranes and gastrointestinal tract and acute renal failure are features of the second week. Survivors enter a recovery phase in the third week. The kidneys are more severely affected in most patients. Though deep jaundice may occur in the most severely ill patients it is disproportionate to the relatively mild hepatocellular necrosis viewed histologically.

Diagnosis. May be difficult in the early stages though leptospira may be detected in thick films of the blood. Later leptospira may be seen in the urine with dark background microscopy, and serological studies show rising titres of antibody. If infected fluids are injected into guinea-pigs or hamsters they produce an acute, often fatal, illness.

Treatment. Benzyl penicillin in high doses may confer benefit if given within the first week of illness. Supportive measures, especially fluid and electrolyte balance including renal dialysis when necessary are most important.

Prognosis. Deep jaundice, acute renal failure and widespread haemorrhage may prove fatal in 10–20% of cases diagnosed. Most infected patients have a much milder illness. A clinical relapse is common during the early convalescent stage but those who survive the acute illness always make a complete recovery.

Jaundice in pregnancy

When jaundice occurs in pregnancy, correct early diagnosis is of vital importance for both mother and fetus.

Viral hepatitis. This is commonest. The incidence and course of the illness is no different from that in a non-pregnant control population. If the mother is HBsAg-positive at the time of delivery, the baby should be immunized soon after birth. This is most important for mothers who had acute hepatitis B in the third trimester and for chronic carriers who are HBeAg-positive.

Gallstones. These have a high incidence in pregnancy and can give jaundice, usually associated with biliary colic. There are also causes of jaundice more specifically related to pregnancy.

Cholestasis of pregnancy

Cholestasis of pregnancy produces pruritus progressing sometimes to jaundice usually in the last trimester; it is the second commonest cause of jaundice in pregnancy. Liver function returns to normal within 3 weeks following parturition. In predisposed individuals there is a strong tendency for cholestasis to recur in subsequent pregnancies or if the patient takes contraceptive steroids, suggesting that sex hormones are important in its pathogenesis. Particularly high incidences of this condition which may be familial are seen in certain countries, notably Chile and Scandinavia. It is essentially benign.

If cholestasis has not resolved completely within 1 month of childbirth, an underlying disorder such as primary biliary cirrhosis which has been unmasked by the pregnancy should be suspected.

Acute fatty liver of pregnancy

Acute fatty liver of pregnancy is a rare but serious condition. It usually presents as hyperemesis in the third trimester and is commoner in obese primigravida patients. Early encephalopathy occurs out of proportion to the jaundice which is seldom deep, but the clinical picture of liver failure progresses via spontaneous haemorrhage and coma to death in up to 80% of cases. Disturbances of serum bilirubin, transaminase and alkaline phosphatase are relatively mild in comparison with the marked prolongation of the prothrombin time and hypofibrinogenaemia even before signs of disseminated intravascular coagulation occur.

The serum uric acid is markedly elevated and thrombocytopenia with normoblasts are usually visible in the peripheral blood. Acute renal failure and disseminated intravascular coagulation develop unless the disease is arrested. The histological picture shows microvesicular fatty droplet degeneration of liver cells. Fetal distress culminating in stillbirth is the rule unless early Caesarian section is undertaken. Early diagnosis, with rapid delivery of the fetus, almost certainly has a profoundly favourable effect on the prognosis in both the mother and baby.

Toxaemia of pregnancy

Toxaemia of pregnancy may also be associated with jaundice, but this is probably related more to haemolysis than to liver disease and is a late feature of the illness.

Nevertheless in fatal cases the liver shows marked fibrin deposition and necrosis in peri-portal areas. There is also danger of spontaneous rupture of the liver in toxaemia.

Reye's syndrome

Reye's syndrome is typical in its clinical manifestations of all the diseases associated with microvesicular fatty degeneration of the liver (Table 13.2). In Reye's syndrome children develop vomiting and clouding of consciousness leading to coma within a few days of a febrile illness (often due to influenza B though other viral causes are also seen). It is the disproportionate severity of encephalopathy when compared to jaundice which characterizes these conditions and explains why Reye's syndrome is often mistaken for a viral encephalitis. Analysis of the blood usually shows very high levels of ammonia. Other common findings are of hypoglycaemia, raised creatine phosphokinase, lactic acidosis and prolongation of the prothrombin time.

Liver biopsy shows characteristic microvesicular cytoplasm surrounding centrally placed nuclei with prominent nucleoli; the appearances are quite different from the more common large droplet fatty changes which is a feature of liver diseases such as those caused by alcohol.

Death has occurred in about 50% of reported cases. Those who die usually have marked cerebral oedema.

Table 13.2. Causes of microvesicular fatty degeneration of the liver.

Acute fatty liver of pregnancy
Reye's syndrome
Sodium valproate
Tetracycline (high doses given intravenously)
Congenital defects of urea synthesizing enzymes
Vomiting disease of Jamaica

Chronic hepatitis

Although chronic hepatitis is usually defined as hepatitis of 6 months or longer duration it is important to realize that the diagnosis may pertain from the first day of clinical illness; a prolonged asymptomatic phase is then assumed. There are three types:

1 Chronic active hepatitis.
2 Chronic persistent hepatitis.
3 Chronic lobular hepatitis.

Chronic active hepatitis

Chronic active hepatitis can be diagnosed clinically or histologically on the basis of the following. The aetiology is shown in Table 13.3.

Clinical. Hepatitis, evidenced by raised serum transaminase, raised serum gammaglobulin and prolongation of prothrombin time after vitamin K. Unless disturbed coagulation precludes liver biopsy, the diagnosis should be confirmed histologically.

Histological (Fig. 13.5). Piecemeal necrosis at the periphery of liver lobules, where chronic inflammatory cells and fibrous tissue produce progressive expansion of the portal tracts by surrounding dying hepatocytes. Cirrhosis may or may not be present at the time of diagnosis, and unchecked the condition leads to cirrhosis.

Clinical presentation. This may be by any of the following:

1 Acute hepatitis with non-resolution.
2 Acute hepatitis with incongruous features from the outset indicative of long standing asymptomatic chronic liver disease, e.g. portal hypertension.
3 Relapsing jaundice.
4 Bruising, acne, hirsutism, facial mooning.
5 Primary or secondary amenorrhoea.

Table 13.3. Aetiology of chronic active hepatitis.

Causes	Diagnostic features
Lupoid	Smooth muscle antibodies Anti-nuclear factor (LE cells in 15%) Absence of causal markers listed below
Hepatitis B virus	HBsAg. Anti-HBc
Hepatolenticular degeneration (Wilson's disease)	Low serum caeruloplasmin; raised liver copper concentration Kayser–Fleischer rings

Drugs
  Isoniazid
  Methyldopa
  Nitrofurantoin
  Oxyphenisatin
	
	Resolution following withdrawal of the offending agent

Non-A Non-B hepatitis	Presumptive relationship to point source (i.e. blood transfusion or contact)
Ulcerative colitis	Rectal biopsy. Barium enema
α_1 antitrypsin deficiency	Low serum α_1 antitrypsin levels. PAS-positive globules on liver biopsy

Normal

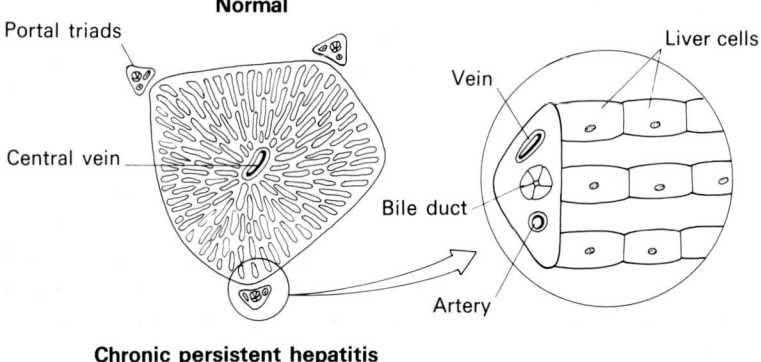

Chronic persistent hepatitis

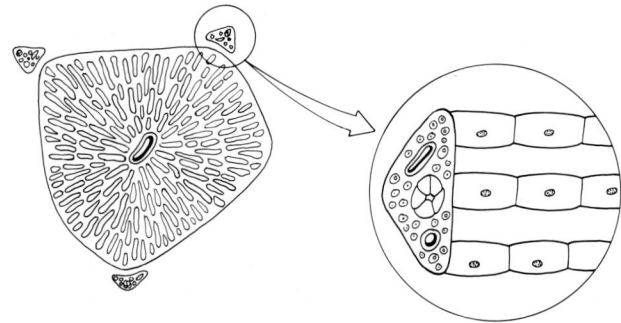

Chronic active hepatitis

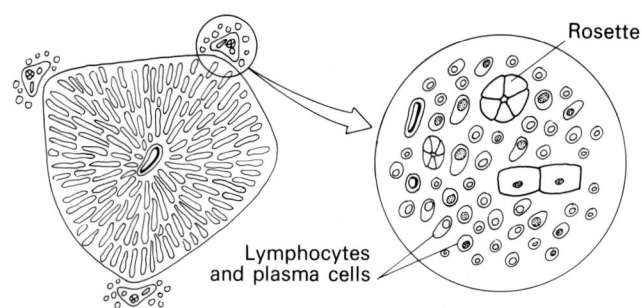

Cirrhosis

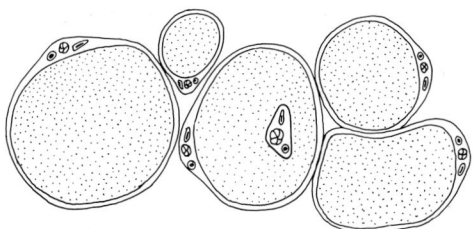

Fig. 13.5. Histological patterns in chronic hepatitis.

6 Ascites, ankle oedema.

7 Haemorrhage from oesophageal varices.

8 Abnormalities on routine biochemical (e.g. ↑AST) or haematological (e.g. ↓platelets↑ESR) screening.

9 Detection of hepatitis B in a volunteer blood donor.

Treatment. Lupoid hepatitis: corticosteroids definitely improve the course and prognosis. Azathioprine, though of no value alone, permits reduction of corticosteroid dosage without loss of effect. If treatment is commenced before cirrhosis has developed, progression to cirrhosis may be prevented. Aim at restoring biochemical tests to normal unless steroid dosages and side-effects are unacceptable. Histological remission probably takes a year longer. Withdrawal of therapy at this stage is associated with a 50% relapse rate. Hepatitis B virus: none known. Wilson's disease: penicillamine. Drugs: withdrawal. Non-A Non-B: none known. α_1-antitrypsin: none known (transplantation corrects biochemical defect).

Complications. Chronic active hepatitis tends to progress to cirrhosis. *Cirrhosis* may already be present when the patient is first seen, suggesting that the disease has been active for several years before producing any symptoms. The histological diagnosis should therefore always include reference to the presence or absence of established cirrhosis. Other complications include hepatocellular failure with jaundice, ascites, encephalopathy and haemorrhage; portal hypertension; complications of therapy, e.g. vertebral collapse due to corticosteroids.

Chronic persistent hepatitis

Chronic hepatitis is evidenced by raised serum transaminases of more than 6 months duration in a patient whose liver biopsy shows chronic inflammation confined to the portal tracts.

Clinical presentation. The patient may present with the following:

1 Acute hepatitis with non-resolution after 6 months.

2 Abnormalities on routine biochemical screening of serum.

3 Detection of hepatitis B in a volunteer blood donor.

Differential diagnosis. The importance of this diagnosis is in its differentiation from chronic active hepatitis. It is rare for chronic persistent hepatitis to cause jaundice. Serum globulins and prothrombin time are usually within normal limits.

Occasionally, other conditions, e.g. primary biliary cirrhosis, may produce a similar histological picture.

Treatment. None required.

Prognosis. Generally very good; only a few patients appear to develop progressive liver disease. It is unclear whether this is a true transition from chronic persistent hepatitis to chronic active hepatitis or whether the histological appearances of the portal tracts on which the original diagnosis was based were unrepresentative due to sampling error with a small needle biopsy specimen.

Chronic lobular hepatitis

Definition. Chronic hepatitis in which the biopsy shows spotty necrosis of hepatocytes similar to that seen in acute viral hepatitis. The marked portal tract inflammation characteristic of active and persistent chronic hepatitis is not seen.

Treatment and prognosis. Corticosteroids are usually effective in producing prompt remission but relapses on withdrawal of therapy may recur for several years. Progression to cirrhosis is rare.

Alcoholic liver disease

The possibility of an alcoholic aetiology should always be considered in patients with liver disease. Many alcoholic patients are evasive and prepared to lie about their drinking habits. Close relatives may be unaware of secret drinking or may even enter into a conspiracy with the patient to deceive the doctor. In more cooperative patients it is advisable to approach interrogation slowly by asking about drinks (a) at night, (b) at lunchtime, (c) early in the day.

There are three main categories of alcoholic liver disease:
1   Fatty liver.
2   Alcoholic hepatitis.
3   Cirrhosis.
    Be alert to the following:
1   Facial plethora, tremulousness, smell of ethanol on breath.
2   Character change, dissolution of mental capacity, absenteeism or other work problems.
3   Accident proneness.
4   $\uparrow\gamma$GT, $\uparrow$MCV, $\downarrow$Na$^+$, $\uparrow$lipids, $\downarrow$urea, $\uparrow$AST.
5   Early morning vomiting.
6   The patient who unaccountably becomes violent or psychotic (due to alcohol withdrawal), e.g. following admission to hospital.
7   Multiple rib fractures visible on chest X-ray without historical explanation.
    If suspected take blood for (4) and blood for ethanol estimation.

Fatty liver

Symptoms. None specific.

Examination. The liver is enlarged, smooth and a little tender.

Liver histology. Many hepatocytes contain large fat droplets but there are no features of alcoholic hepatitis or cirrhosis.

Laboratory investigations. ↑γGT and ↑AST, are commonest. Bilirubin usually normal. ↑MCV↑ serum lipids may also be present.

Treatment. Withdrawal of alcohol.

Prognosis. Excellent. The changes usually regress to normal within weeks.

Alcoholic hepatitis

Symptoms. Jaundice is frequent. Ascites may be present.

Examination. Facial plethora, spider naevi, firm, tender, marked hepatomegaly. Arterial bruit over liver, fever, jaundice, encephalopathy may be present.

Laboratory investigations. Neutrophil leucocytosis. ↑MCV, ↑bilirubin, ↑AST, ↑γGT. Hypertriglyceridaemia may give lipaemia and apparent hyponatraemia.

Liver histology. Hepatocellular necrosis. Polymorphonuclear cell infiltration. Mallory's hyaline. Fine pericellular fibrosis. Central vein sclerosis. Note that a similar histological picture may be seen with hepatotoxic reactions to perhexilene maleate and in some patients following jejuno-ileal bypass for obesity.

Treatment. Calorie substitution during alcohol withdrawal. High protein diet. Vitamin B supplements. Potassium repletion. Initially sedation to avoid delirium tremens (DTs). Corticosteroids have not been shown to be of benefit in most controlled trials. Propylthiouracil has also been tried but is of unproven benefit.

Prognosis. Extremely guarded; when alcoholic hepatitis is associated with encephalopathy the mortality is approximately 50%.

Alcoholic cirrhosis

Symptoms. These as for all causes of cirrhosis. Alcoholic hepatitis may coexist.

Examination. Dupuytren's contractures. Parotid enlargement. Gynaecomastia. Testicular atrophy. Feminization with loss of body hair, Fig. 2.4. These signs of cirrhosis are particularly common when cirrhosis is due to alcoholism.

Histology. May show features of fatty infiltration and alcoholic hepatitis as well as the nodular regeneration of cirrhosis (Fig. 13.5).

Treatment and prognosis. Encourage abstinence. The long-term outcome of alcoholic cirrhosis is generally better than cirrhosis due to other causes (Ch. 14) provided the patient ceases to imbibe.

Primary biliary cirrhosis (PBC)

The disease is more accurately described as chronic non-suppurative destructive cholangitis. The diagnosis is often made many years ahead of the development of cirrhosis.

Diagnostic criteria. The following are features of primary biliary cirrhosis, though it is not essential to find all three to make diagnosis in each patient.
1   Diagnostic (or compatible) liver biopsy (*most* are compatible rather than diagnostic).
2   Positive mitochondrial antibodies (present in 95%).
3   Normal cholangiography (to exclude bilary obstruction).

Clinical features. There is a preponderance of females; F:M ratio=9:1. Presentation is rare before 30 years of age and it peaks between 40–65. Liver function tests show features of cholestasis with high levels of serum alkaline phosphatase. Serum IgM levels are elevated in 60% of cases. Jaundice does not occur until the hepatic lesion is well advanced. Pruritus is a common first symptom and may be present for many years before the onset of jaundice. Occasionally PBC is unmasked by pruritus simulating cholestasis of pregnancy or that in patients on oral contraceptives. Portal hypertension occurs relatively early and hepatosplenomegaly is usually present. Hepatocellular function is well preserved until the terminal phase of the disease. Either the patient or close relatives have a high incidence of other autoimmune disorders, including Hashimoto's thyroiditis, Addison's disease, pernicious anaemia, vitiligo and systemic sclerosis. In patients with PBC, keratoconjunctivitis sicca and xerostomia (sicca syndrome) frequently occur. In the late stages the patient is usually deeply pigmented and deeply jaundiced, and xanthelasmata and xanthomas are common.

Histopathology. The diagnostic finding on liver histology is a 'florid bile duct lesion' in which the epithelial cells of the septal and larger interlobular bile ducts show swelling, proliferation, crowding and rupture in relation to an inflammatory cell infiltration clusters of epithelioid cells, granuloma and lymphoid follicle formation. Scheuer has staged the histological appearances according to the extent of fibrosis:
1   Intact limiting plate.
2   Expansion of portal tracts.
3   Extensive portal fibrosis.
4   Cirrhosis.
The diagnostic lesion is visible on needle liver biopsy in only about 40% of stage (1) and (2) biopsies and 20% of those in stages (3) and (4). In stages (3) and (4) it is

helpful to note extreme paucity of interlobular bile ducts and intense staining for copper and copper-associated protein. Retention of copper within the liver is a feature of chronic cholestasis; hepatic copper concentration frequently reaches levels found in active Wilson's disease. When only some of the diagnostic features are present, the biopsy is described as compatible with PBC and the onus then rests with the clinician to make the diagnosis in the light of the overall clinical picture. Occasionally patients show mixed features of PBC and chronic active hepatitis.

Treatment. Symptomatic: relief of pruritus with cholestyramine. Nutritional replacement: vitamins A, D, E and K as required; occasional calcium and phosphate supplements.

Complications such as ascites, bleeding varices and portosystemic encephalo-pathy are treated in the usual way. Immunosuppressive: it is generally thought that corticosteroids are contraindicated because of the risk of bone thinning which is a notable complication. Penicillamine has been used to suppress inflammation, and to prevent fibrosis and eliminate copper. Because of its potential toxicity its use is usually restricted to patients in stages (3) and (4). The drug may confer benefit but its use cannot be generally recommended until further confirmatory evidence accrues. Liver transplantation: as this treatment becomes available for terminal liver disease, patients with PBC may constitute one of the largest eligible groups. There may be a risk of disease recurrence in the transplanted organ.

Prognosis. This is extremely variable. Many are currently being diagnosed at a pre-cirrhotic stage. Then it is reasonable to predict a life expectancy of more than a decade. This makes it difficult to justify trials of new drugs in stages (1) and (2) of the disease, firstly on the grounds of the untreated patient's general well being, and secondly, the duration of such trials and longevity of the patients studied would probably exceed that of many an interested doctor!

Granulomatous liver disease

Occasionally a liver biopsy shows granuloma formation. Rarely the diagnosis is apparent from the biopsy when schistosomal pigment, acid-fast bacilli or other diagnostic features are present. More commonly, other avenues of investigation have to be pursued in the search for a cause, and often none is found (Table 13.4).

Some aspects of therapy in patients with liver disease

Pruritus

In the treatment of pruritus cholestyramine is the mainstay. It should be given with breakfast to coincide with the maximum expulsion of bile acids into the intestine from the gallbladder. Drugs whose absorption is hindered by cholestyramine, e.g. digoxin, warfarin, vitamin D, etc. should be given in the evening. When cholestyramine produces diarrhoea the cause is usually steatorrhoea, and will

Table 13.4. Causes of hepatic granulomas.

Common
    Tuberculosis
    Schistosomiasis
    Sarcoidosis
Occasional
    Brucellosis
    Primary biliary cirrhosis
    Drug reactions including phenylbutazone, allopurinol
        and many others
    Q fever
Rare
    Parasites including *Strongyloides stercoralis*,
        Ascaris lumbricoides
    Crohn's disease
    Syphilis
    Foreign bodies (especially talcum crystals in drug addicts)

---

usually respond to a low fat diet; otherwise a second cause such as pancreatic or intestinal disease may be suspected. Antihistamines are best avoided if possible, since they may increase drowsiness and lethargy to an intolerable degree. Nevertheless chlorpheniramine is useful at times. Corticosteroids may occasionally be of benefit in the cholestatic phase of acute viral hepatitis but are not advised for chronic forms of cholestasis since they aggravate the already serious tendency in such patients to metabolic bone disease. Phenobarbital is occasionally of benefit in the relief of intrahepatic cholestasis.

If a patient with irreversible pathology has severely distressing pruritus which cannot be relieved by any of the above methods, treatment with the androgenic steroid norethandrolone may be justified. This not only produces hirsutes but also deepens the jaundice; even so in the terminally ill patient this may be an acceptable price to pay for relief of pruritus.

Correction of haematologic disorders
Anaemia in liver disease, especially in the alcoholic patient, may be due to deficiency of haematinics; iron, folic acid, pyridoxine and ascorbic acid are the commonest deficiencies. Intravenous polyvitamin replacement (with parenterovite) may be necessary in the severely malnourished individual but more specific oral replacement usually suffices. Macrocytosis is found in alcoholism and is also a feature of advanced liver disease when target cells are seen on the blood film. It is unresponsive to folic acid or vitamin B_{12} therapy.

Deficiency of clotting factors in pure cholestasis usually results from vitamin K deficiency and can be corrected rapidly by its parenteral administration. The prothrombin time falls to within 3 sec of control values within a few hours. An inadequate response indicates either defective synthesis due to hepatocellular dysfunction or consumptive coagulopathy. In severe hepatocellular failure the prothrombin time is prolonged and unresponsive to vitamin K. When the PT ratio is greater than five, spontaneous haemorrhage is the rule and direct replacement of clotting factors is required. Fresh frozen plasma is effective but has the disadvantage of having a high salt content. If clotting factor concentrates are preferred they must be monitored to exclude high concentrations of activated Factor IX which can produce a dangerous hypercoagulability state. If bleeding occurs in patients with severe hepatocellular failure and transfusion is required, then fresh blood should be used to maximize the amount of clotting factors and platelets that are transfused.

Monitoring of haemostatic function is essential before invasive tests such as liver biopsy. This consists of a minimum of PT, PTT and platelet count and should ideally also include a bleeding time. If after parenteral vitamin K administration the PT exceeds control by more than 3 sec or the PTT is greater than 45 sec (control 30–35 sec) the invasive procedure must not be performed without prior transfusion of fresh frozen plasma or its equivalent. If the bleeding time is significantly prolonged and the platelet count low, fresh platelet transfusion is necessary. Pancytopenia including thrombocytopenia is commonly found in association with splenomegaly in portal hypertension. However, it is seldom a clinically significant problem and therefore the hypersplenism of portal hypertension is virtually never an indication for splenectomy.

Fat-soluble vitamin deficiency states
Chronic cholestasis may produce clinically important deficiencies of the fat-soluble vitamins A, D, E and K.

Vitamin A deficiency produces night blindness, xerodermia and xerophthlamia. Vitamin D deficiency produces osteomalacia. In chronic cholestatic conditions such as primary biliary cirrhosis, osteomalacia is often compounded by coexistent osteoporosis. Vitamin E deficiency has recently been reported to be associated with spinocerebellar degeneration (ataxia, areflexia, ophthalmic paresis) when severe vitamin E deficiency has been present for many years following neonatal bile duct hypoplasia and severe cystic fibrosis. Vitamin K deficiency is usually the first fat-soluble vitamin deficiency state to be detectable clinically. Easy bruising and prolonged bleeding following trauma are reflected by a prolonged prothrombin time and deficiency of the vitamin K dependent coagulation factors (II, VII, IX and X) in the circulation. The presence of micellar concentrations of bile acids within the intestinal lumen is essential for fat-soluble vitamin absorption. If cholestasis is partial, oral supplements of the vitamins may correct the deficiencies. If cholestyramine for relief of pruritus and oral supplements of the fat-soluble vitamins are being prescribed concurrently, they must be distanced as far as possible in time to prevent interaction within the intestinal lumen. If cholestasis is severe, or there is inadequate response to oral therapy, vitamins A, D, E and K should be given parenterally. Steatorrhoea may prevent normal calcium and phosphate absorption and should be palliated by a low fat diet. Supplements of oral calcium and phosphate may be given on alternate days. Very rarely when bone pain is severe, calcium infusions may be required for symptomatic relief.

Chapter 14
Cirrhosis and Other Disorders
of the Liver

Cirrhosis

Cirrhosis may arise as a consequence of many chronic liver diseases (Table 14.1). It is the result of necrosis and regeneration of liver cells with scarring, and is characterized by regeneration nodules. Individual cells within these nodules may appear normal but their typical relationship to portal tracts and hepatic venules within a lobular architecture is lost (Fig. 13.5). Distortion of architecture interferes with blood flow through the liver and handicaps hepatic function. Symptoms and signs of cirrhosis then result from impaired liver cell function and portal hypertension.

Table 14.1. Causes of cirrhosis.

Common
    Alcohol
    Hepatitis B
Occasional
    Chronic active hepatitis
    Primary biliary cirrhosis
    Secondary biliary cirrhosis
Rare
    Haemochromatosis
    Hepatolenticular degeneration (Wilson's disease)
    Cardiac cirrhosis
    Glycogenosis
    Galactosaemia
    Alpha-1 antitrypsin deficiency

Portal hypertension

Clinical findings which support a diagnosis of portal hypertension include splenomegaly, prominent veins on the anterior abdominal wall, oesophageal varices, ascites and fetor hepaticus. Important complications of portal hypertension are the development of ascites, bleeding gastro-oesophageal varices and porto-systemic encephalopathy.

Measurement of portal pressure. Portal hypertension is present when the hydrostatic pressure in the portal vein or its collaterals is greater than 12 mmHg (15 cm H_2O).

Normal portal pressure is 5–10 mmHg. When indicated, measurement of portal pressure can be obtained in the following three ways:

1   Wedged hepatic venous pressure (WHVP) can be measured via brachial or femoral vein catheterization (p. 85).

2   Direct transhepatic approach with a 'skinny' needle used for percutaneous cholangiography (p. 83).

3   Splenic pulp pressure at the time of splenic portography (Fig. 6.13).

Portal hypertension may be classified according to the site of abnormal resistance to portal blood flow (Table 14.2). In pre-sinusoidal portal hypertension the WHVP is normal or low, but splenic pulp pressure is elevated. In alcoholic cirrhosis WHVP is an accurate measure of portal pressure. However, in practice the classification is by no means as clear-cut as suggested by theory.

Ascites

Ascites represents free fluid in the peritoneal cavity and its aetiology is shown in Table 14.3. When ascites is gross the abdomen is protruberant and there is fullness in the flanks when the patient lies supine. Shifting dullness and a fluid thrill may be

Table 14.2. Aetiology of portal hypertension.

Site of obstruction	Cause
Sinusoidal	Cirrhosis
	Alcoholic hepatitis
	Congenital hepatic fibrosis
Pre-sinusoidal or mixed	
Intrahepatic (patent portal vein)	Schistosomiasis
	Non-cirrhotic portal hypertension
	arsenic induced
	vinyl chloride induced
	tropical splenomegaly (Banti's syndrome)
	Sarcoidosis
	Myelosclerosis
	Partial nodular transformation
	Gaucher's
Extrahepatic	Portal vein thrombosis
Post-sinusoidal	
Intrahepatic	Hepatic vein thrombosis (Budd–Chiari syndrome)
	Veno-occlusive disease
Extrahepatic	Web of hepatic vein or IVC
	IVC obstruction by tumour or thrombus
	Constrictive pericarditis

Table 14.3. Aetiology of ascites.

1 Portal hypertension
2 Infection: Tuberculous; following perforation of a viscus; 'spontaneous' infection occurs in cirrhosis; pneumococcal in young girls
3 Malignancy
4 Pancreatic ascites

elicited. In the presence of ascites umbilical or inguinal herniae protrude. The umbilicus is usually displaced down with ascites but up with an ovarian mass. Percussion in the flanks gives a dull note with ascites but is resonant with an ovarian mass.

Diagnostic paracentesis (p. 89). This yields fluid which may be sent for:
1 Total and differential white cell count.
2 Protein estimation.
3 Bacteriological culture.
4 Cytological examination.

'Spontaneous' infection of ascites is diagnosed if a polymorphonuclear leucocyte count greater than 500 cells/mm^3 is found in a patient with cirrhosis. There may be no fever, abdominal tenderness nor systemic leucocytosis. It may explain deterioration with encephalopathy in such a patient, and antibiotic therapy should be commenced immediately rather than await bacteriological confirmation. Gram-negative bacteria from the bowel are the usual contaminants. The fluid may appear turbid. A lymphocytosis suggests tuberculosis.

An ascitic protein concentration of less than 10 g/l in clear straw-coloured fluid represents a transudate due to portal hypertension though higher levels are also often encountered in uncomplicated portal hypertension. When the protein concentration exceeds 40 g/l it usually indicates an exudate due to infection, malignancy or pancreatic ascites. However, this may also occur with post-sinusoidal portal hypertension in the Budd–Chiari syndrome.

Haemorrhagic ascites. In a cirrhotic patient this often indicates the presence of primary hepatocellular carcinoma. In a young woman it may be due to a ruptured ectopic pregnancy or contraceptive steroid-induced hepatic adenoma. Very rarely it occurs because of spontaneous interperitoneal rupture of a dilated venous collateral in portal hypertension and may be secondary to abdominal trauma.

Chylous ascites. This usually represents obstruction of the main lymphatic duct in the epigastrium or thorax by invasive malignancy, or may be due to their rupture following abdominal trauma. If chylous ascites is allowed to stand, chylomicrons float as a creamy lipid layer to the top.

Pancreatic ascites. This is diagnosed by finding an extremely high level of amylase in the fluid. The commonest cause is alcoholic pancreatitis. There is often free communication between the main pancreatic duct and the peritoneal cavity so that pancreatic secretions enter the ascites directly. Patients are notable for rapid, progressive weight loss and muscle wasting.

Ascites in liver disease

Ascites in liver disease occurs in the presence of:

1   Portal hypertension.
2   Hypoalbuminaemia.
3   Renal salt and water retention (one of the earliest detectable changes which precedes ascites).

Renal pathophysiology in ascites of liver origin. This results from:

1   Excessive reabsorption of sodium from proximal nephron; cause unknown.
2   Hyperaldosteronism giving increased sodium reabsorption from the distal convolute tubule. If this mechanism is operative natriuresis occurs in response to spironolactone therapy.
3   Defective free water clearance.

The normal mechanism for excreting a water load depends on water being carried to the distal convoluted tubule by sodium, where removal of sodium without water under the control of aldosterone produces very dilute urine which enters the collecting tubule (where water absorption is regulated by antidiuretic hormone). In ascites with advanced liver disease all available sodium may be absorbed before it reaches the distal convoluted tubule. No mechanism remains for effective excretion of excess water. If the patient drinks freely, hyponatraemia is the likely result.

Therapy. Relief of ascites is seldom urgent and it is often unnecessary to treat mild or moderate ascites in patients with cirrhosis. Indications for its treatment include distress due to discomfort or respiratory embarrassment. There is a limit to the rate at which salt and water can leave the peritoneal cavity; this approximates 1 litre/day. Ideally, therefore, the patient should lose 1 kg/day during diuresis. More rapid weight loss in the absence of peripheral oedema leads to depletion of intravascular volume and pre-renal uraemia. The aim in treating the patient with ascites is to produce a negative sodium balance, i.e. net loss of sodium from the body. During the period of accumulation of ascites very little sodium (usually less than 10 mmol/day) escapes in the urine. Urinary sodium concentration on any urine sample gives an indication of whether a therapeutic diuresis can be anticipated. There is virtually never any indication for giving sodium supplements, e.g. saline infusion, to a patient with ascites, as this will normally aggravate the problem. Giving sodium is an inappropriate response to hyponatraemia in liver disease with ascites since a low serum sodium concentration in this situation merely indicates that accumulated total body water is in even greater excess than the salt. Hyponatraemia is therefore corrected by water restriction and any appropriate measures which may increase renal free water clearance.

Management. A patient admitted to hospital for treatment of ascites should initially be confined to bed and given a diet of salt and water restriction.
1   Monitor body weight daily.
2   Measure urine sodium concentration on first sample of each day (discontinue when Na^+ exceeds 40 mmol/l).
3   Check blood urea, electrolytes and creatinine twice weekly
   If urinary sodium concentration remains low it is advisable to introduce a diuretic which is potassium sparing and acts on the distal convoluted tubule. Spironolactone is an aldosterone antagonist which if effective works very satisfactorily. In men it may induce painful gynaecomastia which regresses on substitution of the drug by amiloride or triamterene. There is a latent period of 48–72 h before the full effect of a given dose of spironolactone can be assessed. At this stage a thiazide may be added with benefit. Treatment is aimed at loss of 1 kg/day body weight (more is acceptable only if peripheral oedema coexists with ascites).

Paracentesis and drainage. These are ill advised and contraindicated except for emergency decompression to alleviate (a) discomfort due to tense distension, and (b) symptoms and signs due to distension, e.g. respiratory failure. These indications are usually confined to ascites of malignant disease. When the measures recommended above fail, venous reinfusion of ascites after its ultrafiltration extracorporeally ('Rhodiascit' apparatus) or a 'Leveen' (peritoneo-jugular) shunt may be attempted. Both techniques have high morbidity and should be used very conservatively if at all. Before commencing ultrafiltration and venous reinfusion of protein-rich ascites, first check that the fluid is sterile, low in protein and free of malignant cells. Beware bacteraemia, overload of the circulation giving congestive cardiac failure or haemorrhage due to rapid distension of oesophageal varices.

The hepato-renal syndrome (or 'hepatic nephropathy')
The development of uraemia in a patient with cirrhosis and ascites carries a grave prognosis. The situation soon becomes irreversible with death an almost certain outcome. The kidneys do not appear intrinsically diseased—if transplanted they function normally. The condition is often iatrogenic—usually diuretic induced or a consequence of paracentesis.
   Significant progressive elevation of blood urea or creatinine during treatment of ascites constitutes a contraindication to further diuretic therapy.

Porto-systemic encephalopathy (PSE)
This (also called hepatic encephalopathy) is due to impaired brain function

secondary to liver disease. It may be aggravated by a porto-systemic collateral circulation or due entirely to this bypass.

Pathogenesis. No single neurotoxic agent has been identified. PSE is probably caused by several factors, some of which may potentiate one another. Postulated factors include ammonia, false neurotransmitters (octopamine), free fatty acids, mercaptans, and a disturbed ratio of branch-chain amino acids to others.

Normally ammonia absorbed from the intestine is efficiently removed from portal blood by the liver and converted into urea via the urea cycle. Increased amounts of ammonia enter the systemic circulation when hepatocellular function is markedly deranged (e.g. acute liver failure) or when blood is shunted past the liver by a porto-systemic collateral circulation. Potassium depletion (which may be severe though hypokalaemia is slight or absent) favours intracellular partition of ammonia by increasing the pH gradient which normally exists between intra- and extracellular fluid (intracellular fluid is the more acid) (Fig. 14.1). K^+ depletion is

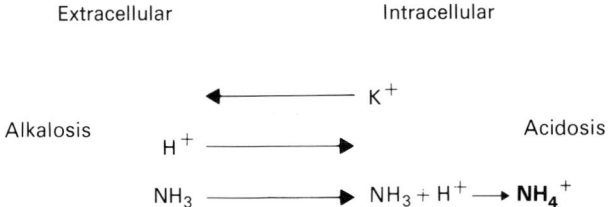

Potassium depletion

Extracellular   Intracellular

Alkalosis   Acidosis

K^+

H^+

$NH_3 \longrightarrow NH_3 + H^+ \longrightarrow NH_4^+$

Fig. 14.1. Ammonia in porto-systemic encephalopathy (PSE). Ammonia tends to partition on the acidic side of a diffusion barrier. Potassium depletion due to diarrhoea or diuresis produces an extracellular alkalosis and intracellular acidosis, thus favouring the partitioning of ammonia into the brain cell. Similarly by acidification of colonic contents, lactulose helps to trap ammonia within the colon lumen and reduce its absorption.

common in cirrhosis (especially in alcoholics) due to hyperaldosteronism, diarrhoea and other factors. As body potassium stores are depleted K^+ diffuses out of cells in exchange for H^+. Though this produces an extracellular metabolic (hypokalaemic) alkalosis, the intracellular fluid becomes more acid and thus favours intracellular sequestration of ammonia in its non-diffusable cationic form of NH_4^+. In addition to reduction of ammonia production it is imperative to maintain normal body potassium stores in patients subject to hepatic encephalopathy. Therefore avoid diuretics, especially K^+-wasting ones wherever possible.

Factors which may precipitate PSE are shown in Table 14.4.

Pathology. Characteristic changes in the brain consist of a proliferation of enlarged astrocytes with distorted nuclei. They are seen in PSE and other hyperammonae-mic syndromes.

Clinical types

Acute. Clouding of consciousness and coma resulting from acute liver failure. Beware of hypoglycaemia which can also produce unconsciousness in these patients.

Chronic. Manifestation of longstanding, usually large porto-systemic collateral circulation. This may be a result of surgical therapy, e.g. porto-caval anastomosis, or arise as a result of naturally occurring porto-systemic shunts. Manifestations are protean and can be easily mistaken for primary neuropsychiatric or neurologic disorders, e.g. Parkinson's syndrome, dementia, cerebellar syndrome.

Acute on chronic. An intercurrent event supervenes on a background of chronic PSE to make it worse. Common causes are listed in Table 14.4.

Table 14.4. Factors which may precipitate porto-systemic encephalopathy (PSE)

Heavy protein meal⎫ Constipation ⎬ Gastrointestinal haemorrhage⎭	By increasing absorption of bacterial products of nitrogen metabolism
Hypokalaemia ⎫ Overdiuresis ⎬	By affecting acid base balance
Drug therapy	Especially narcotics; there is increased sensitivity to opiates together with a decrease in their metabolism
Intercurrent infection	
Infected ascites	(Often spontaneous and asymptomatic)

Clinical features

Disturbances (amounting to inversion) of sleep rhythm occur early. Other symptoms and signs of mental impairment and clouded consciousness vary from mild forgetfulness and irritability to drowsiness, stupor and coma. During examination of the patient asterixis (wing-flapping tremor) may be demonstrated. A characteristic breath odour of fetor hepaticus is often easily detected as the patient breathes deeply to facilitate palpation of the liver and spleen.

An objective record of change in mental impairment may be obtained by simply getting the patient to sign their name or copy a star at each consultation.

Diagnosis. Constructional dyspraxia is usually demonstrated by inability to copy a five-pointed star (Fig. 14.2) or trace numbers sequentially in a timed 'trail test'. Electroencephalography (EEG) shows slowing of the dominant waves, and delta waves (3–4 cycles/sec) are characteristically found with PSE. Showing an elevated

Star chart

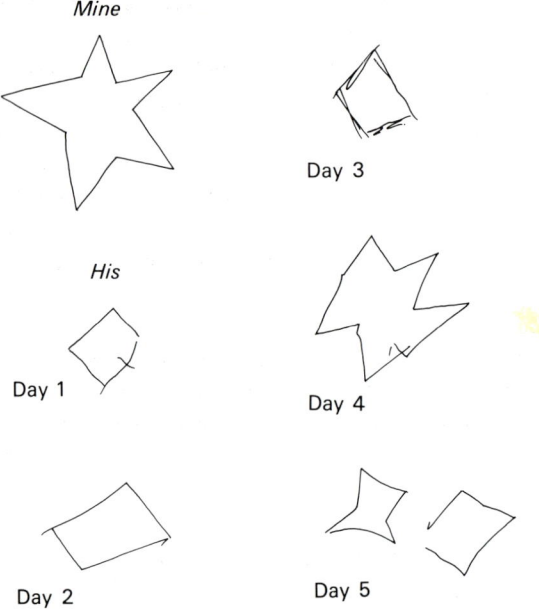

Mine

Day 3

His

Day 1

Day 4

Day 2

Day 5

Fig. 14.2. Star chart. A five-pointed star (upper left) was drawn by the doctor and the patient was asked to copy it. The patient demonstrated constructional apraxia due to porto-systemic encephalopathy. Serial testing showed some improvement during treatment with lactulose and neomycin.

blood ammonia concentration by laboratory measurement is seldom required clinically. There is poor correlation between the blood ammonia concentration and clinical measures of PSE.

Management. This should first be directed to correcting the precipitating factors such as bleeding or infection. Also all sedative medication should be discontinued. The aim of treatment is to decrease production and absorption of ammonia and other toxins produced by bacterial metabolism of nitrogenous substances in the intestine.

Lactulose is a non-absorbable disaccharide which is extremely useful in the treatment of PSE. It is usually combined with restriction of dietary protein. The patient must be instructed that the correct dose cannot be estimated in millilitres, but is the amount required to provide two, three or four loose bowel actions daily. Purported mechanisms of action include (a) purgation, (b) alteration of colonic bacteria flora, and (c) trapping of ammonia within the colon (see Fig. 14.1). Both (a) and (c) are the result of acidification of the colon when bacteria metabolize the lactulose to short chain fatty acids, e.g. acetic acid. Neomycin given orally is also effective in relieving symptoms of PSE. Although often termed a non-absorbable antibiotic, its long-term use carries the hazard of ototoxicity due to finite absorption, and the risk is greater when renal function is impaired. These measures are combined with a low protein diet. Restriction may be to 60, 40, 20 or 0 g/day and can be monitored by clinical testing or electroencephalopathy. Magnesium sulphate or other acidic enemas are useful in treatment of severe PSE with pre-coma or coma. By washing out the colon they remove the source of noxious substances in the same ways as stated for lactulose above. In comatose patients all protein is withdrawn and all calories are usually supplied as carbohydrate. Constant feeding is recommended because of the concurrent risk of hypoglycaemia in severe hepatocellular failure.

Bleeding varices

Haematemesis and melaena due to rupture of oesophageal varices carries a poor prognosis. Of all patients admitted to hospital with bleeding varices only a third leave alive; this contrasts with an overall mortality of about 9% for hospital admission due to upper gastrointestinal haemorrhage from all causes.

Pathogenesis. Many factors may contribute to a bleeding tendency in patients with liver disease including portal hypertension, poor general nutrition and capillary fragility, impaired blood coagulation due to impaired synthesis of clotting factors by the liver; disseminated intravascular coagulation and excessive fibrinolysis, and hypersplenism-induced thrombocytopenia.

The risk of bleeding is broadly related to the size of the varices and to the height of portal pressure, but the precipitating event is often unknown. Sudden increases of portal pressure such as may occur from rapid blood transfusion or during reinfusion of ascites after extracorporeal ultrafiltration or insertion of a peritoneo-jugular shunt may cause bleeding from varices. Occlusion by thrombus or tumour of the portal or hepatic veins also causes a sharp rise of portal pressure. The presence of ascites also increases portal pressure and its formation often precedes and may precipitate upper gastrointestinal bleeding from varices.

Diagnosis. Oesophageal varices can be seen by barium swallow (Fig. 14.3) but endoscopy is the only reliable way of determining the source of bleeding in patients with liver disease. In a population of patients known to have alcoholic liver disease and oesophageal varices, only 50% were actually bleeding from their varices. Other common lesions included chronic peptic ulcer, gastric erosions and Mallory–Weiss tears. In a non-alcoholic population of patients with chronic liver disease and oesophageal varices upper gastrointestinal bleeding originates from varices in about 80% of instances.

Management. Resuscitation: Acute blood loss is best replaced by whole blood transfusion. If the patient's coagulation is poor, fresh blood is better. To correct

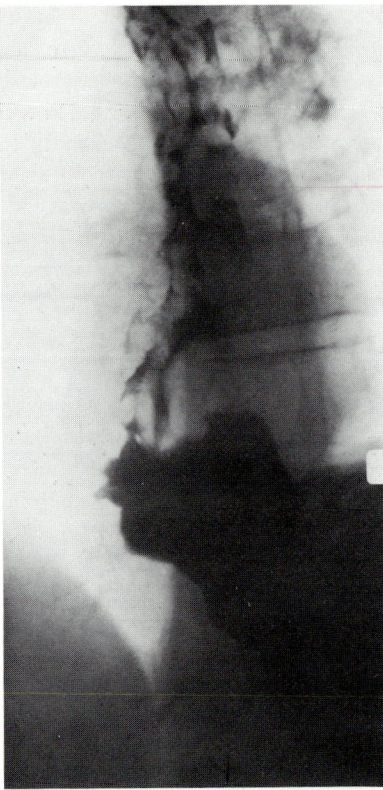

Fig. 14.3. Demonstration of oesophageal varices on barium swallow. The varices can be seen as filling defects thinly coated with barium within the oesophageal lumen.

anaemia due to chronic blood loss in cirrhotic patients with a normal circulating volume, packed cells should be transfused slowly in order to avoid distension of varices and formation of ascites by plasma salt and water.

PSE precipitated by bleeding is treated with lactulose orally and magnesium sulphate enemas. Haemostatic deficiencies are corrected when possible, e.g. with vitamin K injections. Fresh frozen plasma may be required if the prothrombin time is markedly prolonged, but this has the disadvantage of giving large amounts of salt and water which may produce ascites.

Lowering portal pressure: Vasopressin 20 u/100 ml of 5% dextrose given intravenously over 20 min helps to stem the tide of severe variceal bleeding. An effective infusion of vasopressin makes the patient blanche and causes smooth muscle contraction so that the patient usually experiences abdominal colic with evacuation of a large melaena. Peripheral vein infusion of vasopressin can exacerbate myocardial ischaemia and should not be given to patients with known coronary artery disease. If an intra-arterial cannula has been sited in the superior mesenteric artery portal pressure may be reduced by continuous intra-arterial infusion of vasopressin at a rate of 0.4 u/min. This avoids the risk of coronary insufficiency but still has the risk of producing ischaemic necrosis of the intestine locally. Another theoretical risk with vasopressin is that it increases tissue plasminogen activator and thrombolytic activity.

Alternative therapies for reducing portal pressure are currently under evaluation, including triglycylvasopressin (a synthetic analogue of vasopressin which has a longer half-life), vasoactive nitrates, β-adrenergic blockers and somatostatin, but their efficacy has not been adequately assessed.

Balloon tamponade: This is reserved for patients in whom brisk bleeding continues despite the above measures.

Procedure. Check that all four channels are correctly labelled (Fig. 14.4).

Inflate the gastric balloon to the required volume (400–500 ml) recording the pressure on a sphygmomanometer with every 50 ml increment before intubating

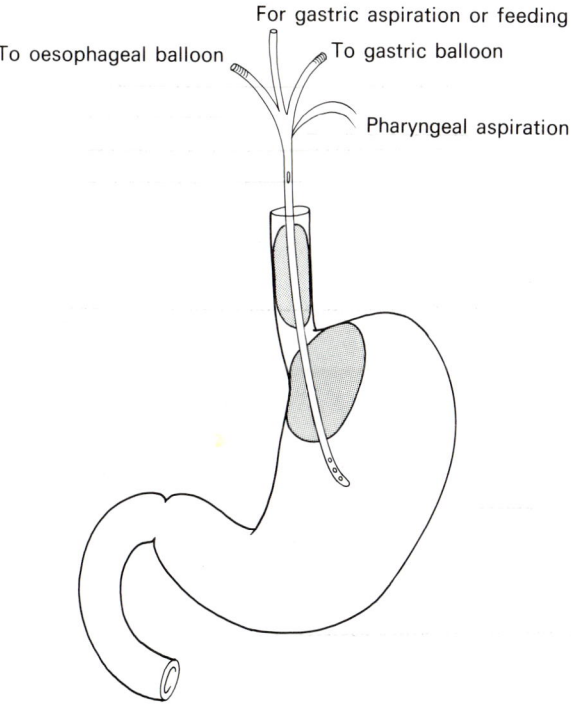

For gastric aspiration or feeding

To oesophageal balloon

To gastric balloon

Pharyngeal aspiration

Fig. 14.4. Balloon tamponage. The Sengstaken–Blakemore tube is illustrated. It has four lumens. Two permit inflation of a gastric balloon (which compresses the stomach at the gastro-oesophageal junction) and an oesophageal balloon. In addition gastric contents and pharyngeal secretions can be aspirated.

the patient and use the readings for comparison after intubation. This ensures that excessive pressure causing rupture of the oesophagus due to faulty balloon placement cannot occur.

Ensure that the gastric balloon is adequately filled within the stomach before applying traction. Check position of the balloon with X-ray.

Maintain constant traction by weight and pulley or a similar device. This should stop the bleeding. Inflation of the oesophageal balloon is thereafter optional with the Sengstaken–Blakemore tube, but not possible with the Linton–Nachlas tube. If insufficient traction on the balloon is exerted at the gastro-oesophageal junction blood continues to enter the oesophageal varices and inflation of the oesophageal balloon may then only serve to increase the rate of the variceal blood loss.

Aspirate pharyngeal secretions to prevent aspiration pneumonia; avoid trauma due to strong suction—this can cause pharyngeal bleeding. Endotracheal intubation with occlusive balloon then becomes necessary to avoid aspiration pneumonia.

Release the pressure in the oesophageal balloon (if present) and the traction on the gastric balloon at a planned moment within 16–24 h. This is essential to avoid pressure-necrosis of the oesophagus. If the gastric balloon is allowed to lie loose, though inflated, within the stomach for a few hours before its final removal it remains available for instantaneous haemostasis by re-application of traction should bleeding recur.

Sclerotherapy: (a) Endoscopic: injection of sclerosant solution (e.g. ethanolamine oleate) into oesophageal varices results in their occlusion and when successful diminishes the risk of rebleeding. Several sessions at weekly or longer intervals are usually required before all varices can be obliterated. Prior to this the risk of continued or recurrent bleeding persists. Recanalization is also likely to occur so that check endoscopy at 3–6 monthly intervals is essential to allow further obliterative therapy for early recurrent varices. (b) Transhepatic: this procedure is occasionally used to arrest an episode of severe bleeding unresponsive to other non-surgical measures. It is not recommended as a measure for the long term control of bleeding varices because of its difficulty and morbidity and the tendency of obliterated porto-systemic collateral vessels to recanalize.

Early studies suggest that long-term treatment with oral propranolol may reduce the incidence of rebleeding from oesophageal varices.

Surgical treatment of bleeding oesophageal varices
Surgery has been used in three situations of which only the first two are now permissible:

Emergency: as a life-saving procedure to stop an episode of bleeding from varices.

Elective: i.e. in a patient who has previously bled from varices but in whom bleeding is not an active problem.

Prophylactic. This category is definitely contraindicated, i.e. operating in patients who have never bled in an attempt to remove the risk of bleeding.

Operative procedures. Local therapy: These procedures are designed to stop bleeding without reducing portal pressure, e.g. oesophageal transection or gastric transection with porta-azygous disconnection.

Advantages are rapid cessation of blood loss, and maintenance of portal blood supply to the liver. Disadvantages are high morbidity and mortality, especially when done as an emergency procedure and recurrence of varices with attendant risk of bleeding after about 1 year.

Shunts: These procedures are designed to reduce the risk of bleeding by lowering portal pressure. Advantages are lower mortality than oesophageal transection when done as either emergency or elective procedure, and the permanent effect (provided shunt remains patent) in lowering portal pressure and diminishing risk of bleeding. The disadvantage is that by reducing portal blood flow, liver failure with PSE is produced more rapidly and frequently than is seen in a comparable group without shunts.

Assessment of benefits versus risks of shunt surgery. The disadvantage of advancing death due to liver failure incurred by performing shunt surgery has produced the following results in controlled clinical trials:

1 Survival was shorter in the shunted group when prophylactic shunting was performed.

2 There has been no significant prolongation of life by elective shunting, although there is a statistically insignificant trend for the shunted group to fare better.

Selection of patients for shunt surgery. In most recorded series Child's selection criteria (Table 14.5) have been applied, group A being regarded as 'good risk' patients and group C as 'poor risk' patients. However, although a good indication of immediate (operative) mortality, this classification correlates poorly with long-term survival in shunted patients and new better methods are required to permit selection of those patients (who undoubtedly exist!) who have previously bled from varices and whose life expectancy would be increased by shunt surgery.

Table 14.5. Child's classification of patients with cirrhosis in terms of hepatic functional reserve.

	A	B	C
Degree of impairment	Minimal	Moderate	Severe
Serum bilirubin (μmol/dl)	<35	35–50	>50
Serum albumin (g/l)	>35	30–35	<30
Ascites	None	Easily controlled	Poorly controlled
PSE	None	Minimal	Advanced; 'coma'
Nutrition	Excellent	Good	Poor; 'wasting'

Iron storage diseases

Physiology. Absorption of dietary iron is normally regulated to balance body losses. About 10 mg daily is taken in the diet of which 1 mg (2 mg in menstruating women) is absorbed. Total body iron amounts to 3–4 g.

Absorption is stimulated in response to erythropoiesis, hypoxia and depletion of body iron stores. Iron is transported in the blood bound to transferrin and stored in tissues bound to ferritin.

Pathophysiology. Total body iron stores may be increased due to:
1   Excessive intake of oral iron, e.g. in alcoholic drinks.
2   An inherited defect in the normal mechanism regulating absorption, i.e. idiopathic haemochromatosis.
3   A chronic stimulus to intestinal absorption, e.g. chronic anaemia due to hereditary thalassaemia or hereditary spherocytosis.
4   Parenteral administration, e.g. blood transfusion in thalassaemia.

Definitions. Haemochromatosis involves iron overloading of the parenchymal cells of the liver and other organs which may be sufficiently severe to damage that tissue. In idiopathic haemochromatosis there are no recognizable stimuli for excessive iron absorption. Secondary haemochromatosis can be attributed to an obvious cause, e.g. chronic anaemia. Haemosiderosis describes excessive tissue iron deposition which may or may not have the intensity or distribution to constitute haemochromatosis.

Interactions of hepatic iron overload states with other hepatic disease
Idiopathic haemochromatosis may be very difficult to diagnose if the patient also has features of alcoholic liver disease. In alcoholic cirrhosis there is usually an excessive amount of iron in the liver (haemosiderosis). However, it is usually less than that seen in typical haemochromatosis and is not as easily mobilized by venesection.

Several factors appear to increase intestinal iron absorption in cirrhotics including (a) increased intake, e.g. in alcoholic drinks, (b) stimulation of iron absorption by alcohol, (c) porto-caval shunting, (d) chronic pancreatitis and (e) folate deficiency.

Alcoholism and hepatic siderosis are common in patients with porphyria cutanea tarda, who suffer blistering and scarring of their hands in response to sunlight and minor trauma. Symptoms often improve with venesection and abstinence from alcohol.

Idiopathic haemochromatosis
First described by Troisier, this disease was later called bronze diabetes by Hanot and haemochromatosis by von Recklinghausen.

Definition. A rare genetic disease usually with an autosomal recessive pattern of inheritance. Lifelong excessive intestinal absorption of iron leads to its heavy deposition within parenchymal cells of the liver, pancreas, gut, heart and endocrine glands where it produces anatomical and functional disturbances.

Clinical features. The typical patient is male with deep brown or slate grey pigmentation of the skin due to increased melanin production and atrophy of the skin, particularly of exposed areas. Firm, smooth hepatomegaly is usual. Signs of hepatocellular disease are usually absent until the late stages of the disease. Patients have an increased risk of primary liver cancer. Diabetes mellitus (bronze diabetes) occurs in two-thirds and may be complicated by typical retinal, renal, neural and peripheral vascular complications.

Anterior pituitary function is impaired due to iron deposition giving low gonadotrophin levels, testicular atrophy, loss of secondary sex characteristics, loss of libido and impotence.

Polyarthropathy, often affecting metacarpophalyngeal joints and chondrocalcinosis of the larger joints (ankles, knees and wrists) also occur.

Cardiomyopathy produces a flabby dilated heart with risk of arrhythmias, right heart failure or sudden death. It is more prominent in children with secondary haemochromatosis.

Diagnosis. In haemochromatosis the saturation index of serum total iron binding capacity is usually greater than 80% (normal less than 50%). Serum ferritin levels, with rare exceptions, are proportional to total body iron stores and therefore can be used to monitor progress during iron depletion therapy. In haemochromatosis total body iron stores as high as 20–60 g are common (normal 3–5 g). Liver histology shows excessive iron deposition mainly in periportal hepatocytes. The iron is associated with aggregated ferritin known as haemosiderin. Progression of the disease produces periportal fibrosis and culminates in cirrhosis.

Hepatic iron determined directly, is the single most reliable diagnostic test and in idiopathic haemochromatosis usually exceeds one per cent of dry liver weight (i.e. 1 g Fe/100 g dry liver).

Treatment. Venesection of 1–2 pints of blood per week is effective. One 500 ml unit of blood contains about 250 mg of iron; to deplete the body of a 40-g iron store would therefore require removal of 500 ml twice weekly for more than a year. Anaemia does not develop until the body's iron stores have been depleted. Subsequently venesection is continued 3 monthly.

Chelation therapy is less effective than venesection and more troublesome and is not indicated in idiopathic haemochromatosis. Nevertheless when injections of desferrioxamine are given with blood transfusion to thalassaemic patients liver disease is attenuated. Continuous subcutaneous infusion of desferrioxamine is also effective. Oral ascorbic acid supplements increase urinary iron excretion.

Prognosis. Typical 5-year survival figures are 90% for those efficiently venesected and 30% for the untreated. However, the risk of primary liver cancer does not appear to be diminished by venesection.

Screening for idiopathic haemochromatosis is necessary in all male and postmenopausal female siblings. A blood sample should be taken for estimation of serum iron, total iron binding capacity and ferritin and if either the saturation index or serum ferritin is high, biopsy of the liver is indicated for direct measurement of hepatic iron.

In other generations of the family, especially the young, comparison of HLA types with the proband traces the haemochromatosis gene (often HLA A3 B7) before other features of non-overload are detectable.

Wilson's disease (hepatolenticular degeneration)

Wilson's disease is a familial disorder of copper metabolism with autosomal recessive inheritance which classically presents in the teens or twenties as either hepatic or neurologic disease. The major symptoms and signs result from excessive copper accumulation in the liver and basal ganglia. It was first described by Kinnear Wilson in 1912 in an article entitled 'Progressive lenticular degeneration: a familial nervous disease associated with cirrhosis of the liver'. A similar disease occurs in the Bedlington terrier.

Clinical features

Liver disease may present as acute hepatitis, chronic active hepatitis or cirrhosis. CNS disease produces rigidity, tremor, dysarthria, choreo-athetosis and other extra-pyramidal manifestations. Kayser–Fleischer rings (see below) and blue lunulae may be present. Haemolysis may accompany hepatitis due to Wilson's disease. Renal tubular damage results in amino aciduria, phosphaturia, glycosuria and hypercalcuria, sometimes with metabolic bone disease.

Diagnosis

The typical diagnostic features of Wilson's disease include:

1   Kayser–Fleischer rings (produced by copper deposited at the rim of the cornea). Though always present when Wilson's disease has produced abnormalities of the CNS they may be absent in the younger patient with liver disease. They are virtually diagnostic of Wilson's but very rarely occur in other conditions in which chronic cholestasis leads to heavy accumulation of copper within the liver. K–F rings cannot be ruled out except by a slit-lamp examination of the eye.

2   Low serum ceruloplasmin and copper concentrations are found in 95% of all Wilson's disease, 85% of those presenting with liver disease and 10% of disease-free heterozygotes. A low ceruloplasmin can also occur due to the nephrotic syndrome, protein-losing enteropathy, fulminant hepatitis, active chronic hepatitis, and as a non-Wilsonian hereditary characteristic.

3   Raised urinary copper. This also occurs in other forms of chronic liver disease,

but the increase of 24-h urinary copper excretion during ingestion of D-penicilla-mine (1 g/day) is greater than in any of the other conditions in which baseline values are raised.

4   Liver histology reveals fatty change and nuclear vacuolation in the early stages, but extensive inflammation and fibrosis culminating in cirrhosis develops later. Special staining with rhodamine may detect excess copper but is less reliable than direct physiochemical determinations of the *hepatic copper concentration*. This is usually greater than 250 μg/g dry weight in Wilson's disease and less in heterozygotes (normal less than 50). Significantly elevated values are also seen as a consequence of chronic cholestasis.

5   Radio-copper studies involving administration of the radio active isotopes ^{64}Cu or ^{67}Cu, show that patients with Wilson's disease have (a) reduced hepatic incorporation of Cu into ceruloplasmin; (b) decreased hepatic uptake of Cu, and (c) prolonged turnover of Cu in the body. These tests are extremely complex and are seldom indicated clinically.

Treatment. Dimethylcysteine (D-penicillamine) in an initial dose of 20 mg/kg per day chelates copper and enhances its urinary excretion. By maintaining a negative copper balance this therapy usually arrests the disease and many features regress. If penicillamine is not tolerated, alternative treatment is with triethylenetetramine or zinc.

Prognosis. This is good once treatment is established. The disease is entirely preventable if diagnosed in presymptomatic siblings. Therefore suspect Wilson's disease if there is:

1   A family history of liver disease in a sibling.
2   Associated neurologic disease.
3   Hepatitis and haemolysis.
4   Chronic active hepatitis in a patient aged under 35 years.
5   Liver disease in the offspring of consanguineous parents.

Alpha$_1$-antitrypsin deficiency

Deficiency of serum α_1-antitrypsin (which normally constitutes 90% of the α_1 band on electrophoretic strips of serum protein) is associated with liver disease in early life and predisposes to pulmonary emphysema, especially in smokers, later. It is unknown why some individuals sharing the same deficiency may be entirely healthy while others suffer such widely differing diseases.

Clinical features. Classically cholestatic jaundice occurs in the neonatal period but fades spontaneously over subsequent months. It may be wrongly assumed that liver disease has resolved until 5–15 years later when the patient may present with recurrent jaundice, a variceal bleed or other signs of advanced chronic liver disease. In other patients cirrhosis occurs in adulthood with no previous episode of jaundice.

Still others have no history of liver disease and normal liver histology apart from the presence of characteristic inclusions.

Diagnosis. (a) Serum α_1-antitrypsin concentrations are subnormal. (b) Liver biopsy reveals periodic acid Schiff (PAS)-positive, diastase resistant globules of α_1-antitrypsin within hepatocytes, especially in periportal zones. Immunodiagnostic techniques confirm that these globules consist of immunoreactive α_1-antitrypsin. (c) Acid starch gel electrophoresis reveals a slow moving band of glycoprotein: these are characterized according to mobility as M=medium, S=slow, Z=very slow. Seriously affected individuals are usually homozygous for the protease inhibitor (Pi) type PiZZ though heterozygotes with SZ phenotypes may also be at increase risk of developing clinically apparent disease.

Treatment. No antidote is known to prevent progression of liver disease. Transplantation of the liver corrects the biochemical abnormality, confirming that the abnormality resides in the diseased liver. Affected relatives are counselled against tobacco smoking.

Non-viral infections and infestations of the liver

Liver abscess
In some patients with a liver abscess there may be no localizing signs which hint at liver involvement. It is, therefore, one of the causes one should seek to exclude early in investigating a patient with pyrexia of unknown origin. An amoebic abscess should be excluded if the patient has lived in or visited tropical and subtropical areas. The abscess commonly produces a large liquefied space in the upper and outer quadrant of the right lobe of liver. Needle aspiration produces material resembling 'anchovy sauce', but the infecting organism, *Entamoeba histolytica*, may be difficult to find unless material from the lining of the abscess cavity is available.

Bacterial infection is usually secondary to metastatic spread from infection elsewhere especially within the abdomen, such as from a peri-colic or appendix abscess. Ascending cholangitis may also lead to liver abscess formation, especially when cystic dilatation or obstruction of the bile ducts is present.

Primary bacterial causes of a liver abscess are rare but are particularly prone to occur with *Streptococcus milleri*. This organism may produce multiple liver and brain abscesses without any apparent source of the infection.

Diagnosis. It should be suspected in a patient with a swinging pyrexia who complains of right hypochondrial pain and who, on examination, has tender hepatomegaly and may be jaundiced. The abscess cavities may be demonstrated by ultrasonography or scintigraphic scanning. Amoebic serology may be valuable in areas where a rapid laboratory service exists. Otherwise needle aspiration of the cavities is recommended to provide material for a microbiological diagnosis.

Treatment. This involves effective antibiotics, coupled in some instances with drainage either at open surgery or by percutaneous needle aspiration. Amoebic abscesses usually respond satisfactorily to metronidazole combined with needle aspiration of the largest cavities, but occasionally additional amoebicidal drugs are required.

Helminthic infestation

Helminthic infestation of the liver in man may be due to the adult form of trematodes (fluke) and nematodes (roundworm) or to the larval stage of the cestode (tapeworm) which causes hydatid disease (Table 14.6). *Ascaris lumbricoides* usually produces symptoms confined to the gut or respiratory system but may rarely obstruct the bile ducts or pancreas.

Table 14.6. Parasites which may affect the liver.

		Host for	
		Adult stage	Ova or Larva
Protozoa (unicellular organisms)	*Entamoeba histolytica*		
Trematodes (flukes)	*Fasciola hepatica*	Sheep, man	Snail
	Clonorchis sinensis	Fish or man	Snail
	Schistosoma mansoni	Man	Snail
Nematodes (round worms)	*Ascaris lumbricoides*		
Cestodes (tapeworms)	*Echinoccus granulosus*	Dog	Sheep or man
	Echinococcus mutilocularis		

Fasciola hepatica

The adult worm inhabits the biliary tract of cattle, sheep and rarely man and sheds eggs which hatch in water where the snail *Lymnaea truncatula* provides the intermediate host. A typical way for human infestation to occur is by eating watercress picked from near a pond in a sheep field.

Clinical presentation. With heavy infestation a generalized systemic illness with fever, weight loss and jaundice with hepatitic features occurs during the initial migratory phase. Subsequently a cholestatic jaundice without systemic illness develops.

Diagnosis. A high eosinophilia should suggest the diagnosis. Confirmation is by detection of ova in the stool and by a strongly positive fasciola complement fixation titre.

Treatment. Bithionol has been used with success. Emetine hydrochloride has also been used successfully but has marked toxicity.

Clonorchis sinensis

This trematode infests more than 25% of the population of certain countries in the Far East. The adult worm inhabits the bile ducts and releases eggs which complete their life cycle via water snails. Human infestation is thought to result from eating raw fish.

Clinical presentation. Symptoms and signs of initial infestation are frequently mild or absent. The major problems involve the late complications of intrahepatic sclerosing cholangitis, intrahepatic biliary calculi, bacterial cholangitis, and cholangiocarcinoma.

Schistosomiasis (Bilharzia)

Infection by *S. mansoni* and *S. japonicum* may lead to features of intestinal and hepatic disease. *Schistosoma haematobium* most commonly produces haematuria by involving the genito-urinary tract. *Schistosoma mansoni* is endemic in many parts of Africa, the Middle East and South America; in Egypt the infection rate has been estimated to be as high as 80%. *Schistosoma japonicum* is confined to the Far East.

Life cycle. The intermediate host is a water snail. Cerceriae leave the snail and penetrate the human skin. Worms mature and form sexual pairings in the liver. They swim against the portal stream to lie in the veins of the splanchnic circulation. Eggs laid in the submucosa of the gut enter the faeces to complete the life cycle. Each worm pair may produce 300–3000 eggs per day for many years.

Clinical features. Acute: infection is usually symptomless. About 1 month later lymphadenopathy, hepatosplenomegaly and pruritus with rash, fever and diarrhoea may occur. Chronic sequelae: (a) Hepatic fibrosis occurs around ova deposited in the portal tracts to produce pre-sinusoidal portal hypertension. The severe peri-portal fibrosis was noted by Symmers (1904) who likened the portal tracts to a number of white clay pipe stems pushed through the liver at various angles ('pipe-stem fibrosis'). Patients with portal hypertension frequently present with bleeding varices as a primary manifestation of their disease. At this time splenomegaly is readily palpable. Jaundice and other signs or symptoms of liver disease are usually absent and hepatocellular function is well preserved. However, it is important to note that porto-systemic shunt operations are poorly tolerated by these patients and carry an unacceptably high risk of subsequent porto-systemic encephalopathy. Therefore local measures, e.g. sclerotherapy, to prevent recurrence of variceal haemorrhage are currently favoured.

(b) Intestinal: *S. mansoni* has a predilection for the inferior mesenteric vein and therefore affects the sigmoid colon and rectum, whereas *S. japonicum* migrates to the superior mesenteric veins and has a more marked effect on the small intestine. Migration of worms and deposition of ova within the intestinal wall may produce acute inflammatory and late fibrotic reactions. Bloody diarrhoea (dysentery) may be seen in the acute phase. Later, fibrosis may lead to small intestinal stricture formation and symptoms of subacute obstruction.

Diagnosis. Ova in the stool or in rectal biopsy tissue. Liver biopsy. Serological testing (detection of circulating antibody).

Treatment. Detection of ova in the stools of subjects in an endemic area is not regarded as sufficient indication for treatment because of the inevitability of re-infestation. When disease is symptomatic and progressive, treatment is recommended with praziquantel 50 mg/kg as a single dose initially. Niridazole is also effective, and well tolerated by children, but in adults with a significant porto-systemic collateral circulation its use carries an unacceptably high risk of toxicity to the central nervous system and liver. In patients who have established portal hypertension complicated by ascites and bleeding varices, it is probably best regarded as too late for anti-schistosomal chemotherapy.

Hydatid disease

Hydatid disease is caused by infection with the tapeworm *Echinococcus granulosus*. The disease is endemic in certain areas of the world, notably the Middle East, southern Europe, South America and Australasia. In Britain most cases occur in Wales.

Life cycle. Man (more commonly sheep and cattle) becomes infested by ingestion of embryophores eliminated in the faeces of dogs. The larva burrows through the intestinal mucosa to reach the portal vein and localizes in the liver where it proliferates by exogenous budding to form cysts. Less commonly cysts occur in the lungs or elsewhere. Dogs become infected when they eat viscera of sheep or cattle, offal or carcasses left in fields.

Clinical presentation. Cysts are usually asymptomatic for long periods before diagnosis. They may first be detected incidentally as hepatomegaly or an upper abdominal mass on physical examination. Alternatively the patient may become aware of abdominal discomfort or become jaundiced. Rarely cysts rupture into the peritoneal cavity, bile ducts or through the diaphragm into the lungs. Secondary infection with abscess formation may then follow. Rupture of the cyst may be accompanied by hypersensitivity reactions including anaphylactic shock.

Diagnosis. Hydatid disease should be considered when there is:
1   Calcification of round lesions in the liver on plain radiograph in a person who has visited an endemic area (Table 14.7).

Table 14.7. Differential diagnosis of calcified area(s) in the liver on plain radiograph.

Occasional
    Hydatid disease
    Primary liver cancer
    Secondary adenocarcinoma (pancreas, colon, apudomas)
Rare
    Haemangioma
    Amoebic abscess
    Gumma

---

2   One or more cystic lesions in the liver on ultrasonography or CAT scanning (Table 14.8). Calcification within the wall can be clearly seen on CAT scanning and the diagnosis is virtually certain if cysts are shown by either of these methods to contain septae or daughter cysts. Arteriography is not usually required; the cysts are apparent only as avascular areas with stretching of the vessels in surrounding parenchyma. Liver biopsy or needle aspiration is absolutely contraindicated because of the risk of inducing anaphylaxis and further dissemination of the disease.
3   Serological testing (detection of circulating antibody).
4   The Casoni test, involving intradermal injection of hydatid antigen, is insufficiently reliable and seldom used.

Prevention and treatment. Prevention is better than cure and since it requires only simple de-worming of dogs, its neglect by the farming community can hardly be excused. Often cysts appear harmless and can be left alone. Medical treatment is with albendazole or related antihelminthic agent. Since the cysts develop a thick wall, penetration by drugs is generally poor. Surgery is occasionally necessary for large cysts causing significant symptoms. A cryosurgical technique, whereby a funnel is frozen on to one wall of the cyst prior to its evacuation, has proved very successful in the prevention of intraoperative spread.

Table 14.8. Differential diagnosis of a cystic intrahepatic space-occupying lesion.

Common
    Simple cyst occurring in isolation or in association with renal and pancreatic cysts in
    familial polycystic disease
Occasional
    Hydatid cyst
    Neoplasm with liquefaction of necrotic centre
Rare
    Congenital cystic dilatation of the bile ducts (Caroli's disease)

Neoplasms of the liver and biliary system

The liver is commonly involved by metastatic carcinoma from all parts of the gastrointestinal tract (especially stomach, colon and pancreas) and also by carcinoma of other origins, especially breast and bronchus. Primary neoplasms are much rarer except in those parts of the world where primary liver cancer is common. The types of neoplasm and possible causes are listed in Tables 14.9 and 14.10.

Table 14.9. Hepatobiliary neoplasms.

Malignant		
Primary	occasional	Hepatocellular carcinoma (primary liver cancer)
		Hepatoblastoma (in children)
		Cholangiocarcinoma
		Carcinoma of the gallbladder
	rare	Angiosarcoma
		Endothelial haemangioendothelioma
Secondary		Neoplasm by metastasis
Benign		
		Hepatic adenoma
		Focal nodular hyperplasia
		Haemangioma

Hepatocellular carcinoma (primary liver cancer)

Although seemingly rare in Western society this is the commonest form of cancer in the world. Areas of high incidence are those in which a carrier status for hepatitis B is common. Cirrhosis is present in 70–80% of patients. Conversely, the risk of hepatocellular carcinoma in a patient with cirrhosis is 15–20%, and is probably higher when cirrhosis is due to hepatitis B or haemochromatosis.

Table 14.10. Inducing agents and promoters of hepatobiliary neoplasms.

	Tumour type
Hepatitis B	
Cirrhosis due to alcoholism, haemochromatosis	
Aflatoxin	Primary liver cancer
Androgenic steroids	
Arsenic (inorganic)	
Oestrogenic steroids	Adenoma
Thorotrast	
Clonorchiasis	Cholangiocarcinoma
Vinyl chloride	Angiosarcoma

Development of a primary liver cancer may present as a general clinical deterioration and weight loss in a patient with cirrhosis or the patient may have noticed a mass or pain in the right upper abdomen. The finding of an arterial bruit over liver or of blood-stained ascites should immediately suggest the diagnosis to the doctor.

Diagnosis. The following may be found helpful in diagnosis:

1 Alpha fetoprotein is a normal secretory product of human fetal liver, but serum levels fall rapidly after birth to normal adult levels (1–10 ng/ml). Derepression of the fetal genome in primary liver cancer is thought to be responsible for its reappearance in the serum. Extremely high levels (1000 ng/ml) in patients with known liver disease are virtually diagnostic of primary liver cancer, though they are also seen with germinal cell tumours of the testis and ovary. Slightly lower levels can also be seen in non-malignant liver disease. Unfortunately diagnostic elevations of fetoprotein occur in only 40% of Caucasians though in 80% of Africans with primary liver cancer.

2 Liver biopsy is the most direct method. It is useful to have a prior ^{99}Tc liver scan or ultrasound of the liver to assist in correct direction of the needle biopsy.

3 If needle biopsy is precluded a presumptive diagnosis of primary liver cancer can be based upon arteriographic findings (Fig. 6.14). or the pattern of scintigraphic scanning: a negative ('cold spot') filling defect on ^{99}Tc-colloid scan is frequently positive ('hot spot') on subsequent scanning with gallium or selenomethionine.

Treatment. Surgical resection: this is rarely possible because of late presentation. If a partial hepatic resection is feasible with complete tumour removal this is the treatment of choice.

Following transplantation, recurrence of the hepatic tumour often occurs despite apparent absence of spread at the time of organ replacement. Nevertheless in suitable candidates it may be the treatment of choice. Doxorubicin (adriamycin) has been used with some benefit in about 25% of treated cases. However, the overall results with both chemotherapy and radiotherapy are very disappointing.

Prognosis. Except when surgical removal of the tumour is achieved patients seldom survive more than 6 months from diagnosis.

Hepatocellular adenoma

This benign tumour is markedly more common since the advent of oral contraceptive therapy. The risk of developing hepatic adenoma is estimated to increase twenty-five-fold in a woman who has been 'on the pill' for 9 years. The patient who is quite well in other respects may develop pain in the right hypochondrium or become aware of a mass there.

Bleeding either into the tumour or into the peritoneum is a potentially serious complication. There may also be an extremely small risk of malignant transformation.

Diagnosis. This is done by a combination of ultrasound, scintigraphy, arteriography and biopsy.

Treatment. Withdrawal of contraceptive steroid will usually lead to spontaneous regression of the adenoma. If emergency surgery is essential to arrest bleeding, the minimum necessary should be done and the temptation to remove all the adenomata, which may be multiple, should be resisted.

Storage diseases causing hepatomegaly

Because of a deficiency of a degradative enzyme, there is excessive accumulation of its substrate. The nature of the accumulating substance determines the classification of the disorder. There are three main categories of which only the sphingolipoidoses and mucopolysaccharidoses primarily involve the spleen.

Glycogen storage disease

One of the enzymes required for normal breakdown of glycogen to glucose-1-phosphate and glucose is deficient. Glycogen accumulates in a variety of organs.

Von Gierke's disease (Type I glycogen storage disease)

Severe hepatomegaly (without splenomegaly) is present from the first few months of life. Hypoglycaemia occurs if feeding is delayed and necessitates continuous nocturnal intragastric feeding. Surgically created porto-caval shunts have conferred long-term benefit.

Sphingolipidoses

Sphingolipids occur as structural elements within membranes throughout the body. There are at least *ten* inherited disorders which have in common excessive accumulations of lipids containing ceramide. Heterozygotes can be identified and amniocentesis permits diagnosis in early pregnancy. Examples include Gaucher's disease, Niemann–Pick disease, Tay–Sachs disease and Fabry's disease.

Gaucher's disease

Described by Phillipe Gaucher (1882) as an 'epithelioma of the spleen', this is the commonest of the lipidoses. It is inherited as an autosomal recessive trait and is especially common among Ashkenazi Jews. It is caused by a deficiency of the enzyme glucocerebrosidase which catalyses the reaction:

$$\text{Glucocerebroside} + H_2O \xrightarrow{\text{glucocerebrosidase}} \text{glucose} + \text{ceramide}$$

Glucocerebroside is derived from catabolism of cell membranes, especially senescent erythrocytes and leucocytes. Deficient catabolism results in their accumulation within lysosomes to produce the characteristic 'Gaucher cells'.

Clinical features. The spleen and liver enlarge and there may be erosion of the cortices of the long bones and pelvis. In certain subtypes there is also cerebral involvement. The patient may first become aware of an abdominal mass due to splenomegaly. Investigations may show a marked thrombocytopenia and elevation of serum acid phosphatase. Bony involvement leads to pain and spontaneous fractures. X-ray of the femur may show the classical appearance of expansion of the cortex resembling an Ehrlenmeyer flask. Pingueculae occur in the eye. Portal hypertension is rarely troublesome.

Diagnosis. Adult: microscopic examination of cells aspirated from bone marrow, liver or spleen shows large cells of the reticuloendothelial system which have a fibrillar cytoplasm, described as 'wrinkled tissue paper' (Gaucher cells), in contrast to the 'foamy' cells seen in other lipidoses. Assay of glucocerebrosidase activity can be performed on liver biopsy cells or leucocytes from peripheral blood.

Antenatal detection of heterozygotes and homozygotes can be achieved by amniocentesis.

Treatment. No effective treatment is currently available. Preliminary experimental work suggests that infusions of glucocerebrosidase may be able to compensate for the inherited deficiency.

Transplantation of the liver and pancreas

Liver transplantation has been successfully established as an important form of treatment in a few centres in the world. Each candidate has to be assessed individually but the best candidates are young, have disease confined to the liver, good cardiovascular and pulmonary function, a strong desire to live, and a prognosis which is otherwise hopeless. Thus children with inborn errors of metabolism such as α_1-antitrypsin deficiency or young mothers with primary biliary cirrhosis are examples of potentially good candidates. Malignancy is generally regarded as a contraindication, although for primary hepatocellular carcinoma with no evidence of extrahepatic spread it can achieve acceptable results.

The outcome depends on the selection of patients, the skill of the surgeon and his supporting staff, the resilience of the patient, and careful monitoring of postoperative immunosuppressive therapy. Because of the need for good compliance with medical advice and drug treatment after transplantation, patients who have suffered from alcoholism during the previous 2 years are generally regarded as unsuitable candidates.

About 40–60% of patients survive more than 1 year but the proportion varies considerably between centres.

Pancreatic transplantation is at an earlier phase of development. Although some grafts survive and function for more than 1 year these are generally used for their endocrine activity, as in diabetics with renal failure who have combined kidney and pancreas transplantation. Pancreatic exocrine insufficiency is not a sufficient indication for attempted pancreatic transplantation.

Chapter 15
Malabsorption

The small intestine is indispensable, whereas life is possible without the stomach or colon. One third of the small intestine can be removed and one half is usually the upper limit of safety, though patients where two-thirds have been excised have survived. The length is variable: it is longer in races who eat much roughage but shorter in females. The length of the living bowel is different from the toneless gut of the operating theatre or dissecting room where it averages 6 m (20 ft). In the living, it is about 2.6 m, and a tube 3 m (10 ft) long may protrude from the mouth and the anus simultaneously. The surface area of the small intestine with the valvulae conniventes and villi each lined by about 600 microvilli is the size of a tennis court.

Certain segments have special functions (Fig. 15.1): that the jejunum is the main site of absorption is suggested by its anatomy, by the surface area being greater, the mucosal folds more numerous and villi better developed, and its increased motility especially of non-propulsive segmental movements; being first reached by food, it absorbs most substances. The ileum acts as a reserve when large amounts of fat or other substances are fed and when the upper gut is damaged by disease; it is also the special site of absorption of bile salts and vitamin B_{12}. The normal function of the small intestine depends upon the conditions shown in Table 15.1 and these are considered elsewhere.

Disease or surgical resection leads to steatorrhoea and also metabolic consequences: loss of weight, anaemia due to deficient absorption of iron, folic acid and vitamin B_{12}, water and electrolyte disturbances and loss of sodium and potassium, oedema of the legs due to a low serum albumin, rickets in children and osteomalacia in adults due to defective absorption of fat-soluble vitamin D and perhaps haemorrhage from defective absorption of vitamin K—also fat soluble. Many diseases cause malabsorption (Table 15.2); diarrhoea is not always present and some present with one of the nutritional or metabolic consequences just mentioned. The prototype and probably commonest form of malabsorption is adult coeliac disease (non-tropical sprue; idiopathic steatorrhoea; primary malabsorption syndrome).

Morphology of the small intestinal mucosa
Normal villi (Fig. 7.3) are long and slender, varying in height between 320 μm and 510 μm. Their formation is a cause of wonder, for the columnar epithelial cells which cover them are formed by dividing cells in the glands of Lieberkühn and ascend from the crypts like steps of a moving staircase. Their span of life is probably

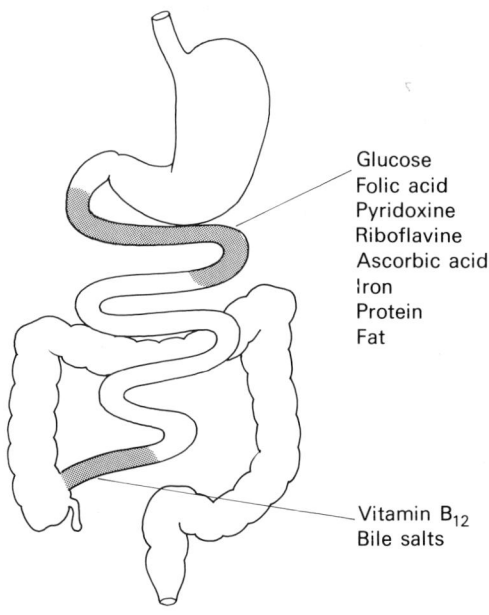

Glucose
Folic acid
Pyridoxine
Riboflavine
Ascorbic acid
Iron
Protein
Fat

Vitamin B$_{12}$
Bile salts

Fig. 15.1. Absorption in the small intestine.

2–3 days before being cast off at the tip of the villus. These cells, passing up the villi to die at their tips, are the essential functional units and not only absorb nutrients but also synthesize protein and other substances. Between these are the goblet cells, shaped like a brandy glass, secreting mucus which lubricates the food and protects the surface from damage. At the base of the crypts are the Kultschitzky cells, the granules of which contain 5-hydroxytryptamine; carcinoid tumours originate from these endocrine cells. Other cells are of more speculative origin. The Paneth cells are confined to the small intestine and contain numerous rather coarse granules but their purpose is unknown. Similarly, mast cells are a mystery and may secrete heparin and histamine and may perhaps be concerned with intestinal motility.

The morphology of the small intestinal mucosa varies according to the part of the bowel. Duodenal villi are broader (leaf-shaped) and more branched than the long slender finger-like villi seen in the jejunum and Brunner's glands may be seen in the duodenal biopsy specimen. Villi are shorter and broader in the ileum and relatively more goblet cells are present; there may be more collections of lymphoid tissue and sometimes the villi may be absent.

The shape of the normal jejunal villus (Fig. 7.3) may vary from being finger-like to leaf-like in the normal. The lamina propria forms a structural support for the villi and contains plasma cells, lymphocytes, macrophages, fibroblasts and capillaries. The immune mechanism of the gut originates here, for the B-lymphocytes are conceived and the plasma cells produce IgA. IgA precursor cells are also elaborated in the Peyer's patches and other lymphoid tissue. Intestinal IgA provides an

Table 15.1. The function of the small intestine depends upon the following.

Normal structure
Normal movement
Normal flow of bile, bile salts and pancreatic juice
Freedom from bacteria
An intact stomach
Intestinal hormones

'immunological barrier' at the mucosal surface and so has an important protective function.

The microvilli (brush border) are digestive units containing enzymes such as disaccharidases (e.g. lactase hydrolyses lactose to glucose and fructose). They increase the surface of the epithelial cells by a factor of 40 and the half-life of the brush border is 6–14 h. The conception of digestion taking place at or within the brush border has replaced the idea of a special enzyme-containing 'succus entericus' causing digestion in the gut lumen. Disorders of the microvilli cause a number of diseases: amino acid malabsorption, cystinuria and Hartnup's syndrome, familial vitamin B_{12} and malabsorption.

Table 15.2. Causes of malabsorption.

Common
    Coeliac disease
    Crohn's disease
    Stagnant bowel syndrome
    After gastric operations
Occasional
    Pancreatic disease
    Hepatobiliary disease
    Drugs, e.g. neomycin, cholestyramine
    Tropical sprue (in UK)
    Dermatitis herpetiformis
Rare
    Whipple's disease
    Lymphoma of small intestine
    Giardia lamblia
    Mesenteric ischaemia
    Thyrotoxicosis
    Hypogammaglobulinaemia and other rare disorders
        of the small intestine (Chapter 16)

Coeliac disease

Coeliac (from the Greek meaning belly) disease has undergone much renaming, having previously been called coeliac sprue, idiopathic steatorrhoea, coeliac syndrome, idiopathic sprue and non-tropical sprue, and gluten-induced entero-pathy.

It occurs in 0.1–0.2% of the population and often presents in children as soon as they start eating gluten; however, it commonly starts in adult life, equally in men and women; only about one-third give a history of coeliac disease in childhood. It is sometimes familial.

The small intestine looks normal, except for a constant change in the jejunal mucosa—sometimes involving the ileum as well (Fig. 15.2). There is partial or

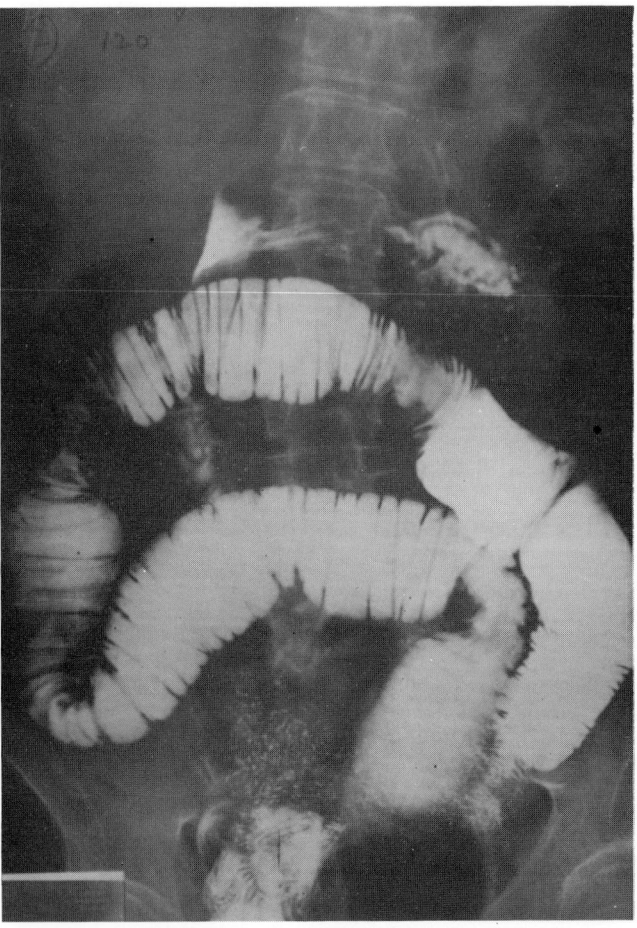

Fig. 15.2. Dilated jejunum (width greater than 3 cm) in adult coeliac disease.

complete atrophy of the villi (Fig. 7.3d). This damage to the epithelial cells and to the microvilli of the brush border where enzymes are synthesized causes defective absorption of all nutrients—fat, protein, carbohydrates, vitamins, minerals and also water.

Pathogenesis

Discovery of the cause of coeliac disease is one bonus to balance the disasters of the Second World War; for Dutch workers (Kamer and Weigers) noticed that children with coeliac disease improved when the Dutch were unable to get bread and relapsed when bread was eaten again. Wheat or rye flour is usually the cause and the offending portion of the flour lies not in the starch but in the protein fraction, gluten. Gluten, from the chemist's point of view, is a vague term applied to the tenacious almost tasteless substance obtained by washing flour in water. Several different types of gluten occur in nature and it is curious that wheat and rye flour which both cause coeliac disease also make dough suitable for bread-making. Rice and maize, although containing gluten, can be eaten by coeliac children without ill-effect and do not make dough; without dough, bread loses its elastic quality and becomes crumbly like cake.

The cause of the toxicity of gluten is unknown. Allergy is possible, although no other allergic tendencies occur. Intestinal infusion of α-gliadin (a breakdown product of gluten) certainly provokes a reaction in patients where gluten withdrawal has restored the jejunal mucosa to normal; however, nothing is seen before 4 h and mucosal damage usually occurs by 18 h; this excludes immediate hypersensitivity and is too soon for delayed hypersensitivity; the timing suggests a local Arthus type of reaction.

That the disease is due to an abnormal immunological response is also indicated by the following: the jejunal plasma cells are defective in producing IgA—an immunoglobulin which normally protects the gut against bacteria and toxic substances; antibodies to some fractions of the gluten are found in the serum and faeces; serum complement levels may be low; there is atrophy of lymphoid tissue as in the spleen, which may be reduced to a small fibrous organ; and malignant lymphomatous change may take place in the bowel.

Clinical features. Defective function of the small intestine not only results in fatty diarrhoea, but has widespread effects throughout the body from nutritional, haematological and electrolytic disturbances. The spectrum of symptoms is therefore wide (Table 15.3) and it may mimic many diseases (Table 15.4) and, where diarrhoea is minimal or absent, escape detection until especially considered. Patients may present with any of three groups of symptoms.

Diarrhoea. The frequency of defaecation may not be more than two or three times daily and so longstanding that the patient has accepted this as normal; he will reply yes when asked if his bowels are normal, so the question about the number of actions

Table 15.3. Symptoms of coeliac disease.

Common
    Anaemia: macrocytic; microcytic; dimorphic
    Glossitis
    Weight loss
Occasional
    Rashes
    Pigmentation
    Oedema (due to hypoproteinaemia)
    Tetany
    Osteomalacia
    Purpura
Rare
    Spinal cord degeneration
    Peripheral neuritis
    Psychosis
    Diffuse interstitial fibrosis
    Arteritis
    Malignant change (usually lymphoma)

---

daily must be specific. There may be episodes of severe diarrhoea with prostration. Diarrhoea is painless and an observant patient may have noticed pale, foul-smelling stools, or be surprised by their gargantuan size; they may be seen floating in the lavatory pan and be difficult to flush away, and greasiness may be felt through the toilet paper.

Table 15.4. Malabsorption: the great mimic. Clinical conditions which coeliac disease may resemble.

Pernicious anaemia
Rheumatic disorders (due to pains from osteomalacia)
Addison's disease
Colitis
Nervous diarrhoea
Skin conditions
Neurological problems
Behaviour disorders
Intestinal obstruction
Malignant disease
(It may also present as a problem of amenorrhoea, infertility, or
    hypothermia.)

General ill-health. Lassitude, loss of weight, sore tongue, and symptoms of anaemia often dominate the clinical picture. The anaemia is often macrocytic like pernicious anaemia, but due to lack of folic acid rather than vitamin B_{12}. A dimorphic picture is seen when iron deficiency is present as well.

Systemic disease. Tetany, symptoms associated with osteomalacia, or neurological disorders resembling subacute combined degeneration of the cord sometimes are the main concern.

Signs of disease

No abnormal signs may be found, but most are undernourished and some are pigmented and small, particularly if it followed coeliac disease in childhood. The tongue may be smooth and glazed from glossitis, usually from deficiency of the vitamin B group such as nicotinic acid, riboflavine, folic acid, or B_{12}. Rashes, either eczema or dermatitis herpetiformis, are occasionally seen and pellagra may be provoked by the sun. The blood pressure is often low, and dehydration occurs when diarrhoea is severe. The abdomen may be distended in the presence of excess fluid, and gas in the small gut may result in a doughy feeling on palpation. Sigmoidoscopy is normal or shows slight erythema suggestive of proctitis, due to irritation from fatty acids.

Diagnosis

Coeliac disease can easily be missed especially if no-one looks at the stools from patients with diarrhoea. It must be considered in patients with chronic ill-health especially with any history of glossitis or anaemia. Diarrhoea is a helpful pointer but not necessary; a few have a normal bowel action and may be constipated. The criteria for diagnosis are given in Table 15.5.

Proof of gluten sensitivity is essential. The patient should be re-assessed after 3 or 6 months and preferably another biopsy done to show improvement. Sensitivity to gluten can be proved by arranging a xylose test (p. 95) and/or jejunal biopsy before and after reintroducing gluten (or gliadin). Deterioration in both occurs within a few days.

Differential diagnosis

Many patients with coeliac disease are wrongly labelled as it can mimic so many other disorders (Table 15.4) and there are many causes of malabsorption (Table 15.2). Some or all of the symptoms are seen with structural abnormalities of the gastrointestinal tract such as Crohn's disease, stricture or fistula, but then abdominal pain is often marked.

Chronic pancreatitis may resemble it but the glucose tolerance test is often abnormal whereas the curve may be low or flat in adult coeliac disease.

Table 15.5. Criteria for diagnosing coeliac disease.

Specific
1   A flat jejunal biopsy.
2   Response to the gluten-free diet.
Non-specific
1   The serum folate is low (below 3 ng/ml) (other incidental causes for
     this, apart from disease of the jejunum where it is absorbed, are
     dietetic as stores of folic acid in the body only last a few weeks, drugs
     and systemic diseases like rheumatoid arthritis or neoplasm).
2   Wide coils of jejunum (more than 3 cm) seen by barium progress
     meal or floculation of barium due to excess of mucus (rare with
     modern barium suspension) within 2 h (Fig. 15.3).
3   Abnormal xylose excretion test.
4   Daily faecal fat excretion of more than 7 g (25 mmol).
5   Serum gluten antibodies are present in 90% coeliacs but also in 20%
     normals.
6   IgG and IgM are sometimes low.

Treatment

The basic therapy is dietetic. Exclusion of wheat and rye flour eliminates bread, cakes, pastry, gravy and soups thickened with flour, together with buns and biscuits and so on. Gluten is separated from wheat on a commercial basis and the product, pure wheat starch, can readily be obtained. The bread, though palatable, is less easy to make than ordinary bread, being more crumbly and heavier because of the lack of the dough-making property of gluten; it goes stale sooner than ordinary bread, though keeps fresh in a deep freeze for months. Some make their own bread and cakes; others arrange for a local bakery to do it. Gluten-free foods (already made) can be bought. In the UK, National Health Service patients can be prescribed the following: wheat starch and other gluten-free flours, gluten-free bread, and gluten-free biscuits.

The diet is easy in the home, for all natural foods can be eaten and the special flour is used only for baking bread and cooking. Difficulty arises in restaurants as flour is used in cooking in so many ways. Processed foods and drinks frequently contain flour and the list of ingredients on the label should be scrutinized. Commercial names are not infallible and one patient failed to respond to the diet because of a taste for so-called arrow-root biscuits; after many months it was discovered that these consisted mainly of wheat flour.

The gluten-free diet is successful in 80% of patients or more and those that will not respond cannot be distinguished at the time of diagnosis. Sometimes the reason for failure is dietetic, as gluten may not have been completely excluded or the patient may not have dieted long enough (3 or 6 months). Other reasons are given in Table 15.6.

Table 15.6. Reasons for failure to respond to gluten-free diet.

Faulty diet
Extensive mucosal involvement (including ileum)
Pancreatic atrophy
Malignant change
Wrong diagnosis
Unknown

Response to the gluten-free diet is noted by the return of normal colour to the stools, disappearance of diarrhoea and increase in weight—a most important sign. The jejunal biopsy appearance improves and may become normal. Fat absorption becomes normal and also the small intestine as seen later by barium meal. If no response, admit the patient to hospital for assessment. This will avoid depriving him unnecessarily of the pleasures of the table by prolonging a useless diet.

Those who fail to respond to the diet should be treated by a diet high in protein, usually 100–120 g, and low in fat, 50 g or less; also folic acid 5 mg once daily by mouth. Calcium salts have a constipating effect and the following mixture can be given: calcium phosphate 2 g, calcium lactate 2 g, calcium carbonate 2 g. This is prescribed as a powder, 6 g or more being taken three times daily, or as often as necessary. Occasionally a short course of a broad spectrum antibiotic may result in improvement with some increase in weight, perhaps because the small bowel is cleared of bacteria. Corticosteroid drugs improve the function of the small intestine and prednisolone up to 15 mg daily can be tried if all other measures fail.

Multiple vitamin and other deficiencies are so common that adult coeliac disease provides one of the few rational indications for 'shotgun' therapy. These patients might therefore be given iron, calcium, vitamin preparations and so on. However, this is unnecessary if the diet is successful and prescribing is tempered by the knowledge that few take drugs regularly and conscientiously. The better policy is to see patients regularly in follow-up clinics and to check their blood counts, the levels of calcium, alkaline phosphatase, folic acid and B_{12}, and to prescribe only when the need arises. Otherwise a false sense of security may be given. Patients may be helped by joining the Coeliac Society (PO Box 181, London NW2 2QY).

Prognosis
Mortality was 20% before the gluten-free diet but is now almost nil in gluten-sensitive cases. Death was caused by haemorrhage from vitamin K deficiency, or volvulus of the large and redundant sigmoid colon; respiratory and other infections including tuberculosis were also a hazard. Some have died from hypothermia, easily missed with an ordinary thermometer. Malignant change in the

small intestine may develop in longstanding cases though fortunately rarely; raised IgA levels sometimes accompany a lymphoma.

Tropical sprue

Tropical sprue is a malabsorption syndrome with no discoverable cause, occurring in people living in or visiting the tropics; the main endemic areas include the Indian subcontinent, South-East Asia, Indonesia and certain islands of the Caribbean. The cause is environmental and is consistent with the initial lesion being an infection of the jejunum, complicated by a progressive folate deficiency.

Symptoms

The onset may be sudden with acute watery diarrhoea, vomiting, colic and fever, but often is insidious. There is then fatty diarrhoea with stools that are frothy and difficult to flush away. Loss of appetite followed by loss of weight occurs with a striking lethargy, often with depression. Glossitis presenting with crops of small painful ulcers involving first the edge and later the whole of the tongue and inside of mouth is seen in many after 2 months. Megaloblastic anaemia usually from folate, but sometimes B_{12}, deficiency is common. Spontaneous remission usually occurs after leaving the tropics but sometimes symptoms persist for many years in a temperate region.

Diagnosis

This is made by three criteria after excluding intestinal parasites:
1   Abnormal jejunal biopsy. Occasionally, there is villous atrophy but more often the changes are less severe—partial villous atrophy—compared with adult coeliac disease. Eosinophils may be present.
2   The presence of malabsorption (increased faecal fat and abnormal xylose excretion).
3   Nutritional deficiencies such as low serum folate and vitamin B_{12}.
    The barium meal shows changes similar to adult coeliac disease with thickened transverse mucosal folds and dilatation of the small bowel.
    Diagnosis may be confused because malnutrition and minor abnormalities of jejunal biopsy are common in the tropics, perhaps due to diet, bowel bacteria or parasites. The suggestion has been made that tropical sprue is not a distinct entity but merely one end of a spectrum, but epidemiological evidence is against this. Malabsorption may occur in heavy infections with *Giardia lamblia*, intestinal moniliasis, and helminthic infections like strongyloidiasis, ancylostomiasis and intestinal capillariasis, but in these xylose absorption is usually normal; mucosal changes are less severe and folate deficiency is not a feature.

Treatment

The effect of folic acid is dramatic with early relief of symptoms and improvement in intestinal function and structure. Vitamin B_{12} deficiency must be excluded and the vitamin given if necessary, otherwise subacute combined degeneration of the cord could be induced. Folic acid 5 mg daily is sufficient and could be continued for 6 weeks. A wide-spectrum antibiotic such as tetracycline must also be given for at least two weeks. A complete remission is expected in most patients.

The stagnant bowel syndrome (Blind loop syndrome)

The small intestine is almost sterile, for most organisms swallowed with food are destroyed by the acid gastric juice. The normal clearance mechanisms are:

1 A changing pH (due to hydrochloric acid and the alkaline pancreatic juice).
2 Peristaltic sweeps.
3 Immune defence mechanisms.

Any resident microflora increase in concentration on the way down the small intestine and both aerobic and anaerobic organisms are present in the ileum. These and other antigens stimulate the immune mechanisms of the gut and may have beneficial effects by synthesizing nutrients such as folate and vitamin K, but in excess may harm the patient by taking up nutrients or deconjugating bile salts.

Stagnation of bowel contents, as occurs above a stricture, encourages a luxuriant growth of these bacteria; such infection also happens when other hollow tubes such as the ureter or bile ducts are obstructed. A similar situation arises when peristalsis is defective as in systemic sclerosis and occasionally in an apparently normal small bowel in the elderly. Bacterial excess in the small bowel may cause a clinical picture like that of adult coeliac disease except that deficiency of vitamin B_{12} is characteristic; the cause for this is not clear as there is no evidence of enteritis, and jejunal biopsy is normal. Bacteria either compete for vitamin B_{12} or produce metabolites which interfere with its absorption.

Causes (Fig. 15.3)

Strictures: These are usually due to Crohn's disease or to tuberculosis (usually secondary to lung lesions, but less common since effective chemotherapy of this disease). Tablets, like enteric-coated potassium chloride can damage the small bowel and cause strictures.

Blind loops: These usually result from fistulae or operations which bypass loops of bowel, and both are often due to Crohn's disease.

A blind loop may form after a Polya partial gastrectomy due to obstruction at the exit of the afferent loop from narrowing due to fibrosis.

Gastro-jejuno-colic fistula: This nearly always occurs after operations on the stomach by perforation of a stomal ulcer into the colon; other causes are malignant growth, Crohn's disease, or foreign bodies. Food does not, as once thought, pass directly from the stomach into the colon. It goes the usual way, as does barium; a barium meal rarely shows the fistula because a flap of mucosa prevents it entering

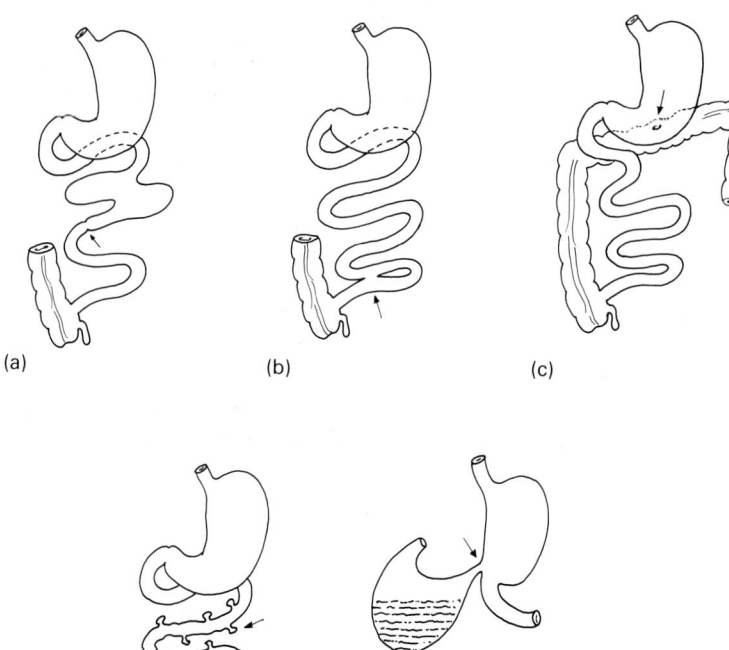

(a)   (b)   (c)

(e)

(d)

Fig. 15.3. Causes of stagnant bowel syndrome: (a) stricture; (b) fistula; (c) gastrocolic fistula; (d) diverticulosis of small intestine; (e) obstruction to outlet of afferent loop after Polya gastrectomy.

the colon. Diagnosis is made by barium enema when the barium immediately enters the stomach or jejunum, and symptoms are caused by the jejunum being contaminated by colonic bacteria. The breath sometimes has a faecal odour. An operation to close it is usually necessary.

Diverticulosis of the small intestine. This occurs in middle or old age and the diverticula are often small and multiple; their narrow mouths lead to stagnation so that bacteria flourish and infect the small intestine. It is often symptomless though may cause vague dyspepsia. Complications as with other diverticula are infection, haemorrhage or perforation, but are unusual. Sometimes the only symptom is megaloblastic anaemia.

Diagnosis

1 Barium progress meal usually shows the structural abnormality.

2 The serum B_{12} should be low. Absorption of radioactive B_{12} (p. 44) is depressed and this can be temporarily improved by an antibiotic.

3 Tests for detecting the presence of bacteria in the small intestine are described on p. 101.

Prevention and treatment

The surgeon, now aware of the complications from blind loops and stagnant areas, does his best to avoid causing them when operating upon the bowel. Steatorrhoea may be controlled by a high protein, low fat diet, but the gluten-free diet is useless. A small dose of an antibiotic taken continuously or intermittently may help and the anaemia responds to injections of vitamin B_{12}. Fortunately only a few patients with a stagnant bowel develop symptoms and the reason for this is unknown.

Chapter 16
Occasional and Rare Disorders of the Small Intestine

Protein-losing enteropathy (PLE)

Protein-losing enteropathy may complicate a number of diseases (Table 16.1). The fact that protein can be lost into the bowel from inflammatory and other lesions previously escaped notice because albumin is digested and amino acids formed from it are reabsorbed, so faecal nitrogen is not raised. A small amount of protein leaks into the normal bowel and PLE only develops when the loss in the stool is so great that the liver is unable to synthesize new protein rapidly enough, so a low serum albumin results. The proteins most affected are those where the molecule is small (Fig. 16.1); this together with the slow turnover especially applies to albumin. Rarely, if the leak is severe and especially if the small intestinal lymphatics are blocked as in lymphangiectasia or nodular lymphoid hyperplasia, an immunodeficiency syndrome is caused. A guide to this is lymphocytopenia; there may be a low IgG and IgA but a normal IgM and skin anergy. Impaired homograft rejection also results, and tying the thoracic duct has been suggested as a preliminary to transplant in humans.

Symptoms. Patients usually present with oedema and ascites—the result of hypoproteinaemia. Otherwise there will be the symptoms of the underlying disorder.

Investigations. Protein loss can be demonstrated by giving a variety of radioactive—labelled agents intravenously and then measuring radioactivity in the stool. Those commonly used are radioactive chromium chloride and polyvinylpyrrolidone.

Measuring the faecal excretion rate of α_1-antitrypsin can be used as a simple guide to the severity of PLE; as its name and function suggests, it is resistant to digestion by pancreatic protease and when leaking into the gut appears unchanged in the stool.

Treatment. The first problem is to treat the underlying disease. Symptomatic measures consist of a low salt diet, diuretics and perhaps intravenous albumin.

Disaccharide intolerance

Certain patients with abdominal distension and diarrhoea have been found to lack specific enzymes in the intestinal cells. These enzymes split disaccharides to monosaccharides (Fig. 16.2) which are then absorbed. Lactase deficiency is the

Table 16.1. Causes of protein-losing enteropathy.

Common
    Ulcerative colitis
    Crohn's disease
Occasional
    Coeliac disease
    Carcinoma of stomach or colon
    Congestive cardiac failure
    Acute infectious enteritis
    Dysentery
Rare
    Whipple's disease
    Lymphangiectasia
    Ménétrièr's disease (large gastric folds)
    Allergic gastroenteropathy
    Constrictive pericarditis
    Nodular lymphoid hyperplasia

---

commonest example; lactose taken in milk cannot be split into glucose and galactose so that it remains unabsorbed in the small intestine where it causes diarrhoea either by osmosis, like magnesium sulphate when used as a purgative, or by providing a nutrient for bacterial growth which causes irritant products from sugar fermentation; hence the terms osmotic and fermentative diarrhoea. A similar deficiency

Loss from gut depends upon molecular size

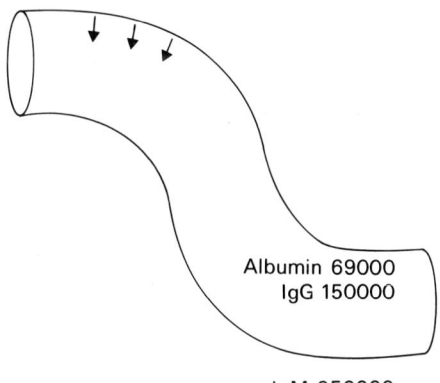

Fig. 16.1. Protein-losing enteropathy. Albumin is mainly lost because of its smaller molecular size.

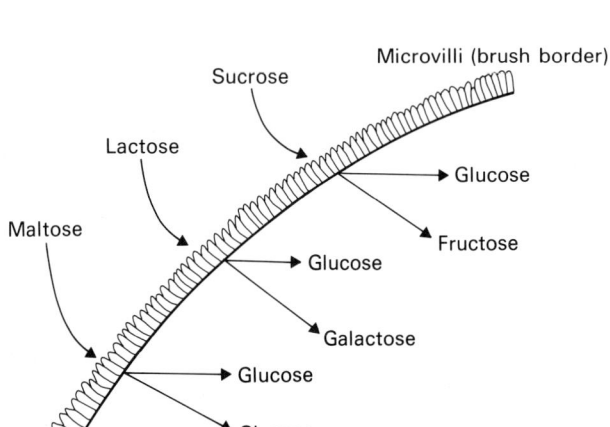

Fig. 16.2. Disaccharides are split into monosaccharides at the brush border.

may very rarely affect enzymes which split sucrose to fructose and glucose, and maltose to two molecules of glucose.

It is usually seen in infants and causes failure to thrive, dehydration, and frequent watery and frothy stools; secondary sugar (usually lactose) malabsorption may follow recovery from another illness like coeliac disease which damages the mucosa, or (temporarily) after simple gastroenteritis in infants. In adults the watery diarrhoea with distension, pain and borborygmi can be mistaken for the irritable bowel syndrome. Some have noticed that milk upsets them.

There is a marked racial variation; lactase activity in the brush border of the intestinal cell persists into adult life in northern European populations, perhaps because they continue to drink milk—life-long suckling by remote control—whereas it is the exception in tropical populations. Adult Asians may develop symptoms when changing to a Western (e.g. milk) diet.

Diagnosis. In infants and childhood stool pH (less than 5.5) and the presence of reduced substances, where testing with Clinitest tablets shows 0.5% or more reducing substances, is strongly suggestive.

In adults a simple screening test is to give 50 g lactose in a fruit drink: lactase deficiency is virtually excluded if there is neither abdominal rumblings nor diarrhoea within 6 h. The lactose tolerance test consists of giving 50 g lactose and then measuring the blood glucose as for a glucose tolerance test: in lactase deficiency, the blood sugar (glucose) fails to rise more than 20 mg/100 ml. Another method is to give a mixture of lactose and barium as a barium meal and this shows a rapid passage of barium. Lactase can be estimated in a sample of jejunal mucosa obtained by biopsy but its distribution may be patchy and a deficiency in one specimen does not prove the diagnosis.

Treatment. The offending disaccharide is withdrawn; in lactase deficiency the diet excludes milk and milk products. Lactose-free milk substitutes will be necessary for infants. If diarrhoea disappears, proof that the diagnosis is correct can be obtained when relapse is caused by giving the patient lactose again—preferably without his knowledge. Lactase deficiency explains most cases of milk intolerance.

Diabetic diarrhoea

Some diabetics complain of bouts of diarrhoea for no obvious reason: often mild, but sometimes so frequent as to disorganize the patient's life. The diarrhoea is often nocturnal: then the bowels are quiescent during the day but nights are dreaded because of the risk of incontinence. Pain is unusual and the stools watery and copious. Sometimes there may be mild steatorrhoea. Barium meal may show gastric stasis, but small intestine and colon are normal as is jejunal biopsy. The cause is probably a neuropathy involving the autonomic nerves of the gut, similar to the neurogenic bladder, impotency and postural hypotension. The diarrhoea is intractable to treatment and not often cured by proper control of the diabetes. Antispasmodic drugs and codeine should be tried. An antibiotic such as tetracycline is sometimes helpful, presumably because of some additional infection of the small intestine, and can be continued in a small dose indefinitely.

Meckel's diverticulum

Meckel's diverticulum may be a short stumpy pouch or a long tube resembling a duplication of the bowel, situated 30–100 cm from the ileo-caecal valve. It is a true diverticulum with smooth muscle in its walls and the most frequent malformation of the alimentary tract; it is slightly more common in men and its incidence varies between 1–2%. Sometimes the mucosa contains glandular tissue of gastric or duodenal type which secretes hydrochloric acid; colonic mucosa or pancreatic tissue may also occur. It is due to persistence of the proximal end of the vitelline duct.

It is symptomless unless a complication arises. Inflammation (diverticulitis) is commonest and is usually wrongly diagnosed as appendicitis. Perforation is more dangerous than with appendicitis because it lies freely in the peritoneum and general peritonitis occurs. Intestinal obstruction may develop when the tip is adherent to an adjacent structure, for this creates a snare for loops of bowel. Sometimes it becomes invaginated and causes intussusception of the ileum, which may be diagnosed radiologically as an intralumina elongated filling defect. The secretion of hydrochloric acid may cause a typical peptic ulcer and is subject to the same complications as duodenal ulcer, but haemorrhage causes red blood in the stool and not melaena. However, Meckel's diverticulum is usually a coincidental and unimportant finding at laparotomy. It is often difficult to detect by barium progress meal or rarely by scanning (Fig. 7.8b). In fact, when it causes trouble, it is rarely if ever diagnosed before operation.

Intussusception

A portion of the intestine, usually the ileum near the ileo-caecal valve, is invaginated into the lumen of the bowel immediately below (Fig. 16.3). Infants are more affected than adults, and the symptoms are then acute compared with their chronic nature in adults.

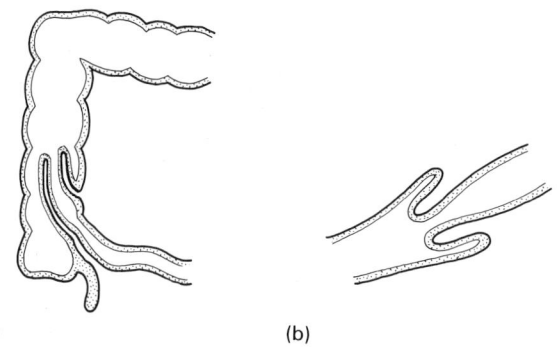

(a)   (b)

Fig. 16.3. Types of intussusception. (a) ileo-caecal, (b) entero-enteric.

Chronic intussusception
This in adults occurs more commonly in men than in women; a growth either benign or malignant usually provokes it and forms the apex of the invaginated gut. Symptoms point to intermittent obstruction, often with blood and mucus in the stools. Sometimes a palpable mass can be felt; this varies in size and may disappear completely when the bowel becomes disinvaginated, only to recur at a later date. Owing to the obstruction, colicky pain recurs and there may be constipation and vomiting, or acute obstruction may supervene. Operation is then indicated and the intussusception may be reduced or resected and careful search made for a cause, such as a polyp.

Congenital abnormalities

The following are usually confined to the newly born: atresia and stenosis affecting the oesophagus, duodenum or small intestine, and imperforate anus. In the adult, malrotation may cause confusion perhaps if the caecum and appendix are in the upper abdomen but generally these abnormalities are symptomless except when bands produce obstruction. Meckel's diverticulum and Hirschsprung's disease are considered elsewhere.

Cholera

This most savage of all intestinal infections is still common in the East and with modern air travel might occur anywhere; this risk is small, however, as carriers of *Vibrio cholerae* are almost unknown. Incubation period is from a few hours to 10 days. The disease results from faulty sanitation and especially occurs where a river acts both as a sewer and supply of drinking water. Outbreaks have occurred in places of religious assembly where pilgrims bathe in holy water, which is also the source of their water supply. Vaccination is compulsory for international travel in the affected areas. Preferably two doses of cholera vaccine should be given at 7 day intervals; this gives partial immunity lasting from 3–6 months.

Stools appear like rice water, the particles consisting mainly of mucus rather than cellular débris; the lack of the usual colour of faecal matter is due not to obstruction of bile flow but to great dilution by the large volume of water, partly because bile pigments are converted to a colourless compound, and partly because of the failure to convert bilirubin to urobilinogen. Surprisingly biopsy specimens taken through the gut show an intact mucosa without significant inflammation. The diarrhoea is largely due to a functional defect of the enterocyte (Table 16.2); cholera exotoxin binds to receptors on the enterocyte, activating adenyl cyclase and producing a profound secretory state in the ileum, and diarrhoea is due to the inability of the colon to reabsorb this quantity of fluid. All the clinical and metabolic features are due to the rapid loss of an electrolyte-rich liquid stool: hypovolaemia, acidosis from base deficit, and hypokalaemia. Absorption from the proximal intestine is more or less normal and provided the patient can take in a sufficient volume of water, glucose and electrolytes, the disease is self-limiting.

Diagnosis. Dark-ground microscopy of the stool should demonstrate the darting vibrios and these can be immobilized by group-specific antisera to confirm that they are *Vibrio cholerae*. Culture of the stool is also done; serological tests such as agglutination are performed mainly for epidemiological studies.

Treatment. This consists of complete replacement of lost water and electrolytes and usually has to be started before the diagnosis is confirmed. The use of glucose orally to potentiate the passage of the sodium ion through the enterocyte (Fig. 16.4) has reduced the need for intravenous fluids. The World Health Organization recommends the following 'diarrhoea treatment solution': sodium chloride 4 g/l,

Table 16.2. The gut in cholera.

---

1   Jejunal biopsy shows a normal structure of villi and enterocytes.
2   Absorption normal.
3   Pore size normal.
4   The copious diarrhoea is due to a functional not anatomical defect.

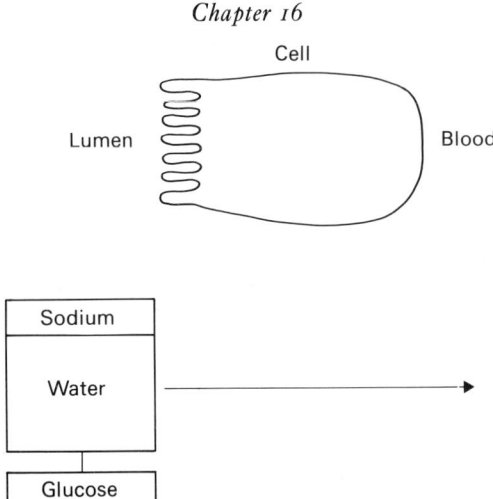

Fig. 16.4. The ionic pump of the bowel.

sodium acetate 6.5 g/l, potassium chloride 1 g/l, and glucose 9 g/l. If the patient cannot drink adequately, this WHO fluid is given intravenously and a large bore needle may have to be used (50–100 ml/min) until the radial pulse is restored. Mortality is almost nil with adequate replacement therapy but in untreated cases reaches over 50%. Antibiotic treatment with tetracycline may be beneficial if given near the onset of an attack.

Tumours of small intestine

Benign tumours
Tumours occur in the small intestine though are rare. Benign tumours are more likely in younger patients and anaemia from occult bleeding may be the first and only sign. Different types occur, such as lipomas, fibromyomas or vascular tumours. In the Peutz–Jeghers syndrome, many polyps, usually minute, occur anywhere from the cardia to the anus, but mostly in the small intestine; these are really a congenital abnormality, hamartoma, and new crops grow when others are removed. The hallmark of the condition is pigmentation especially of the face. Minute discreet dark brown or black macules are grouped around the openings of the face: the eyes, the nostrils and especially the mouth—the last may make the child's life at school miserable because of his 'dirty lips'. Pigmentation affects the tongue and especially the buccal mucosa. The polyps may be missed by routine barium progress meal unless special techniques are used and often cannot be seen at laparotomy. It is usually detected by 'spot diagnosis'. Freckles are seen on the

cheeks and nose and not inside the mouth. No treatment is possible except for the anaemia and malignancy is unlikely.

Malignant tumours

Adenocarcinomata
Adenocarcinomata in the small intestine form only 1% of gastrointestinal tumours and present with colic, weight loss and anaemia. No predisposing factors are known except that there is slightly increased risk in patients with Crohn's disease of the small intestine.

Lymphomata
These develop as primary tumours without evidence of involvement of tissues elsewhere and may be single, multiple or diffuse. These usually arise in healthy people but adult coeliac disease predisposes to them and it is doubtful whether a gluten-free diet protects from this liability. Tumour invasion is usually too widespread for resection and chemotherapy or radiotherapy are the only possibilities.

Lymphoid tumours of the small bowel are more common in the middle-aged and are associated with parasites like worms and protozoa, and the lymphoid overgrowth may occasionally be reversed by treating these. Patients may present with a dysgammaglobulinaemia-like alpha chain disease.

Carcinoid tumours
These are also called argentaffin tumours because of their affinity for silver dyes and are thought to arise from the argentiffin cells of the normal intestinal mucosa; they are most common in the appendix and terminal ileum. Varying in size from small nodules to large tumours of rubbery consistency, they are characteristically bright yellow. They may pursue a somewhat benign course even if secondary deposits are present in the abdominal lymph nodes or liver.

Chemistry
Carcinoid tumours have achieved notoriety because of the effects of the hormone which they secrete: serotonin which is derived from tryptophan, an amino acid in food. Dietary tryptophan is diverted to the tumours to form serotonin and as nicotinic acid (vitamin B_7) is also derived from tryptophan, symptoms of pellagra sometimes occur. The 'carcinoid syndrome' due to the hormone occurs when hepatic deposits are present as serotonin is then released into the general circulation; otherwise it is destroyed by the hepatic enzyme, mono-amine-oxidase, and cannot pass beyond the liver. Carcinoids may also arise elsewhere as from a bronchus and they then cause symptoms whether or not the liver is involved, for serotonin has direct access to the systemic circulation.

Symptoms

Flushing attacks start in the face and spread to the rest of the body. These can be precipitated by a meal, excitement, palpation of the tumour and drugs such as alcohol, adrenaline and reserpine. There may be diarrhoea, borborygmi and abdominal cramps. Asthma has been fatal during induction of anaesthesia. Carcinoid heart disease is usually confined to the right side of the heart, later effects being pulmonary stenosis with tricuspid regurgitation or stenosis—due to a diffuse fibrosis which can be distinguished from results of rheumatic fever, or from the endomyocardial fibroelastosis in the heart of Africans. The site of the cardiac lesion suggests direct damage by serotonin or other substances from the tumour, possibly by stimulating formation of fibrous tissue.

Diagnosis

Diagnosis is made by estimation of the metabolite 5-hydroxyindole acetic acid (5-HIAA), in the urine by chromotography; the normal excretion is from 2–10 mg over 24 h, but in carcinoids, excretion which is variable is rarely less than 50 mg/24 h. Slight increases may occur from eating bananas, and in adult coeliac disease.

Treatment

Simple appendicectomy is usually sufficient for carcinoids of the appendix when discovered incidentally at laparotomy, and the prognosis is excellent. Symptoms of the syndrome are difficult to treat: deprivation of tryptophan from the diet is not practical. Nicotinic acid should be given to prevent pellagra. Serotonin antagonists occasionally relieve symptoms, especially diarrhoea; the drugs being used are methysergide and cyproheptadine. Flushes may be helped by alpha-blockade with phenoxybenzamine. p-chloro-phenylalanine, an inhibitor of tryptophan, also relieves diarrhoea in some patients. After surgery, such as ileal resection, diarrhoea may be due to another cause as in a cholerrheic enteropathy, so treatment with the bile acid binding resin cholestyramine may be needed. When the patient has serious complications (e.g. intractable diarrhoea or valvular heart disease), hepatic involvement should be assessed to see whether partial hepatectomy may remove sufficient tumour to cause regression of the disease. Cure is never possible at this stage since secondary tumour is so widespread.

Intestinal pseudo-obstruction

Most surgeons have had the experience of operating upon a patient with symptoms and signs of mechanical obstruction where no cause is found. The small and large bowel may be very dilated, sometimes with an area of obstruction due to spasm. It can be primary, probably due to a disorder of motility, or secondary to abdominal disease not involving the bowel itself, like carcinomatous invasion of the coeliac plexus. Other causes are neurological disorders like Parkinsonianism, polyneuritis, tabes, or lead poisoning, and it occurs in patients with prolonged hypotension or anoxaemia—and porphyria may mimic it. Treatment is unsatisfactory and drugs have so far had no effect. Operation is occasionally advised to remove a segment where mobility obviously is impaired.

Endometriosis of the bowel

The bowel, usually the colon, is often involved when patients are operated upon for endometriosis. Usually this is superficial and of no significance, but occasionally the bowel wall is invaded and tumour-like masses may lead to obstruction. There are no diagnostic features at sigmoidoscopy or X-ray, and rectal bleeding is rare. Symptoms may be worse at menstruation and lesions regress after bilateral oophorectomy or hormonal therapy.

Whipple's disease

The original description by Whipple (1907) of the 36-year-old American physician who lived with and died from this disease will always remain a testimony to the value of a single case report. Since then little has been added to this detailed clinical, pathological, histological and chemical study. The clinical picture has been widened and more cases are being discovered, as jejunal biopsy has so simplified the diagnosis.

Pathology. The small bowel appears to be the origin of the disease. The mucosa of the jejunum is flecked with little pin-point yellowish white grains from bulbous villi. Microscopically, the villi are distended from masses of large granular histiocytes which contain abundant PAS-positive material and fat deposits. The lacteals may be markedly dilated due to involvement of the mesenteric lymph nodes. The curious rods and granules seen in the lamina propria are encapsulated bacilliform bodies but no one has yet isolated a specific organism.

Symptoms. Men approaching middle age are most prone to it, and fever and bronchitis sometimes ushers in the diarrhoea, and neurological complications may occur. Typically, it causes a triad of steatorrhoea, enlarged lymph nodes (superficial as well as mesenteric) and arthropathy; sometimes the patient is diagnosed as suffering from sero-negative rheumatoid arthritis as the diarrhoea may not appear for some years after its onset. If joint symptoms are absent, it mimics adult coeliac disease. The ESR is raised and a polymorphonuclear leucocytosis is common.

Diagnosis. Jejunal biopsy proves it and the appearance even by naked eye is diagnostic; a hand lens or dissecting microscope will show better the bulbous yellowish villi. The microscopical appearance is unique (Fig. 16.5). Synovial fluid, if arthritis is present, is similar to that of rheumatoid arthritis but a synovial biopsy may show the 'organisms'. Barium studies show coarsening of the duodenal and jejunal folds and widening as in coeliac disease.

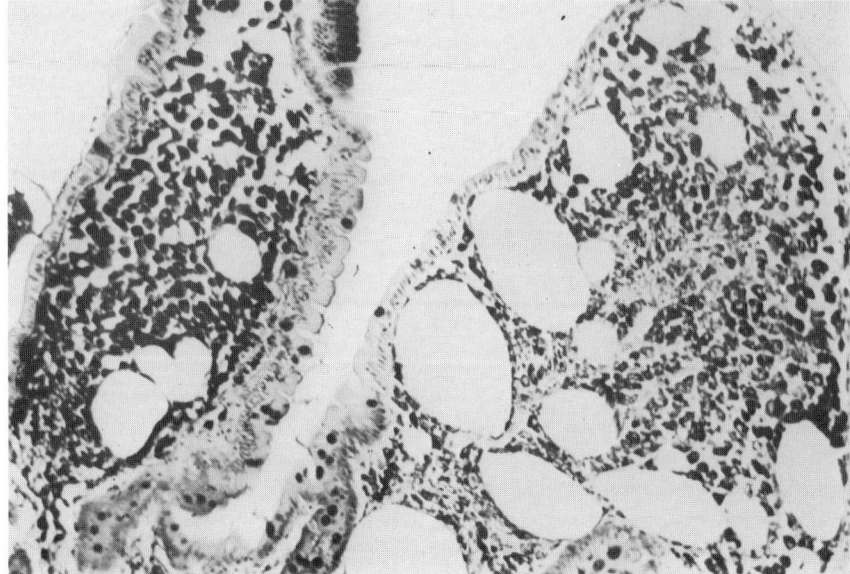

Fig. 16.5. Villi in Whipple's disease (PAS stain, high power). The black cells are PAS-positive macrophages and the empty spaces are dilated lacteals.

Treatment. Long-term antibiotics such as tetracycline cure both the malabsorption and complications like arthritis but will have to be continued indefinitely, either in the minimal effective dose or in courses. The jejunal biopsy will return to normal and the 'organisms' disappear. Previously it was often fatal.

Amyloidosis

Primary systemic amyloidosis is nowadays more common than the secondary type because sepsis is less frequent; amyloid material occurs in the skin and mucous membranes, striated muscles, heart, lungs and gastrointestinal tract. Secondary amyloidosis may accompany chronic inflammatory bowel disease, tuberculosis, or multiple myelomatosis and it is sometimes confined to one organ or tissue.

No part of the gastrointestinal tract is immune. Deposition in the tongue causes the 'scrotal tongue', the oesophagus shows a rigid dilated appearance like achalasia, atrophy of the mucosa and peptic ulceration may occur in the stomach, involvement of the small intestine causes malabsorption and colonic amyloidosis may mimic ulcerative colitis. Biopsy of the rectum is the best method of diagnosis; otherwise from a nodule in the skin, or from the gum, liver or kidney. Proteinuria is often present.

Abetalipoproteinaemia (acanthocytosis)

This rare syndrome consists of a curious spiky appearance of the red blood cells (acanthus means a thorn or sharp point), retinopathy and neurological signs, together with malabsorption. It is due to a hereditary defect of apoprotein synthesis with consequent failure to form chylomicrons. The serum cholesterol is very low, serum beta-lipoproteins are absent, and the very low plasma triglyceride fails to rise after eating triglyceride. Jejunal biopsy is typical with columnar cells covering the villi engorged with triglyceride droplets, even after an overnight fast. Substituting medium chain triglycerides for ordinary triglyceride helps as chylomicron formation and lymphatic absorption are not then involved.

Alpha-chain disease
This rare form of malabsorption may occur in patients with lymphomas. So far, it has been described in patients from the Middle East who present with abdominal discomfort and weight loss from malabsorption and diarrhoea and have mesenteric and small intestinal lymph node involvement from lymphomas. Immunoelectro-phoresis of serum provides the diagnosis (p. 347). Chemotherapy may cause remission.

Primary intestinal lymphangiectasia
This causes intermittent diarrhoea with steatorrhoea and excessive loss of protein into the gut. It is confirmed by jejunal biopsy where dilated lymph vessels are seen in the submucosa with chyle leaking into the intestinal lumen.

Dietary fat should be reduced so as to diminish chyle flow and medium chain triglycerides, which are transported by the portal vessels rather than via lymphatic chyle, can result in clinical improvement and reduction of the steatorrhoea.

Pneumatosis cystoides intestinalis
This curious condition of gas-filled cysts in the bowel wall is usually discovered accidentally. At laparotomy the cysts resemble a cluster of grapes or a hydatidiform mole if they are subserosal. Diagnosis has been made at sigmoidoscopy when cysts like globular masses protrude into the lumen and partially occlude it; they disappear like magic if a biopsy is taken. They can be seen by X-ray. They are caused by air originating from a lesion of the gastrointestinal tract such as intestinal obstruction or a neoplasm, or in asthma or other diseases of the lung, though sometimes there is no other disease.

No treatment is needed if symptoms are absent or mild. Breathing high concentrations of oxygen (70%) using either a head tent or face mask could be tried as the cysts may diminish in size after several days and may not recur; oxygen lowers the partial pressure of nitrogen in the capillary and enables the nitrogen from the cysts to diffuse back into the circulation. Otherwise no treatment is needed except for the primary cause.

Eosinophilic infiltration of the gut
Synonyms include eosinophilic enteritis, Loeffler's eosinophilic infiltration and

allergic regional enteritis. It is a histological diagnosis and the cause is unknown but parasitic infestations, connective tissue disorders or food allergy should be considered. Symptoms depend on the site of involvement and sometimes polypoid lesions occur. Corticosteroid therapy can be effective.

Retroperitoneal fibrosis

In this rare and curious condition, a mat of fibrous tissue gradually spreads over the posterior abdominal wall, usually starting over the sacrum and extending upwards—sometimes even into the mediastinum. It is more common in males, and signs of inflammation—slight fever, loss of weight, anaemia and raised ESR—are often present. The ureters bear the main brunt of the disease and occasionally the gut can be involved so nausea and vomiting result.

It is usually of unknown origin but drugs such as methysergide taken for migraine and the beta-blocker practolol have been incriminated. Occasionally a mass can be felt or it arises secondary to malignant disease. Death is usually caused by renal failure.

Ultrasound is probably the most helpful method of diagnosis, though, in practice, laparotomy with biopsy is usually necessary. Intravenous pyelography shows medial displacement of the ureter and evidence of obstruction usually at the level of the pelvic rim with hydronephrosis.

Progress is slow and life can be maintained by operation to relieve ureteric obstruction. Corticosteroid therapy has been used.

Sclerosing peritonitis has some similarity with retroperitoneal fibrosis. Masses due to areas of fibrosis enveloping loops of bowel may be felt. Practolol has been withdrawn for oral use because it caused it, but so far no other drugs have been incriminated and there is no evidence against other beta-blockers.

Chapter 17
Inflammatory Bowel Disease

Crohn's disease (regional enteritis)

Dr Burrill Crohn of New York put this disease on the map by describing fifty-two cases in 1932. It was first called 'terminal ileitis' because it usually involved the end of the ileum. Its name was soon abandoned, partly because of the depressing effect on the patients who misconstrued the meaning of the word 'terminal', and partly because the position was not always correct. Although the ileum is the commonest site, Crohn's disease may occur anywhere in the alimentary tract from mouth to anus, and so was renamed 'regional enteritis'.

Historical aspects

It is not a new disease, so that environmental factors such as food and its additives or stress are unlikely to be the sole cause. Retrospective diagnosis is easier than for ulcerative colitis as the naked eye appearance (Fig. 17.1) is so typical (the thickened bowel, skip areas, and enlarged lymph nodes), providing tuberculosis has been excluded since ileo-caecal infection mimics it. Probable cases were recorded in the medical literature nearly two centuries ago; they appeared under various synonyms from chronic cicatrizing enteritis to non-specific granuloma of the intestine. A case of stricture and thickening of the ileum demonstrated at the Royal College of Physicians in 1813 by doctors Combe and Saunders was probably an example of Crohn's disease: the ileum was 'contracted for the space of three feet to the size of a turkey quill' and there were skip areas. In 1913 the Scottish surgeon Kennedy Dalziel reported nine patients and wrote that 'the affected bowel gives the consistency and smoothness of an eel in a state of rigor mortis, and the glands though enlarged are evidently not caseous'—an elegant description though few will have handled an eel in this sad state. Crohn's disease, though still unusual, seems to be becoming more frequent; this increase also appears to be a true one and not due to increased recognition.

Aetiology

No pathogen, bacterium, protozoa or virus has yet been found and there is no similar disease in animals. The porcine ileitis in Denmark, in which the terminal ileum is thickened and lymph nodes enlarged, is unlike Crohn's disease histologically for there are no giant cell systems. A disorder primarily of the lymph nodes has been suggested and various substances such as silica have been injected into the mesenteric lymphatics of animals and have sometimes produced a thickened bowel from oedema of the submucosal and muscular layers resembling

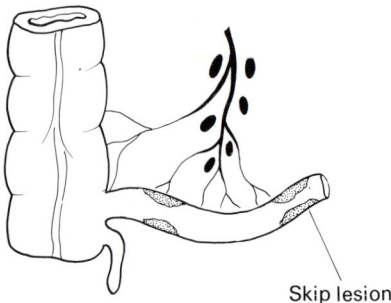

Skip lesion

Fig. 17.1. Crohn's disease of ileum with enlarged lymph nodes.

Crohn's disease; however, this hypothesis is unproved. Disturbances of the immune mechanism are found: circulating immune complexes have been isolated in nearly half the patients and many with both Crohn's disease and ulcerative colitis show signs of activation of the complement sequence. Anergy is found in many patients and T-lymphocyte counts are reduced; also the B cells in the inflamed mucosa are increased together with the number of IgG cells. It is more likely that most of these changes are a response to inflammation rather than the cause of it.

Pathology
Crohn's disease is so distinctive (Table 17.1) that the surgeon can usually diagnose it at laparotomy. Microscopically there are often no specific features, just various degrees of acute, subacute and chronic inflammation. More important are the focal collections of epithelioid cells, lymphocytes, and giant cells without caseation, called granulomas; these also explain why originally many cases of Crohn's disease

Table 17.1. Characteristic appearances in Crohn's disease.

---

1 A segment of bowel has a red, congested oedematous appearance and feels solid and firm like rubber hose.
2 Skip lesions may occur elsewhere in the bowel.
3 Several coils of bowel may be matted together by adhesions.
4 The attached mesentery may be thick, stiff and corrugated and the lymph nodes are enlarged.
5 Fistulae between loops of bowel or organs such as the bladder are common.
6 Strictures and abscess formation are likely.
7 The mucous membrane is red, swollen and ulcerated, and the surface resembles cobble-stones when transverse folds of mucosa are partly destroyed and intersected by longitudinal ulceration.
8 Microscopical appearances are similar to tuberculosis but without caseation.

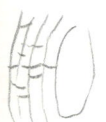

were regarded as tuberculous. Tiny white nodules may be on the surface of the bowel and in the lymph nodes.

Symptoms

The usual complaint is of abdominal pain and diarrhoea; pain may be in the right iliac fossa and a normal appendix is often removed at the start. A curious and inexplicable fore-runner of the disease is a peri-anal lesion, either abscess or fistula. This may antedate the diarrhoea by many years or so dominate the clinical picture that the enteritis is overlooked; microscopically it shows the typical non-caseating giant cell systems.

Pain is often followed by a desire to defaecate and this relieves it. Occasionally discomfort starts 2 or 3 h after a meal when it reaches the ileum and so suggests peptic ulcer.

Crohn's disease has the unique propensity for fistula formation. Perforation into the peritoneum causing peritonitis is rare; the usual course is for the bowel to become attached to some surrounding structure and then for fistula formation to result. A fistula through the wound of an appendicectomy strongly points towards Crohn's disease. When the bladder is involved the patient may pass gas (pneumaturia) or particles of food in the urine and this may be the first symptom.

Many have symptoms of general ill-health with fever and sweating and some present with pyrexia of unknown origin. Extra-alimentary complications cause problems (Table 17.2) Arthritis, erythema nodosum and iritis may occur in 10–15%. Vitamin B_{12} deficiency is likely when the ileum is severely diseased. Protein may be lost from the inflamed bowel (protein-losing enteropathy) and the consequent low serum albumin causes oedema of the legs. Anaemia is usually due to iron deficiency from oozing of blood from the ulcerated mucosa, but the activity of the disease may prevent full response to iron.

Signs

Abdominal examination may be normal. A tender abdominal mass is felt in one third of cases, usually in the right iliac fossa, due to matted loops of bowel or to a walled-off abscess. Rectal examination may show a fissure, fistula, abscess, ulceration, or scars from previous operations (Table 17.3).

Diagnosis

Early diagnosis can be difficult unless the index of suspicion is high; methods are as follows.

Radiological appearance (Figs. 17.2–17.7). Severe disease or even partial obstruction may be present before a barium progress meal becomes abnormal. The outline of the affected loop of bowel may resemble a tubular cast or piece of string—the string sign—being narrowed from oedema or fibrosis. When obstruction is suspected, a barium enema should first be ordered as the barium meal may complete the

Table 17.2. Extra-alimentary complications of inflammatory bowel disease.

	Common	Occasional	Rare
Systemic	Malnutrition Anaemia Water and electrolyte disturbances	Thromboembolism	
Skin	Erythema nodosum Drug rashes	Pyoderma gangrenosum	

Locomotor	Arthropathy and
	    arthritis
		Ankylosing
		    spondylitis	

Eye		Anterior uveitis Conjunctivitis Episcleritis	

Liver	Fatty infiltration
	Pericholangitis
			Sclerosing
			    cholangitis
			Chronic active
			    hepatitis
			Cholangiocarcinoma

Miscellaneous		Clubbing of the fingers	Amyloidosis

obstruction and the terminal ileum can often be clearly seen by an enema; double contrast studies could also detect lesions of the colon. A chest X-ray will be necessary to exclude tuberculosis.

Evidence of inflammation. Pyrexia may be present and the erythrocyte sedimentation rate (ESR) is raised. A neutrophil leucocytosis suggests that an abscess has formed.

Sigmoidoscopy. In contrast to ulcerative colitis, the rectum is commonly not involved even in Crohn's colitis. The early change is the 'aphthoid ulcer' which represents focal necrosis in the mucosa overlying a pathological lymphoid aggregate (Table 17.3).

Table 17.3. Rectal appearances in Crohn's disease.

Mucosal oedema
Patchy inflammation
Ulceration: (i) discrete aphthoid ulcers, and (ii) serpiginous ulcers
Cobble-stone mucosa

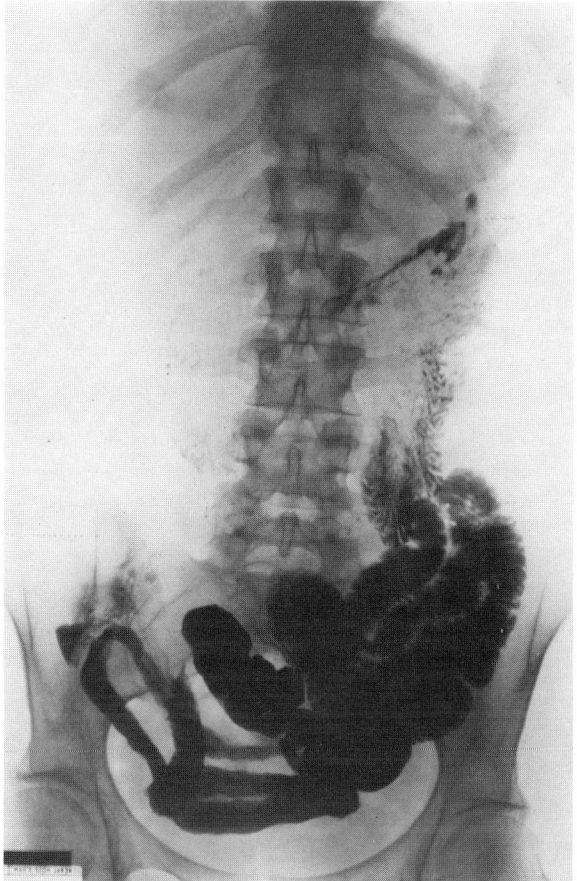

Fig. 17.2. 'Hose-pipe' thickening of terminal ileum as shown by separation of the barium-filled bowel lumen.

Rectal biopsy. Epithelioid granulomata may be found in a biopsy specimen even when there is no visible abnormality, but the chance of this is small.

Colonoscopy. This may detect Crohn's disease of the colon which is beyond the reach of the sigmoidoscope.

Examination of the stools. Stools may look normal, loose or fatty. Occult blood tests are often positive; visible blood is unusual.

Differential diagnosis. (Table 17.4)
Ileo-caecal tuberculosis must be excluded, especially in coloured races, by Mantoux

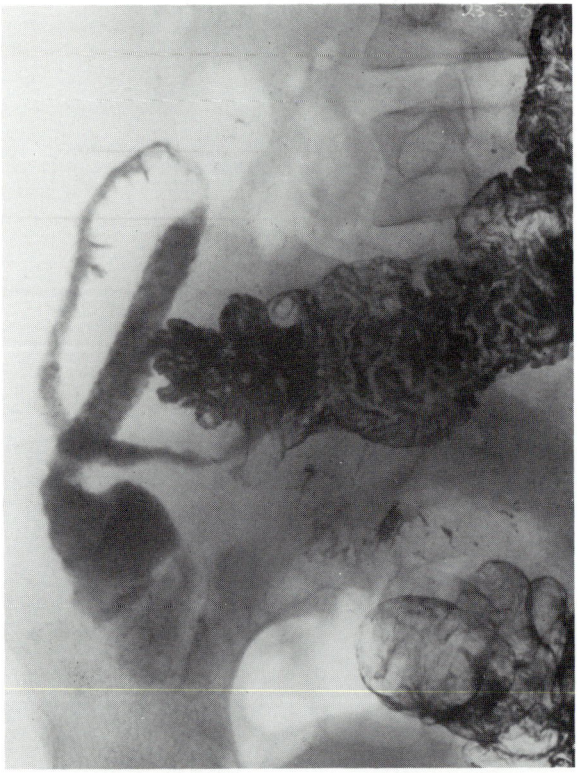

Fig. 17.3. Involvement of ileum after ileotransverse colostomy showing 'rose-thorn' ulcers which could develop into fistulae.

testing, X-raying the chest, and checking the stools for tubercle bacilli. Neoplasms of the ileum can mimic Crohn's disease, especially lymphoma. Crohn's disease of the stomach may resemble carcinoma (Linitis plastica) and diffuse lesions of the small intestine (jejuno-ileitis) can be confused with adult coeliac disease. An ischaemic stricture can cause a 'string-sign' like Crohn's disease (Fig. 17.8). A lump in the right iliac fossa may be an appendix abscess and not Crohn's disease.

Treatment

An important aim is to maintain the general health and this often means regular visits to a special follow-up clinic. Anaemia is treated by iron, either orally or parenterally, or vitamin B_{12} if the serum B_{12} is low. Electrolyte disturbances must be corrected. If there is steatorrhoea, fat should be reduced to 50 g daily or less. Otherwise a diet high in protein and calories is prescribed; trials are being done to assess the effect of the high residue diet as Crohn's disease is more common in industrialized countries. Antibiotics are of no use apart from the treatment of

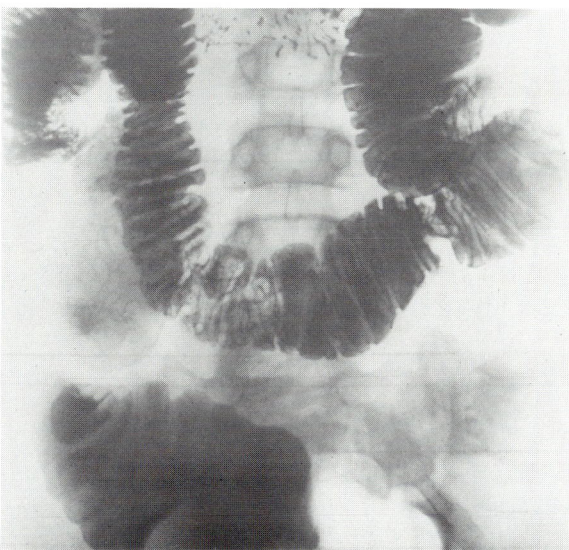

Fig. 17.4. Cobble-stone mucosa in colon.

pyogenic complications. Sulphasalazine is of doubtful effect, compared with its benefit in ulcerative colitis. Corticosteroid therapy, such as prednisolone 10–15 mg daily, can be given when other measures fail, preferably in courses rather than continuously. Immunosuppressives like azathioprine have found support in some controlled trials though not in others.

Surgery is palliative though may be life-saving when complications arise. The enthusiasm of the surgeon to cure the disease by radical removal is tempered by the high rate of recurrences. He is also wary of the serious nutritional consequences that follow a blind loop, or removal of large sections of bowel (p. 297). Indications for operation are shown in Table 17.5 (p. 296).

Prognosis
The outlook depends especially on the site and extent of the disease and these vary greatly. For many patients, the course is benign and fluctuating so that they can live a reasonable life. However, recurrence is usual and the most important factor in determining the recurrence rate is the length of the follow-up period; recurrence is likely in half the patients over a 10-year period. The young are more prone to further attacks than the old and a recurrence often starts within the first year after operation; further trouble is less likely if the patient has remained fit for 5 years. Unfortunately no time interval is a guarantee against relapse and this may occur even 20 years after a radical resection, for example, of the terminal ileum.

The mortality rate is also difficult to estimate because of the protean forms of the

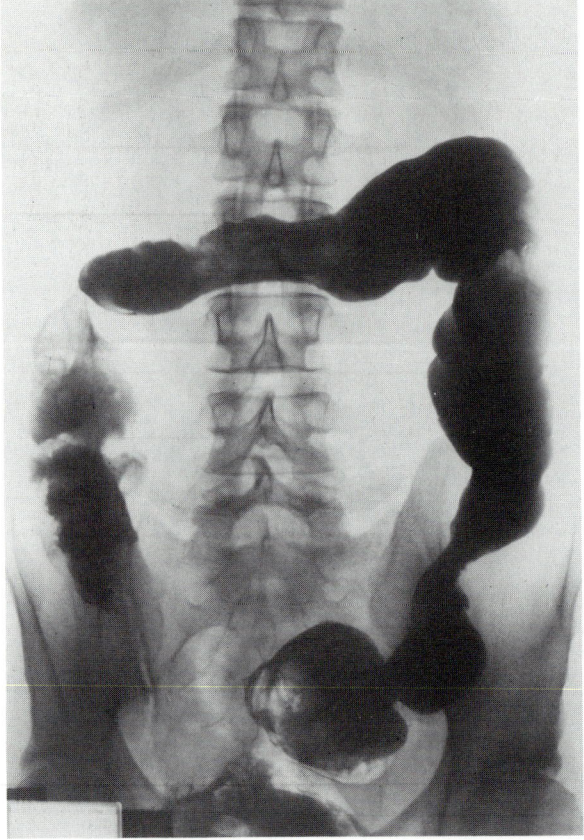

Fig. 17.5. Crohn's colitis. The barium enema shows the irregular involvement and a long asymmetrical stricture with tapering margins in the descending colon. The splenic flexure and rectum were free from disease.

disease. Some reports suggest a two-fold increase in death rate when the small intestine is involved and a four-fold one with Crohn's colitis, compared with the healthy population. Death usually occurs from complications.

Special clinical problems

Diarrhoea

Various factors may cause this:

1 Cholerrheic diarrhoea may occur because the diseased ileum cannot absorb bile salts.

2 A stagnant bowel syndrome may have developed because there is a stricture or

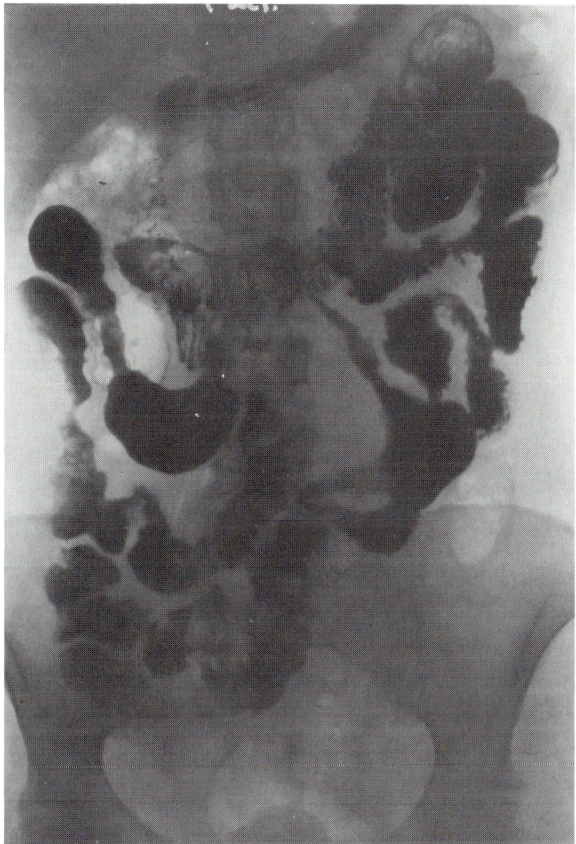

Fig. 17.6. Skip areas in the small intestine.

fistula; so the bile salts will have been deconjugated by the bacterial overgrowth thus preventing fat digestion.

3   There may be very extensive involvement of the small intestine as in jejuno-ileitis causing steatorrhoea.

4   Crohn's colitis may prevent the dehydration of stool.

5   The surgeon may have removed so much gut that the short bowel syndrome has developed.

Intestinal obstruction

This is a common problem and causes colicky pain. Sometimes the obstruction which is partly due to oedema and inflammation responds to corticosteroids and, if acute, drip and suction. This is always well worth trying but operation may become necessary.

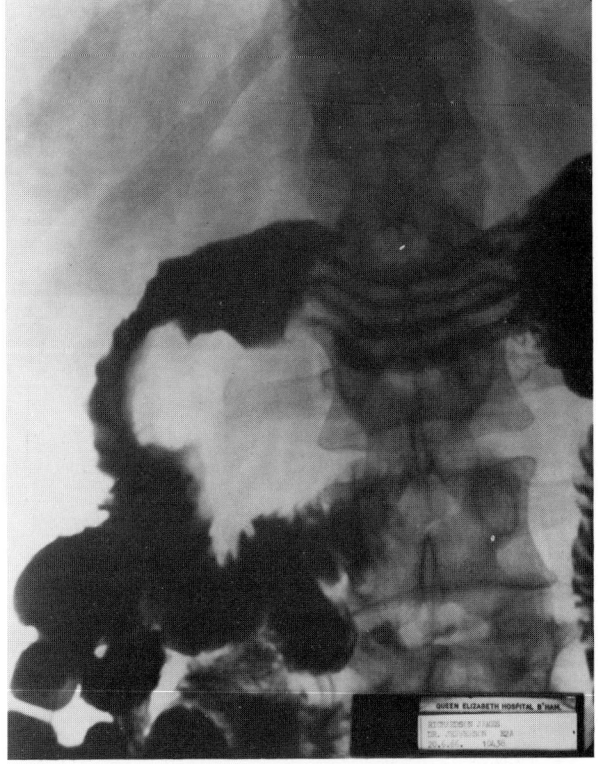

Fig. 17.7. Crohn's disease of the duodenum causing deformity and narrowing.

Fistulae

These may occur anywhere, even from the terminal ileum into the loin, but more commonly they are ileo-ileal, ileo-colic, ileo-vesical or ileo-vaginal. Some cause surprisingly little trouble to the patient but more often operation is needed.

Abscess

An intra-abdominal abscess is often difficult to detect. It sometimes can be felt as a tender mass, or it may lie deep and be concealed. The white cell count may rise. Ultrasound or CT scanning may be needed to detect it. It often fails to respond to antibiotics—though these are worth trying—and a surgeon is needed to deal with it.

Crohn's colitis

The colon may be involved by the ileo-colitis type of Crohn's disease or by skip lesions. Total colitis may occur and this was formerly misdiagnosed as ulcerative colitis. If it fails to respond to medical treatment the same indications for operation arise as for ulcerative colitis (Table 17.11). Ileostomy and total colectomy may have

Table 17.4. Differential diagnosis of Crohn's disease.

	Occasional	Rare
Ileo-caecal disease	Lymphoma	Carcinoids
	Tuberculosis	Drug-induced stricture
	Appendix abscess	
	Yersinia enteritis	
Colonic disease	Ulcerative colitis	Ischaemic colitis
	Irritable colon	Amoebic colitis
	Carcinoma	(in the UK)
	Pseudomembranous colitis	Irradiation colitis
	Campylobacter colitis	
Jejuno-ileal disease	Coeliac disease	Lymphangiectasia
	'Non-specific ulcerative jejunoileitis'	Whipple's disease
	Infective enteritis	Nodular lymphoid hyperplasia
	Lymphoma	Alpha-chain disease
	Infestation (e.g. *Giardia lamblia*)	Irradiation enteritis
		Eosinophilic gastroenteritis

to be done but is less satisfactory than for patients with ulcerative colitis because complications are more common and the small intestine may be diseased or become so later.

Anal lesions

Lesions of the rectum and anus often cause the greatest personal and social distress. Fissure, fistula or peri-anal abscess commonly involve the anus. When infection is present, metronidazole may be helpful. Occasionally the only treatment may be ileostomy and colectomy with removal of the rectum though some surgeons have suggested a benefit from a split ileostomy which defunctions the colon but allows the possibility of re-anastomosis in continuity. But many patients tolerate anal lesions for long periods and the present view is that the surgeon is reluctant to operate unless driven to do so.

Effect on growth

Children with Crohn's disease may fail to grow. If a small segment of bowel only is affected, this would be a cause for removal. Regular and high doses of corticosteroids may also contribute to this failure; prednisolone given on alternate days may have less depressing effects upon growth than if it is prescribed daily.

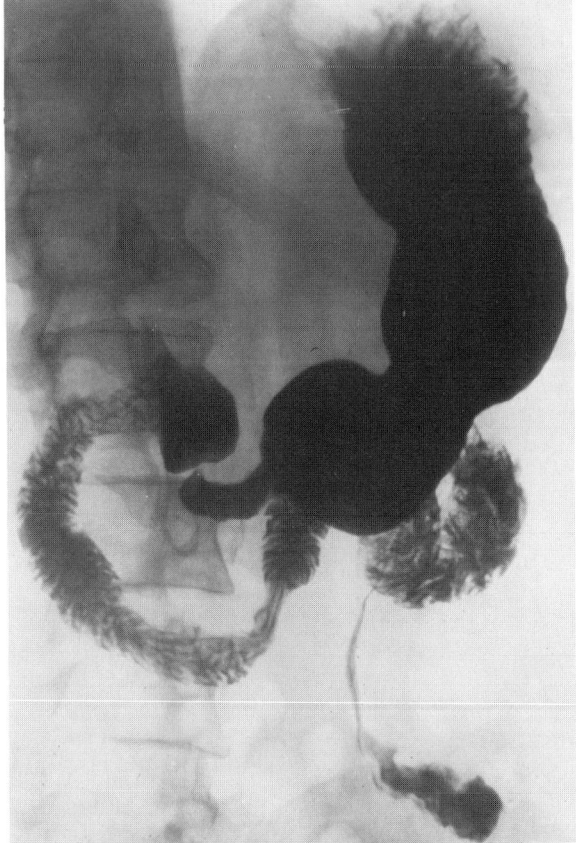

Fig. 17.8. Ischaemic stricture of jejunum after mesenteric embolism in a man suffering from a recent coronary infarction.

Table 17.5. Indications for operation in Crohn's disease.

1	Intestinal obstruction unresponsive to medical measures.
2	To establish the diagnosis in difficult cases.
3	For complications such as fistula, abscess, perforation and haemorrhage.
4	Colectomy and ileostomy for Crohn's colitis.

Pregnancy

The natural history of Crohn's disease seems unaffected by pregnancy. Normal healthy children are expected and the only problem might be local lesions complicating delivery.

Malignant change

The risk of cancer is very small and much less than in ulcerative colitis. The colon and rectum are more likely to be involved.

The short bowel syndrome

Extensive removal of the small gut causes diarrhoea, steatorrhoea, loss of proteins and other nutrients, marked weight loss and inanition, and sometimes death. Removal of the ileum (Table 17.6) is often more troublesome than that of the jejunum because there is loss of bile salts, and a lack of an ileo-caecal valve means that food is not held up in the remaining small intestine. However, the small bowel has the capacity to hypertrophy with an increased diameter, villous height and

Table 17.6. Possible sequelae after resection of the ileum.

1 Diarrhoea due to (i) loss of ileo-caecal valve; (ii) bacterial reflux into ileal remnant; and (iii) colonic irritation from bile salts.
2 Steatorrhoea. Failure to reabsorb bile salts causes reduced micellar formation.
3 Megaloblastic anaemia as vitamin B_{12} is not absorbed (but it is stored in the body for 4 years).
4 Gallstones due to changes in bile.
5 Urinary oxalate stones from increased oxalate absorption.

mucosal enzymes so that some patients tend to improve during the months after resection—providing the remaining gut functions normally and is free from disease.

Treatment includes replacement of fluid and electrolytes and small feeds of a low fat, high protein diet. Additional vitamins, especially B_{12} and folic acid, are necessary. Extra calories can be provided by medium chain triglycerides. Either aluminium hydroxide or cholestyramine may help to bind bile salts and prevent their irritating effect upon the colonic mucosa. Occasionally removal of much of the small intestine results in a reflex rise in serum gastrin with a high gastric output and then an H_2 receptor antagonist could be considered.

Long-term parenteral feeding is rarely required. Operations have been devised to slow up the intestinal passage by reversal of a segment of the small bowel but success is doubtful. Space food (elemental diet), which causes small motions every 5 or 6 days in healthy people, can be used. It is synthetic, consisting of highly purified and discreet chemical constituents like amino acids, and is given as a crystal clear solution with different flavours. It not only reduces the residue but also the bacteria and the stool becomes odourless; there are no indigestible residues.

Extra-alimentary complications

Lesions of the skin, eyes and joints occur in inflammatory bowel disease and could be due to bacterial and toxic products absorbed through an ulcerated bowel or to immune complexes. Studies have shown them to be more common in Crohn's disease—about 15% of patients—than in ulcerative colitis; this may be because the latter is curable by colectomy.

The skin
Erythema nodosum is the commonest skin lesion and occurs in up to 2% of patients, usually during an acute attack. It has occurred before the onset of bowel symptoms. Pyoderma gangrenosum is rare and is not cured by proctocolectomy in ulcerative colitis; no organisms are found and vasculitis is a possibility. Drug rashes occur and the Stevens–Johnson syndrome has been reported, attributed to sulphasalazine. Clubbing of the fingers is more likely with liver involvement.

Eyes
Anterior uveitis has a similar incidence to involvement of the skin; conjunctivitis, keratitis and episcleritis also occur.

Arthropathy and ankylosing spondylitis
The incidence of arthropathy in different studies varies widely and the natural tendency is for rheumatologists who examine these patients to find arthritis more often. These account for the total incidence of the triad of symptoms being as high as 15%. Synovial fluid is similar to that seen in rheumatoid arthritis, with increased inflammatory cells, but it is sterile and the Rose–Waaler test is negative. The arthritis is usually synchronous with bowel symptoms, disappearing during remissions; it responds to the usual measures including injection of corticosteroids into the joints apart from treatment of the bowel disease itself. Ankylosing spondylitis (Fig. 17.9) differs from peripheral arthropathy as it may start long before bowel symptoms and there is a hereditary component as shown by a link with HLA-B27 antigens.

Liver complications
Liver complications are listed in Table 17.2. A fatty liver is common in extremely ill patients, especially in those operated upon for toxic megacolon, and disappears when the patient is better. Pericholangitis is an imprecise term sometimes applied to the appearance of portal tract inflammation in patients with inflammatory bowel disease. The term is probably best avoided and the patient carefully assessed to exclude chronic active hepatitis—rare and more likely with ulcerative colitis than Crohn's disease—and sclerosing cholangitis; the latter is strongly associated with ulcerative colitis and seldom seen in patients with Crohn's disease; both may progress to cirrhosis.

Carcinoma of the bile ducts or gallbladder occurs more often though is rare; when biliary strictures are seen in patients with ulcerative colitis, it may be very difficult to distinguish between sclerosing cholangitis and cholangiocarcinoma.

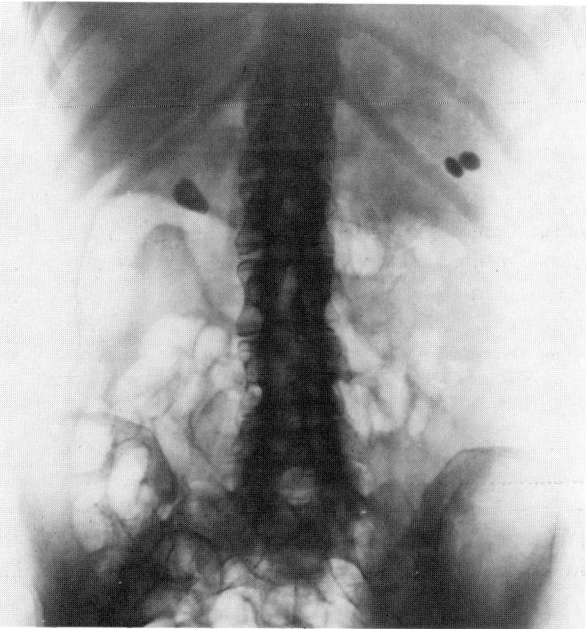

Fig. 17.9. Plain film of abdomen showing air-filled colon with typical appearance of Crohn's colitis, right renal stone and tablets in the stomach. She was 28 years old when Crohn's disease was diagnosed, having been treated for 7 years under orthopaedic surgeons for ankylosing spondylitis; this affected the whole spine and caused complete ankylosis of both hip joints. Rectal bleeding, attributed to piles, started about 3 years after the spondylitis. When Crohn's disease was diagnosed, it involved the entire colon and much of the perineum and vulvae. The perineal disease and arthritis was arrested after ileostomy and total colectomy.

In Crohn's disease, granulomatous hepatitis is occasionally seen and gallstones are more common in those with ileal disease or resection.

Acute ileitis

This is rare. The commonest identifiable cause is infection by *Yersinia enterocolitica* (Gram-negative rods resembling *E. coli*). Clinical features include fever and diarrhoea in children and an acute terminal ileitis with large lymph nodes in adults which mimics Crohn's disease—and some get erythema nodosum and polyarthritis. It is sometimes detected at operation for appendicitis and the appendix should be removed even if it is normal. Often the cause of acute ileitis is unknown but other possible infections are tuberculosis, amoebiasis, and actinomycosis.

Acute colitis

Infection should be the first possibility considered in any colitis of sudden origin.

Priority must be given before treatment to identifying an infecting organism by microscopy or culture either from stool, luminal fluid got at sigmoidoscopy or as scrapings from mucosal lesions. The bacteriologist is now incriminating pathogens not previously considered as a cause of colitis and there are still cases of self-limiting acute colitis with negative findings on bacteriology, which otherwise behave like infective colitis—indicating that other agents so far unrecognized may also cause colitis. Only when infective causes have been reasonably excluded should ulcerative colitis or Crohn's disease be considered.

Salmonella and shigella colitis

Salmonella food poisoning presents either as gastroenteritis or predominantly as colitis with frequent bloody stools and tenesmus; there is a granular proctitis with haemorrhage and serpiginous ulceration. In both infections biopsy shows marked inflammatory change with polymorphonuclear leucocytes and preservation of glandular architecture in contrast to the mainly mononuclear infiltrate and glandular distortion of ulcerative colitis. Patients with chronic colitis may, however, suffer from an intercurrent salmonella infection.

Campylobacter enterocolitis

This is now regarded as the commonest cause of acute bacterial diarrhoea in Britain. The Gram-negative organism escaped detection for so long because of its fastidious growth requirements. It is a zoonosis of low infectivity but poultry workers and puppy lovers should beware because it is much commoner amongst them and in those who drink unpasteurized milk. The incubation period is 2–5 days. It occurs more in children and is usually a self-limiting, mild disease but may present severely with fever and bloody diarrhoea mimicking ulcerative colitis. Erythromycin usually cures it.

Antibiotic-associated (pseudomembranous) colitis

A history of recent antibiotic treatment even if it preceded the onset of colitis by 2 or more weeks strongly suggests an association. Ampicillin, lincomycin and clindamycin are the antibiotics most commonly suspected and the only cause identified so far is the enterotoxin of *Clostridium difficile*. The typical yellow pseudomembranes may be seen at sigmoidoscopy, scattered over an inflamed rectal mucosa, but this diagnostic feature is usually absent. Biopsy specimens show a non-specific acute inflammation with outpourings of epithelial cells, leucocytes and fibrin which form the pseudomembrane. A double-contrast barium enema may show the pseudo-membranes as multiple small round plaques. Vancomycin 500 mg daily by mouth causes the disappearance of the organism and its toxin. Five to seven days is usually sufficient. Toxic effects from vancomycin include decreased auditory acuity and deafness, and metronidazole is often satisfactory as an alternative.

Acute amoebic colitis

Amoebiasis afflicts a large number of the world's population and even more are carriers of the parasite. In the UK, the history is usually of someone who has lived in or visited the tropics, though sporadic cases have occurred. Most have a chronic low grade illness with mild diarrhoea, the stools containing some blood and pus. However, the illness occasionally becomes acute and the patient has bloody diarrhoea and becomes dehydrated with electrolyte depletion. Complications include a mass of granulation tissue, an amoeboma, which may mimic a carcinoma when in the caecum or rectum. A smooth tender enlarged liver together with fever and loss of weight may be caused by a hepatic abscess.

Sigmoidoscopy shows appearances varying from one or two large ragged yellow ulcers to multiple small punched-out ones, commonly in mucosa which seems otherwise normal. Microscopy of a fresh stool may demonstrate motile amoebae (Fig. 17.10) and cysts, many of which contain red blood cells, may be seen and have to be distinguished from those of *Entamoeba coli*. Histologically, there is oedema, vascular congestion, and infiltration with leucocytes, especially eosinophils; a barium enema X-ray may be no different from any diffuse colitis. The gel diffusion precipitin test is positive in most cases.

This condition must not be missed, for if a label of ulcerative colitis is given and the patient treated by corticosteroids, a fatal dissemination of amoebae could follow. Metronidazole has greatly altered the management of amoebiasis since it is effective in all forms. For acute amoebic dysentery, 800 mg orally every 8 h for 10 days is given. It is less effective against cysts and diloxanide (Furamide) 500 mg three times daily for 10 days is preferable. Alternatively, a combination of metronidazole and dilanoxide furate may be given, each for 5 days. A liver abscess may need percutaneous aspiration if large or if the patient is very toxic, but surgical drainage is rarely indicated; aspiration can be aided by ultrasonic or isotopic liver scanning and the response to chemotherapy is now so good that repeated aspiration is rarely required. Emetine is seldom needed.

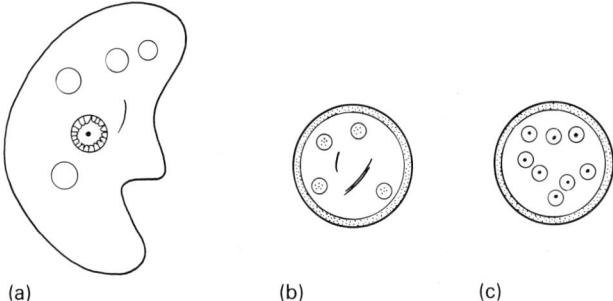

(a) (b) (c)

Fig. 17.10. *Entamoeba histolytica.* (a) Trophozoite with ingested red blood cells; (b) mature cyst with chromatoid bodies and four nuclei; (c) *Entamoeba coli*: mature cyst with eight nuclei.

Schistosomiasis (bilharzia)

Infection with this trematode is most unlikely to be seen except in the Middle East and tropical countries. Ova are deposited in the small tributaries of the portal vein and may be lost in the stool or stay in the bowel wall or pass on to the liver. *Schistosoma mansoni* or *S. japonicum* can both cause an acute distal colitis with mucosal oedema and haemorrhage; this may progress to a chronic phase where the bowel wall is thickened and narrowed from fibrosis and stricture.

Sigmoidoscopy shows an inflamed granular mucous membrane with small minute yellow elevations with surrounding hyperaemia. The diagnosis is proved by finding ova in rectal biopsies; also the complement fixation test may help. Later hepatomegaly develops (ova may be found on a liver biopsy) and then portal hypertension causing splenomegaly, ascites, and oesophageal varices.

Unfortunately these blood flukes which live in the mesenteric vein plexuses are not so amenable to drug therapy as the urinary one (*S. haematobium*). Hitherto the mainstay of therapy has been sodium antimony tartrate but it is most toxic and is being replaced by praziquantel and niridazole; however, the chemotherapy of this disease is difficult and it is probably best to refer patients to a specialist centre.

Acute ischaemic colitis

Abdominal pain and diarrhoea, usually with rectal bleeding, starts suddenly. Patients prone to this are those with arteriosclerosis and (rarely) women taking the contraceptive pill. The splenic flexure is the most vulnerable part of the colon but any segment may be involved, and a barium enema may show a stricture several inches long with 'thumb printing' a sign of mucosal and submucosal oedema. Providing gangrene does not supervene, the condition may resolve leaving a permanent narrowing or develop into chronic colitis. Anticoagulants are indicated for the acute phase though diagnosis is often only made at laparotomy.

Chronic colitis

The differential diagnosis of chronic colitis is wide (Table 17.7), but the usual causes are either ulcerative colitis or Crohn's disease and the distinguishing features between the two are shown in Table 17.8.

Ulcerative colitis

Historical aspects

Some writers have discerned cases of ulcerative colitis reported in the medical literature of bygone days. For example Soranus, a physician from Ephesus, wrote about diarrhoea in AD 130 but apart from his appropriate name, he cannot be regarded as the discoverer of the disease. Similarly Thomas Sydenham, in 1688, is alleged to have used the term 'bloody flux' when reporting a condition which might have been ulcerative colitis—and few patients with this condition would dissent from this description. However, separation from dysentery was only possible when

Table 17.7. Differential diagnosis of ulcerative colitis.

Common
    Crohn's colitis
    Antibiotic-associated colitis
    Irritable colon
    Diverticulitis
    Dysentery and other infection
Occasional
    Coeliac disease
    Ischaemic colitis
    Anorectal gonorrhoea
    Carcinoma of rectum or colon
Rare
    Lymphogranuloma venereum
    Solitary ulcer of rectum
    Irradiation colitis
    Uraemia
    Amyloid disease
    Tuberculosis
    Schistosomiasis
    Behçet's disease
    Systemic lupus erythematosus
    Familial polyposis of colon

---

dysenteric organisms were isolated at the end of the last century and in recent years Crohn's colitis has been found to be the true diagnosis for many patients previously labelled as suffering from ulcerative colitis.

Aetiology

Ulcerative colitis is a disease of unknown origin and is no respecter of persons, for it attacks those in any social strata and in any age group from infancy to old age. It is probably world-wide, but in the tropics it may be difficult to separate from cases due to pathogenic organisms or parasites. It may be one disease or may just represent a non-specific reaction due to various stimuli occurring in predisposed individuals. Much research has gone on to find a causative organism, a search where there is no lack of faecal material available to study. Yet none has been found, and the failure of antibiotics to cure it has dealt a death blow to the bacterial hypothesis. Yet the possibility still exists that the disease is a hypersensitivity reaction to some common, non-pathogenic bacterium or its metabolites; or future work may isolate a virus.

The theory of autoimmunity has been evoked because of clinical features— arthritis, erythema nodosum and eye complications—which may point to hyper-sensitivity or to an altered immune state, and because of the finding of serum

Table 17.8. Comparison between ulcerative colitis and Crohn's disease.

	Ulcerative colitis	Crohn's disease
Stools	Bloody with mucus and pus	Often no visible blood. Steatorrhoea if small intestine involved
Peri-anal lesions	Mild	Often severe
Sigmoidoscopy	Always abnormal. Diffuse inflammation	Maybe normal or patchy inflammation
Rectal biopsy	Non-specific inflammation crypt abscesses	Granulomata with giant cells may be seen
Barium enema	Diffuse changes more marked or confined to distal colon and rectum	Often segmental, perhaps strictures, most marked in proximal colon Ileum involved
Colonoscopy	Extensive superficial ulcers which become confluent and leave pseudopolyps between them	Deep fissured ulcers. Cobble-stone appearance of mucosa. Areas of normal mucosa
Site	Colon only (sometimes last few cm of ileum)	Small intestine, especially terminal ileum

antibodies to human colon. However, the antibody is more likely to be an immunological by-product of no pathological significance, rather than responsible for destructive processes in the colon. Immune complexes do not appear to be relevant.

The fact that fear causes diarrhoea and that attacks of colitis may follow emotional upset has led to the widespread belief that this disease is the response of the colon to a disturbed, anxious mind. Psychiatrists write of the symbolic significance of diarrhoea, yet the importance of this is doubtful as many cases start with constipation and the passage of blood, diarrhoea only occurring later. It is true that victims of ulcerative colitis have often a distinct personality with timidity, lack of aggression, and overdependence on others; they are said to be friendly souls but to have an undercurrent of resentment, frustration and indecision beneath this facade. The cynic will point out that this mentality may be the result rather than the cause of this humiliating complaint, and these characteristics disappear after treatment by colectomy and ileostomy.

Pathology
Ulcerative colitis starts in the rectum so its name, in this respect, is a misnomer; nor is ulceration present in mild cases. Changes are confined to the mucosa and submucosa except in acute fulminating cases where the muscle layer is destroyed

and multiple perforations occur. There is widespread inflammation with ragged superficial ulceration; many mucosal tags project into the lumen and may develop into pseudo-polyps. A strong tendency towards healing and epithelial regeneration is seen, so that the forces of destruction and repair go hand in hand.

Symptoms. The initial symptom is diarrhoea, constipation or rectal bleeding, the last accounting for the frequent diagnosis of 'piles'. Diarrhoea becomes predominant, except when the disease is confined to the rectum. Incontinence and tenesmus, with its urge to empty the bowel, make life intolerable unless there is immediate proximity to a bed-pan or toilet and rectal discharges may occur independently of faeces. Abdominal cramps may be caused by colon spasm, though usually the condition is painless. The clinical spectrum is wide; at one end is the patient with the mild distal type of colitis, whose life may be hardly inconvenienced by the occasional attacks of diarrhoea, at the other end is a dangerous and disabling disease which, unchecked, will result in a profound state of malnutrition and dehydration.

Symptoms depend mainly upon the extent of the colitis, and the following three types (Fig. 17.11), can usually be recognized:

Proctitis. Symptoms are mild and constipation takes the place of diarrhoea; passage of blood is the first and sometimes only symptom and hardness of faeces aggravates bleeding from the fragile mucosa. The patient, though complaining of diarrhoea, often means that he passes mucus, blood and pus throughout the day without faeces. Blood is separate or on the surface of the stool as in piles and not mixed with it as in colitis. The upper limit of the proctitis can be seen at sigmoidoscopy. Some have thought that proctitis is a distinct condition and there are other causes (Table 17.9); allergy may be a factor in some who respond to sodium cromoglycate. However, about 10% develop ulcerative colitis later. Proctitis is a condition that waxes and wanes, often being more an inconvenience than a disability, and subsides altogether in some.

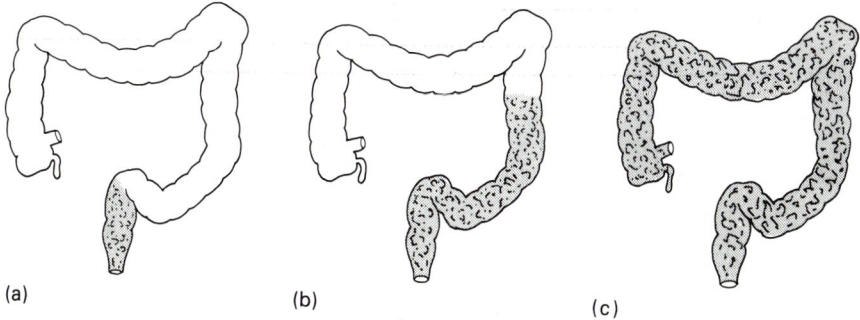

(a)   (b)   (c)

Fig. 17.11. Types of ulcerative colitis. (a) Proctitis; (b) proctosigmoiditis; (c) total colitis.

Table 17.9. Causes of proctitis.

Common
  Ulcerative colitis
Occasional
  Gonococcal
  Syphilitic
  Allergic (?)
  Suppositories
  Crohn's disease
Rare
  Herpes simplex virus
  Lymphogranuloma venereum

Proctosigmoiditis. (proctocolitis Fig. 17.12). Proctosigmoiditis generally pursues a relapsing course with intermittent self-limiting attacks. Patients are treated by the physician rather than the surgeon; they may be well nourished, without anaemia, and afebrile, except during relapses. The usual mildness of the course is no guarantee that, at any time a severe or fulminating episode may not occur, or that the disease may not spread to involve the entire colon.

Total colitis. Involvement of the entire colon causes severe symptoms and can be dangerous especially when toxic dilatation occurs. Indicators of severity are shown in Table 17.10.

    The whole colon bears the brunt of the disease from the onset in some patients, though in others it spreads gradually from the rectum; it is more likely to pursue a continuous than intermittent course, and systemic complications (Table 17.2), including late malignant change, are more likely. Most will eventually require surgery so that if the patient does not soon respond to medical treatment early operation can be advised.

Local complications. Perforation of the colon may be disastrous and is easily missed in patients who are debilitated or receiving corticosteroids. For there may be no rigidity or other abnormal signs even if the peritoneum is filled with faeces; then,

Table 17.10. Indicators of severity in ulcerative colitis.

Fever	> 37.5 C (99.5F)
Tachycardia	> 90 per min
Anaemia	Hb 10 g/dl or less
ESR	> 30 mm in 1 h
Serum albumin	< 30 g/l

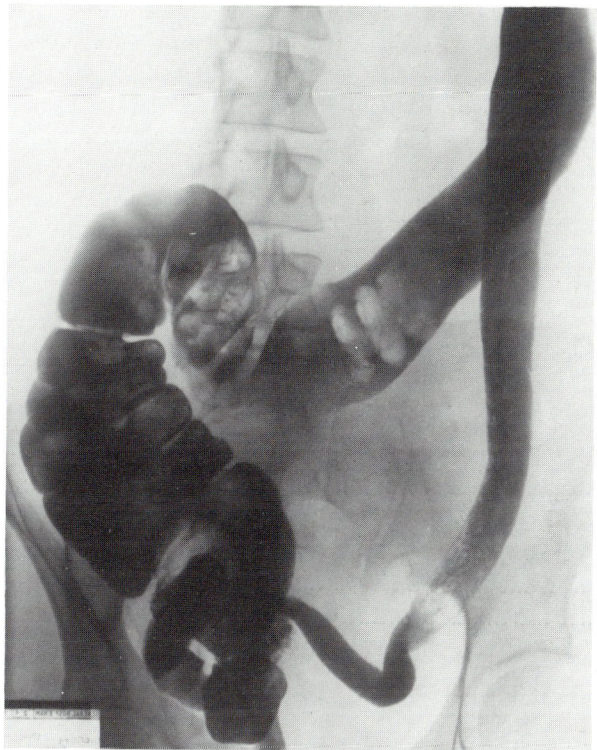

Fig. 17.12. Involvement of distal colon only as in proctocolitis. The proximal colon is healthy and contains normal faeces.

diagnosis is only possible by radiographs to demonstrate air under the diaphragm or in the peritoneal cavity in the lateral position. Perforation must be considered whenever a patient complains of sudden, unexpected pain, particularly if there is shock. Perforation of the rectum is prevented by the surrounding structures and, instead of peritonitis, an ischiorectal abscess or recto-vaginal fistula develops. Rectal complications such as thrombosed piles, fissure, fistula of peri-rectal abscess are less likely than in Crohn's disease; although seldom endangering the patient, they may be so painful as to overshadow other symptoms. Massive bleeding is rare.

Pseudopolyposis (Fig. 17.13) due to regeneration of mucosal tags in the healing phase occurs in more than half the patients. Intestinal obstruction is rare even with a stricture, for the stools are liquid. Cancer may occur in long-standing cases with extensive disease; the most sinister sign on barium enema is the development of the stricture, for this is often malignant.

Systemic complications. Erythema nodosum, arthritis and irido-cyclitis (Table 17.2) occur in ulcerative colitis as in Crohn's disease, usually affecting around 10% of patients. These could be due to bacterial and toxic products absorbed through an ulcerated bowel or possibly to immune complexes. Anaemia is common, due to iron deficiency from occult bleeding or due to the depression of haemopoiesis which accompanies inflammation, and frequently to both. Hypoproteinaemia is often seen, due to loss of protein from the ulcerated bowel (protein-losing enteropathy). The level of liver enzymes may be raised but this seldom indicates any significant damage to the liver; fatty infiltration is the commonest change, but scattered areas of

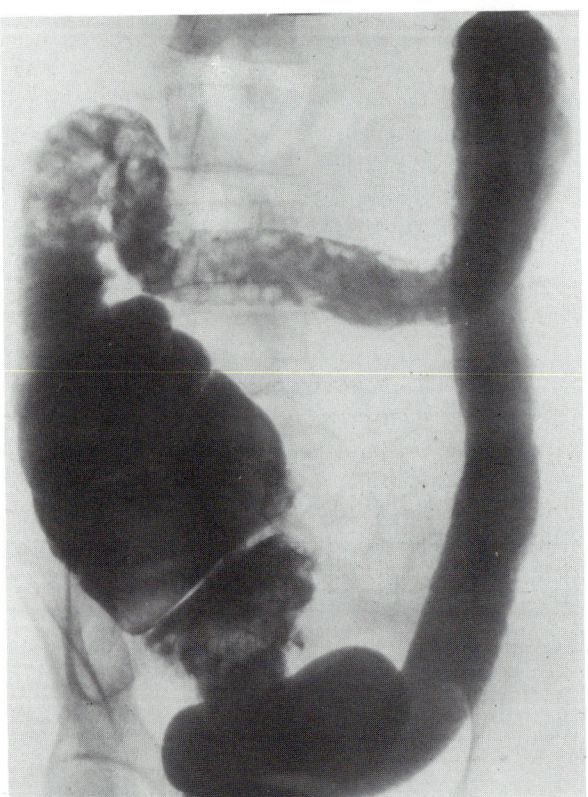

Fig. 17.13. Pseudopolyposis of the colon in ulcerative colitis.

focal necrosis of liver cells with surrounding inflammation also occur; the latter is called peri-cholangitis and has been attributed to bombardment of the liver by bacteria reaching it from the colon via the portal vein. Hepatic lesions are seldom serious. Deep vein thrombosis of the legs is common during attacks. Pyoderma gangrenosum is an uncommon association and also occurs in rheumatoid arthritis and other conditions. Small septic lesions appear usually on the legs and may cause ulcers.

Diagnosis. The stools: these, in the acute phase, consist of blood, mucus and pus only. When blood and mucus predominate, they look like those seen in cancer of rectum or colon; if there is only pus, the creamy stool may mimic steatorrhoea. Stools should always be cultured for pathogenic organisms to exclude an enteric infection.

Proctoscopy. This can easily be done by the inexperienced at the bedside or out-patients; then an immediate diagnosis can be made. In early cases, friability of the mucus membrane which bleeds easily when touched is the best sign; diffuse redness may occur in any type of diarrhoea. Later, the mucosa may be so oedematous as almost to obliterate the lumen and the mucosa is denuded and the surface covered with blood and pus.

Sigmoidoscopy. This can be dangerous in the acute phase because of perforation, either directly by the instrument or in distal parts of the colon from insufflation of air. Rectal biopsy confirms the diagnosis and may be helpful when the disease is quiescent, as the mucosa may look normal in spite of histological changes, and is necessary if Crohn's disease is suspected.

Radiological examination. Early ulcerative colitis may be missed by barium enema and later it does not reveal the extent of the disease. Typically, loss of haustration occurs (Fig. 17.14), and the colon may appear shortened, rigid and tubular like a garden hose-pipe. The descending and sigmoid colon is sometimes ahaustral and narrow in normals, so that an altered mucosal pattern, seen best by double-contrast barium enema, may be the only reliable guide to disease. Barium enema should be undertaken cautiously in severely ill patients, because of the risk of perforation.

Colonoscopy. This allows direct inspection of the whole colon and biopsies can be taken (p. 112). It is essential for assessing the extent of the disease and for detecting early malignant change.

Other techniques. Indium-labelled leucocyte scanning has been used for assessing the extent of colonic disease in ulcerative colitis and Crohn's disease but there is not yet proof that this has any advantage, apart from being non-invasive, over colonoscopy or double-contrast barium meal.

Differential diagnosis. The diagnosis of ulcerative colitis is usually easy in temperate zones and confusion with dysentery or tropical diseases like amoebiasis is unlikely to arise. Crohn's disease of the colon is easily mistaken for ulcerative colitis (Table 17.8), but it more often affects the proximal colon (Fig. 17.15)—sometimes the

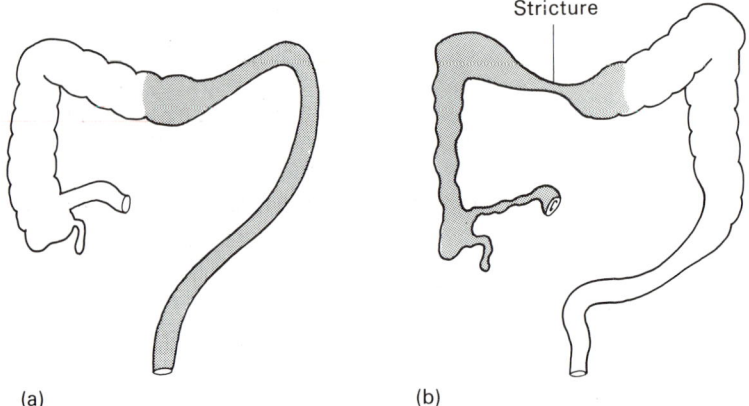

(a) (b)

Fig. 17.14. (a) Ulcerative colitis (distal colon and rectum always involved); (b) Crohn's disease (proximal colon and terminal ileum especially affected).

terminal ileum as well—and causes benign strictures (Fig. 17.5); the rectum may appear normal, but biopsy may show the giant cells of Crohn's disease. Congenital polyposis of the colon can be recognized because haustra are present whereas these have disappeared in the acquired pseudo-polyposis of ulcerative colitis. Other conditions may sometimes be mistaken for ulcerative colitis (Table 17.7).

Treatment. Many cases are adequately treated by medical measurements, especially milder cases where only the distal colon is involved, or where attacks occur with long intervals of slight diarrhoea or normal bowel function. It is in the severe attacks where the whole colon is involved that it is best to share the responsibility with a surgeon especially interested in colitis.

Medical measures comprise: bed rest, a sympathetic physician and confident nursing staff, careful attention to fluid and electrolyte balance, treatment of anaemia by blood transfusion or by oral or parenteral iron, and a diet high in protein and calorie value, though low in residue until the attack subsides. Parenteral feeding is sometimes necessary during the acute phase. Rarely, a patient is allergic to milk, so that a milk-free diet is then advisable.

A bewildering number of therapeutic agents have been used in the hope of aborting an attack, but their effect is difficult to assess, for the course of the disease is unpredictable and spontaneous improvement will foster the bias of the physician in his treatment.

Diarrhoea. This can be treated by: (a) codeine phosphate which is the cheapest and, being an opiate, may help to relieve any pain as well as diarrhoea. Few patients are helped by less than 15 mg thrice daily or by more than 60 mg four times daily if lower doses have failed. (b) Diphenoxylate (Lomotil) is chemically related to opiates, and each tablet of 2.5 mg contains atropine sulphate to discourage abuse. Two tablets three or four times daily are prescribed. (c) Loperamide inhibits peristalsis by antagonizing muscle contraction. The usual dose is 4 mg followed by 2 mg after each loose stool up to a total dose of 16 mg daily. (d) Antispasmodics are occasionally helpful in a patient with inactive disease as diarrhoea may be due to a superimposed irritability of the bowel. Propantheline bromide (Probanthine) 15 mg thrice daily or mebevrine 135 mg three or four times daily can be used. (Note that in total colitis there is a risk of toxic dilatation from motility inhibitors.)

Antibiotics. These are seldom indicated and then only for short periods, unless septic complications have occurred.

Sulphasalazine (Salazopyrine). This has a slight but definite effect in acute attacks but is especially useful in preventing relapses. The large tablets contain 0.5 g and a suitable dose for starting is 1.0 g three or four times daily; if nausea or vomiting occurs the dose should be reduced and then gradually increased. For interval therapy to prevent relapse, a daily dose of 0.5 g three or four times daily can be kept up continuously. Blood disorders such as agranulocytosis or haemolytic anaemia are fortunately rare but indicate the need for occasional blood checks. Rashes sometimes appear and desensitization with small doses may be necessary (Holdsworth 1981). The 5-aminosalicylic acid moiety is probably as effective and does not have the side-effects of Sulphonamide.

Corticosteroid therapy. A 'cortisone' drug is an excellent tonic in any pyrexial illness, for appetitie is improved and a feeling of well-being created. The temperature, whatever the cause, is reduced to normal; this may be dangerous, for symptoms are masked and the disease may progress unsuspected. Corticosteroids, however, help to subdue an attack of ulcerative colitis, and should be given for about 6 weeks, providing immediate improvement is obvious. Prednisolone can be given by mouth in a dose of 50–60 mg daily in divided doses. If parenteral therapy is necessary because of nausea and vomiting, prednisolone 21-phosphate is given as 20 mg twice daily in the intravenous drip or by intramuscular injection. ACTH may be more effective than prednisolone and 40 units can be injected once or twice daily; or the equivalent dose of tetracosactrin zinc phosphate (Synacthen depot 1 mg=80 units ACTH) can be given intramuscularly daily or on alternative days.

Maintenance with corticosteroid therapy has no effect in preventing relapses and is seldom, if ever, justified.

Side-effects of corticosteroids include moniliasis in the pharynx and increased septic complications: they do not affect wound healing or increase risk of perforation. Their greatest hazard is in causing the physician to procrastinate in advising surgery, for the progress of the disease is masked and the patient reaches operation later when a poor risk.

The corticosteroid retention enema was intended as a topical treatment free from the side effects of systemic administration, but all these drugs are absorbed from the colon to some degree, though with most it is the local action that predominates. Retention enemas (Predsol 20 mg) at night should be prescribed and continued for 2 or 3 weeks. The foot of the bed should be raised and retention may be aided by a sedative, or by propantheline 15 to 30 mg given orally or intravenously. Instructions are issued with the disposable plastic bag fitted with a nozzle so that the patient can use the enemas himself at home. For proctitis, suppositories containing prednisolone—21-phosphate (Predsol 5 mg) inserted once or twice daily should be sufficient.

There is as yet no proof that azathioprine or other cytotoxic drugs have any definite effect.

Disodium cromoglycate (Intal) has been used in patients with proctitis where the prominence of eosinophils in the inflammatory exudate or mucosa suggests that allergy may be a factor.

Suppositories containing sulphasalazine 0.5 g have benefited active procto-sigmoiditis. Sulphasalazine is also available in retention enemas of 3 g which may be effective; with a volume increased to 100 ml these enemas may be of value in more extensive colitis.

Surgery. The indications for surgery are shown in Table 17.11. Colectomy and ileostomy is the usual operation; the rectum may be removed at the same time, or later in ill patients. The adherent ileostomy bag (Fig. 17.15) allows a normal life to be lived. Women marry and produce normal children through the usual route, but there is a small risk of impotence in men, because of damage to the presacral nerves. Ileostomy should be performed during a quiescent period preferably instead of as a desperate measure in an ill patient. So, when it is apparent that medical treatment is failing, the subject of ileostomy is cautiously approached and a member of the ileostomy association which all patients should join (Ileostomy Association of Great Britain and Ireland, Amblehurst House, Chobham, Woking, Surrey) is asked to visit and discuss the practical problems with the patient. The ileostomy has to be permanent. A normal diet is allowed though some restrict their food slightly and avoid residue which may form a bolus and cause pain at the stoma. More fluid and

Table 17.11. Indications for operation in ulcerative colitis.

1   When return to normal life is impossible in spite of all forms of medical therapy.
2   Acute severe colitis which has not responded to medical treatment especially if entire colon is diseased.
3   Complications such as perforation, uncontrollable haemorrhage, acute dilatation, or intractable anal lesions such as fissure or fistula.
4   Severe systemic complications like arthritis or iridocyclitis.
5   Prophylactic colectomy when there is a great risk of malignant change.

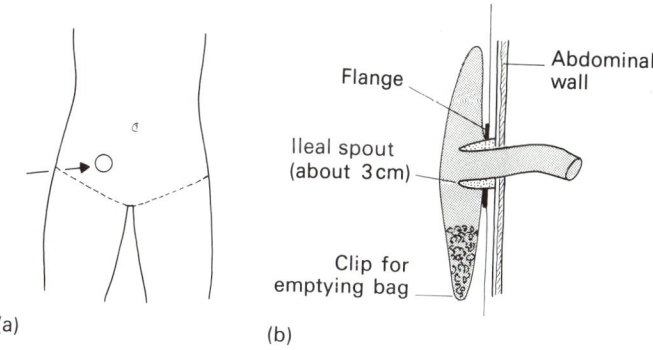

Fig. 17.15. (a) Site of ileostomy stoma; (b) ileostomy bag fixed to abdominal wall by adhesive. The bag may be washable or disposable.

more salt should be consumed as ileostomists may show evidence of mild dehydration and salt depletion. Urinary stones are more common especially in men, possibly due to a low pH in a smaller volume of urine with low solubility for uric acid; gallstones are also more common because of interference with the absorption of bile salts through the ileum.

Ileostomy with colectomy is no bar to life assurance. Complications of the ileostomy itself are excoriation and leakages, sliding recession or prolapse of the stoma, or allergic reactions to the bonding agents used to stick on the appliance. For the last, a trained 'stoma therapist' is especially helpful.

Surgeons strive to develop a stoma which does not need an external appliance. A reservoir fashioned from the last bit of ileum together with a nipple or non-returnable valve can be made: this allows a catheter to be inserted from outside but does not allow the ileal contents to leak out because of the lateral pressure it exerts upon the valve which is then compressed (Fig. 17.16). This can be used for those with conventional stomas suffering from severe skin reactions or for those who have repeated sliding recessions. It is premature to advise a continent ileostomy for younger patients because of complications, such as extrusion of the valve perhaps because the patient has allowed the reservoir to fill excessively, or mucous secretion may collect and exude from the stoma, or difficulties in intubation may be encountered (Gerber *et al.*, 1983).

Total colectomy with ileo-rectal anastomosis is also practised. Many, however, still have diarrhoea because of the diseased rectum and this can be a source of complications and cancer in the future. It is best reserved for those where the rectum is reasonably healthy, for mental cases, or for any who refuse permanent ileostomy.

Prognosis. The extent of colonic disease is the main guide to prognosis. Those patients where the distal colon is involved are often able to lead a normal life because the disease is mild and relapsing, and the risk of malignant change is very small.

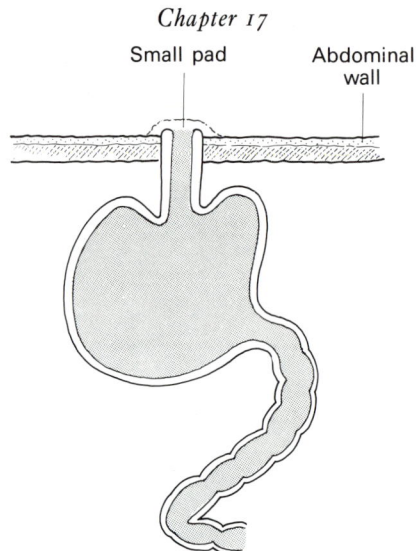

Small pad   Abdominal
                    wall

Fig. 17.16. The Kock continent ileostomy. Reservoir provided with a 'nipple valve'.

With disease of the entire colon, the ability to dehydrate faeces is lost and diarrhoea becomes continuous; occasionally patients make a complete recovery but the outlook for nearly all is poor and early operation is indicated.

Death is more likely in the first attack of ulcerative colitis and during the first year of the disease when the mortality rate may reach 10%. The acute severe attacks carry the greatest risk, the mortality rate being as high as 30%.

Special clinical problems in ulcerative colitis

Acute fulminating ulcerative colitis
This merits special attention because of its dangers. It represents the gravest and most explosive form of the disease. Diarrhoea may vary from six times daily to an almost continuous discharge of blood and pus; toxaemia is often extreme with rapid weight loss; there is tachycardia, anaemia, and a pyrexia sometimes as high as 39.4–40°C. Downhill progress can be relentless and lethal complications such as acute dilatation or perforation of the colon may appear at any time. The physician should treat this type of colitis with the cooperation of the surgeon preferably experienced in this field. Medical treatment, when no improvement has been noticed in 24–48 h, should be abandoned and operation performed. Corticosteroids in particular may mask the signs of a disintegrating colon and make the surgeons task almost insurmountable.

Acute dilatation of the colon (toxic megacolon)
This dangerous and treacherous complication usualy arises in a patient already ill and suffering from acute colitis. The abdomen suddenly becomes distended, tender

and silent, so that a leak may be suspected; indeed, a perforation is often imminent if not actually present. The dilated colon, at operation or necropsy, has a wall so friable and soft that it easily disintegrates on handling. A plain radiograph of the abdomen (Fig. 17.17) is diagnostic and shows an air-filled distended colon with a width greater than 5 cm. The abdominal girth should be measured daily so that the distension can more easily be detected. It is usually an indication for immediate operation.

Ulcerative colitis in children
Its course is similar to that of adults, but there is serious risk of growth being retarded while active colitis persists, and this may be further inhibited if corticosteroids are given. There is no reason to withhold surgery if medical measures fail, and children adjust themselves to ileostomy as well as adults.

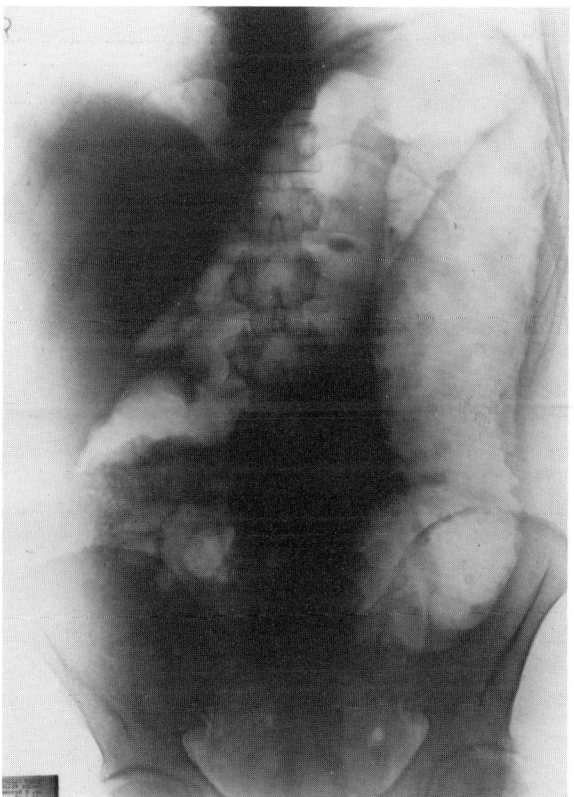

Fig. 17.17. Acute toxic dilatation of colon in ulcerative colitis (width greater than 5 cm). Also pseudopolyposis.

Ulcerative colitis in pregnancy

Fertility is not lessened in ulcerative colitis and, if the disease is reasonably controlled, the chance of delivering a viable infant is good. The effect of pregnancy upon the disease is variable and unpredictable but colitis which begins during pregnancy is more likely to be severe, especially during the first trimester or in the immediate post-partum period. Pregnancy is usually allowed to continue, especially if the desire for a child is great and the colitis not too severe. The colitis should be treated carefully, especially with bed rest. Sulphasalazine can be continued but requires special attention to the newborn since it increases the risk of kernicterus from jaundice. Corticosteroids are not contraindicated. Ileostomy and colectomy are practicable in early pregnancy. When patients with an ileostomy conceive, there is no special reason for Caesarian section and the baby is usually delivered normally at term.

Malignant change

Cancer is a risk in patients with extensive colitis and the longer the duration of the disease, the more likely is malignant change; the young are therefore especially liable to it. Its incidence varies in different series, often according to how the cases are collected. An average figure for those with total colitis is a twenty-fold increase in the second decade and a thirty-fold in the third decade, compared with the healthy population. The cancer occurs in the rectum or sigmoid colon in nearly half the cases and often appears like a stricture. Unfortunately the symptoms are often mild or regarded as a relapse of the ulcerative colitis, so diagnosis is at a late and inoperable stage.

Changes in the mucosa of the rectum and colon such as dysplasia indicate a premalignant phase so screening the patients after perhaps 10 years and those with ileo-rectal anastomosis is practicable—similar to cervical smears for detecting those at risk of developing cervical cancer. Multiple biopsies must be taken and any suspicious area examined most carefully. Suggested programmes advise sigmoidoscopy yearly and colonoscopy every two or three years. However, success will depend upon the following:

1   The cooperation of the patient.
2   Efficiency of the follow-up organization.
3   The skill of the endoscopist.
4   The reliability of metaplasia as a fore-runner of cancer.

Unfortunately none of these is infallible. So, for patients at risk, especially with symptoms, ileostomy with removal of the colon and rectum may be preferable.

Patients may be helped by joining the National Association for Colitis and Crohn's Disease, 3 Thorpefield Close, Marshalswick, St. Albans, Herts. England.

Chapter 18
Motility Disorders of the Colon and Rectum

The colon together with an efficient anal sphincter—the sentinel of social security—allows a social life which would be impossible if, as in the lower species, waste material was discharged at random. Patients with colonic failure in ulcerative colitis are almost like this; life is impossible if they are far from a lavatory as on beaches or motorways. The reserve capacity of the normal colon is great: perfusion studies with a tube in the caecum show that the colon can absorb three litres of fluid daily—six times the normal 500 ml that ileostomies discharge.

The colon absorbs water, sodium and chloride and secretes potassium; in addition bicarbonate ions are secreted into the lumen. Sodium is actively absorbed but chloride absorption is passive. Potassium may be secreted passively into the lumen to maintain electrical neutrality disturbed by the active movement of sodium ions in the opposite direction; or a coupled sodium–potassium pump may exist in the colon, actively transferring sodium ions from the lumen to blood and potassium ions in the opposite direction. Its absorptive function is modified in response to the body's needs; in salt deprivation, stool sodium is reduced because of increased absorption.

Colonic motility
Most contracting waves are of the delayed or segmental type (peristaltic waves are rarely seen) so that contents are kneaded and turned over by non-propulsive churning movements. Annular contractions produce the haustra seen on radiographs and are the chief mixing movements.

The caecum and ascending colon act as a reservoir and movement of colonic contents is imperceptible as far as the hepatic flexure. Mass movements involve the transverse and left colon, the first event being disappearance of the haustra followed by a rapid synchronous contraction of a considerable length (about 20 cm) of the bowel; these occur about three to four times daily, driving contents of the proximal into the distal colon. The rectum is normally empty and faeces accumulate above the recto-sigmoid junction. It takes about 1–8 h for the contents of the stomach to reach the colon. Here matter is stored for varying times until defaecation occurs, perhaps 24 h or longer after eating the food. The frequency of normal bowel action in 99% of the population lies between three times weekly and three actions daily but depends upon habit and the amount of residue eaten.

Food and the colon
Epidemiological and experimental observations suggest that the low fibre intake in

industrialized communities may be a factor in causing several important conditions: constipation, irritable bowel, diverticular disease of the colon, inflammatory bowel disease, cancer of the colon, haemorrhoids and possibly appendicitis.

To function efficiently the colon needs a properly formed stool, so plenty of residue is needed. Fibre consists of a group of carbohydrate compounds including cellulose and the hemi-celluloses, and a non-carbohydrate substance lignin. Although some vegetables and fruit do have a high fibre content, cereal fibre seems to be the most effective. Bran is merely one of the many dietary fibre supplements and is a heterogeneous material supplying from 22–46 g fibre/100 g depending on its source; so a daily course of 20 g bran supplies from 5–8 g fibre. Bran is the outer layer of wheat and other cereal grain which is usually lost in the refining processes.

A high residue diet has the following effect:

1   Colonic transit is accelerated.
2   Stool weight is increased.
3   Intracolonic pressure waves are reduced, usually after 3 months.
4   The bacterial flora of the colon is changed and reduced—noticed by diminished stool odour.

Bran is usually advised as a cheap and natural way of adding residue to the diet. It can be added to cereals, porridge or soup, or in making bread; the amount is gradually increased until a normal soft stool is regularly produced. Coarse is better than fine bran, being more efficient in holding water. Fybranta consists of bran and calcium phosphate, each tablet containing 2 g bran. However, tablets cost more than ten times that of bran and tablets encourage the patient to regard treatment as a medical matter. The fibre content of various foods is shown in Table 18.1.

Faeces
These consist of a cellulose residue and bacteria (15–20% dry weight). The water-soluble fractions contain nitrogen (a by-product of amino acid catabolism), 100 mmol.K./l and 50 mmol.Na/l and the daily excretion of fat in normals is from one to four grams, the upper limit being 7 g, and about half comes from desquamated mucosal cells. The stools are large and pale when disorders of the small intestine cause malabsorption (Fig. 18.1–18.3). In disease of the colon (Fig. 18.4), the stools are usually small and watery and often contain obvious blood.

Irritable bowel

Irritable bowel, like migraine, is a disorder of function rather than of structure. It accounts for up to 50% of patients attending gastroenterological clinics. The term irritable bowel indicates that any part of the alimentary tract may be involved, even the oesophagus. Many have symptoms in the upper abdomen like nervous dyspepsia and aerophagy, and also in the lower abdomen with a change in bowel action. Irritable bowel may start in childhood, 'little belly achers' may grow into 'big belly achers', and it is slightly more common in women. Mild degrees are common in the healthy population who never visit doctors.

Table 18.1. Fibre content of average portions of some foods (28 g = 1 oz).

	Size of portion (g)	Fibre (g)
Vegetables		
Potato (mashed)	120	1.1
Cabbage	75	1.9
Carrots	75	2.3
Peas	75	5.8
Spinach	100	6.3
Fruit		
Grapefruit $\frac{1}{2}$	250	0.7
Apple with skin	120	2.3
Stewed rhubarb	100	2.4
Prunes	25	3.4
Nuts		
Roasted peanuts	25	2.0
Almonds	25	3.6
Bread		
White	40 (1 slice medium loaf)	1.1
Wholemeal	40 (1 slice medium loaf)	3.4
Sunblest Hi-bran	38 (2 small slices)	4.15
Cereals		
Porridge	200 (2 tablespoonfuls oats)	1.6
Cornflakes	25 (4 tablespoonfuls)	2.8
Muesli	50 (3 tablespoonfuls)	3.7
Bran	10 (2 tablespoonfuls)	4.4
Shredded wheat	55 (2 tablespoonfuls)	6.8
All-Bran	50 (4 tablespoonfuls)	13.4

(Note that bran has the highest percentage content of fibre but a smaller portion is usually taken.)

Labels given to it resemble a veritable tower of Babel: spastic colon, dyskinesia, functional enterocolonopathy (a diagnosis which should satisfy any patient), non-specific diarrhoea, lienteric diarrhoea, mucomembranous colic and mucous colitis. The term colitis must be avoided as it causes unnecessary worry: an intelligent patient may become anxious about the need for colectomy and ileostomy.

Aetiology
The cause is unknown but occasionally the following may be relevant:
1 Past infection of the bowel. It may follow amoebic or bacillary dysentery.

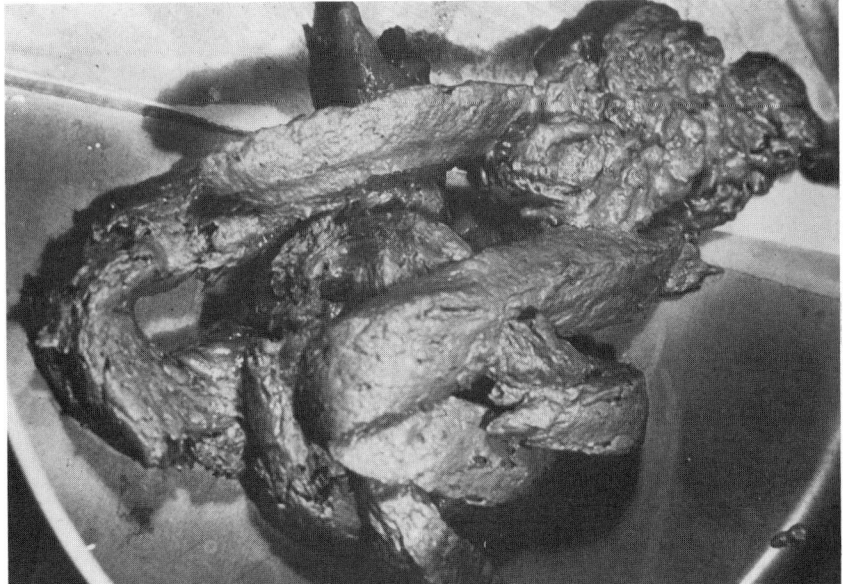

Fig. 18.2. The diagnosis of chronic pancreatitis was made because of a small area of butter-like unsplit fat on the surface of the stool.

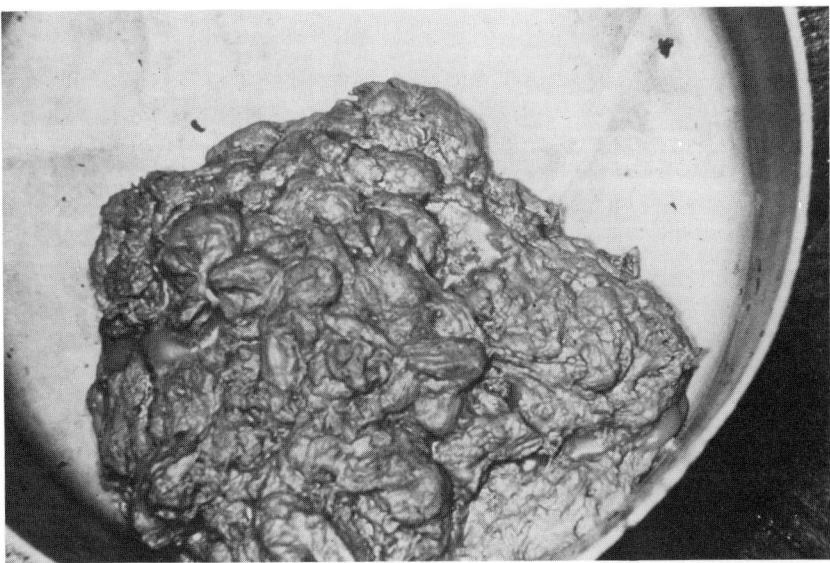

Fig. 18.1. Massive pale fatty stool of patient with adult coeliac disease.

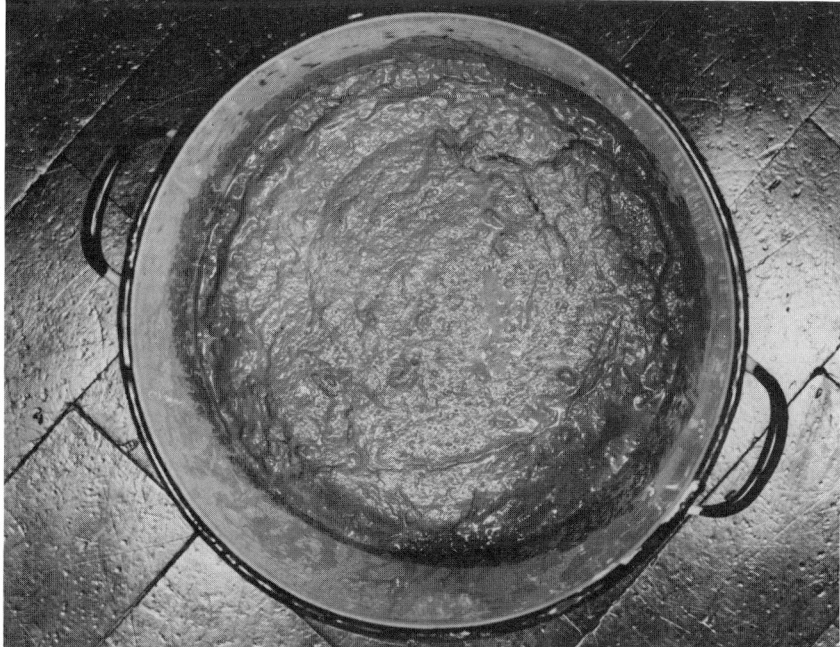

Fig. 18.3. This stool was from a patient with adult coeliac disease who was passing 2–3 litres daily. There was an additional lactase deficiency shown by fermentation producing bubbles on the surface.

2   Purgatives. These were important when it was believed that a daily bowel action was essential for maintaining health; some became obsessed with their bowels and addicted to purgatives which increased colonic irritability. Nowadays some resort to purgatives because of the constipation.

3   Psychogenic factors. Worry may make symptoms worse but this may happen with organic bowel disease and, in the healthy, diarrhoea may be precipitated by taking an examination or suchlike. Experiments also demonstrate the striking effect of emotion upon the human colon, with alterations in its motility and blood supply. Studies of the psychological characteristics of patients with an irritable colon syndrome compared with normals show a good deal of overlap but some series report more anxiety and neurotic traits than in the healthy; however, neurotic traits could have developed as a consequence of the disorder or perhaps from the numerous investigations often undertaken.

4   Diet. 'Westernized' diet is probably important as there is little doubt that a low residue diet is detrimental to bowel function; indeed motility in the colon partly depends upon stimulation by the contents.

5   A disorder of smooth muscle. Some patients may be born with a tendency for

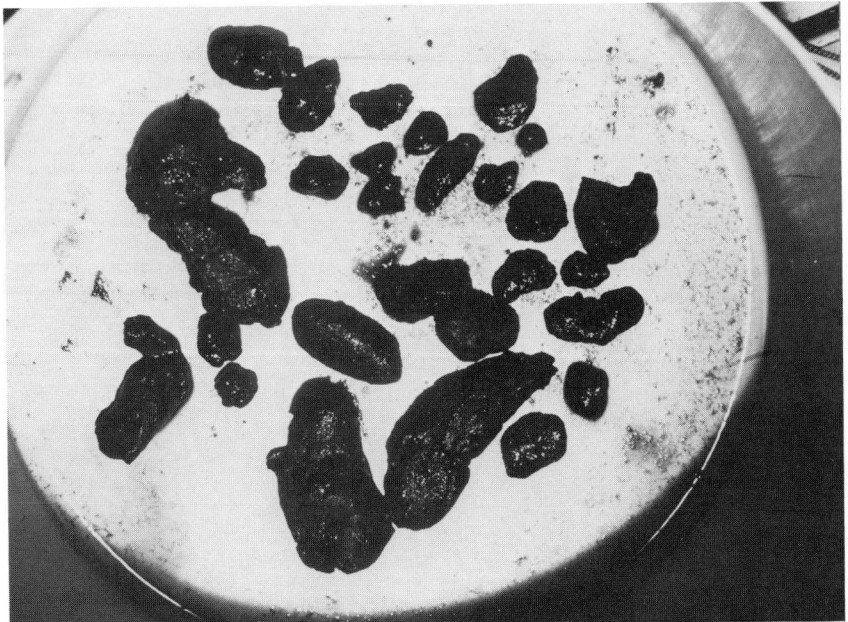

Fig. 18.4. 'Anisocytosis' of stool from man with irritable colon who passed rabbit-like motions and bits of varying size and shape.

their smooth muscle to react abnormally. Many adults date their symptoms to childhood. Also a generalized disorder of smooth muscle could explain other symptoms such as dysmenorrhoea or migraine. Possible genetic factors are suggested by occasional familial occurrences.

6 Lactase deficiency. Failure of lactose to be split into glucose and galactose causes osmotic diarrhoea; these motions may mimic those of irritable colon and a connection with milk or its products may not be noticed. This is sometimes worth excluding (p. 274).

Pathophysiology
This has been partly elucidated by kymographic studies with a latex balloon or photoelectric transducers connected to a pressure recorder. Hyperactive records with increased frequency and force of contraction occur in the spastic group though the painless diarrhoea type show reduced colonic activity. Studies on patients with postprandial symptoms show an exaggerated sigmoid response. Increase in colonic motor activity after a meal could be mediated by humoral agents, perhaps due to an increased sensitivity of colonic musculature to endogenous cholecystokinin. The colon in these patients is certainly over-sensitive to cholinergic drugs.

Clinical features

Some, the majority, complain of pain and constipation whereas others have a painless diarrhoea.

1   Pain. This is usually felt in the lower abdomen especially in the left iliac fossa and defaecation usually relieves it though occasionally aggravates it. It is usually aching though sometimes so severe that patients are admitted to hospital as emergencies and undergo laparotomy. Periods of strain and emotional upheaval often precipitate an attack and fear of cancer tends to prolong the symptoms. Some find that their pain is exacerbated by food and suffer discomfort in the upper abdomen associated with a feeling of bloating.

2   Bowel habit. The constipation of spastic colon often causes small hard stools like 'rabbit droppings'; others describe thin ribbon or pencil shaped stools which vary (Fig. 18.4), unlike those due to a rectal stricture which are persistent. This spasticity of the rectum may account for the feeling that 'the bowel has not been properly emptied'. Such rectal dissatisfaction accounts for some people becoming obsessed about their bowel (Fig. 18.5) and addicted to purgatives. Some mistakenly describe the frequent passage of small constipated stools as diarrhoea.

Diarrhoea is sometimes associated with pain and this may increase in severity, culminating in the urgent passage of a watery or mushy stool with relief of pain. Those who have only painless diarrhoea often complain of urgency, especially in the morning and soon after rising or immediately after breakfast. This sequence of events may repeat itself up to three or four times in an hour, leaving the patient exhausted but needing no further bowel action for the rest of the day. The diarrhoea seldom disturbs the patient during the night and when this happens an organic cause should be suspected.

3   Mucus, blood and other symptoms. Patients often complain of passing mucus in their stools. Formerly large amounts might be seen, indeed so much that mucous casts of the bowel were formed—an example of extreme secretory activity of the colon. This afflicted especially young women at the beginning of this century, particularly after profound emotional upset and the taking of large quantities of

> 5.30 a.m. Urge, wind only
> 6.00 a.m. Normal stool
> 7.45 a.m. Like 'mere shrimps'
> 1.55 p.m. Loose
> 3.45 p.m. Crescent stool
> 6.40 p.m. Mini stool
> 8.25 p.m. Three-pronged stool
> 9.00 p.m. Another mini stool
> 10.30 p.m. Finish with shrapnel neplan stool

Fig. 18.5. Extract from a seven-page letter from a patient who was obsessed about his stools. He suffered from an irritable colon.

purgatives; its disappearance may be due to the emancipation of women and abandonment of purgatives. Rectal bleeding denotes an organic lesion but patients with constipation are liable to develop anal fissures or haemorrhoids which may bleed. Other complaints are common and often nervous: dysmenorrhoea, headaches and dizziness (rarely true vertigo), tiredness, loss of mental concentration, reduced sexual function, depression and anxiety.

Physical examination. Abnormal signs are few. Tenderness may be found in various parts of the abdomen, especially in the left iliac fossa where the colon can be palpated as a firm band. The abdomen may show scars of previous unnecessary operation, such as for a normal appendix.

Diagnosis. Irritable colon is diagnosed from the history and by exclusion of other *likely* causes. Stool-gazing is essential: the small stools with their different shapes, anisocytosis (Fig. 18.4), are typical of the spastic type and make organic disease of the colon unlikely; with diarrhoea the stools are watery and unlike the large volume ones of malabsorption. The following investigations should be done:

1 Rectal examination and sigmoidoscopy: obvious spasm with production of the same pain strongly supports the diagnosis.

2 Barium enema may be necessary except in young women where it can be omitted unless follow-up shows persistence of symptoms. Areas of spasm may be seen coinciding with the same type of pain. Carcinoma of the colon has a wide age range and may occur in the young.

3 Routine blood count. This excludes anaemia and a normal erythrocyte sedimentation rate (Westergren) makes inflammatory disease of the bowel such as Crohn's disease unlikely.

Problems in diagnosis. Confusion often arises as to whether the patient has diverticulitis, usually because a few diverticula are seen on the barium enema.

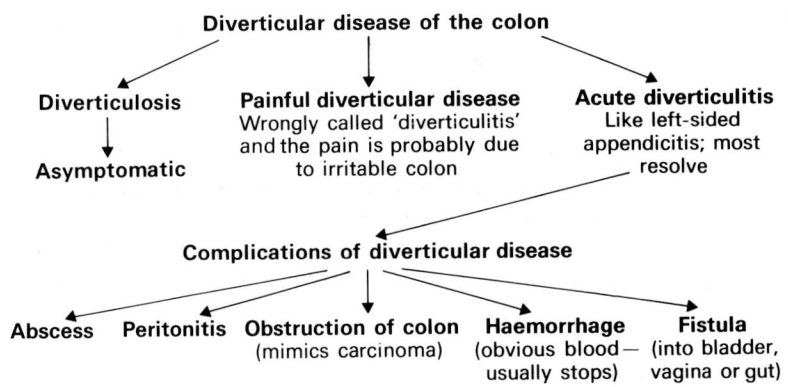

Fig. 18.6. Diverticular disease of the colon.

However, this appearance is a normal symptomless finding and diverticulosis sometimes follows a long history of irritable colon and is probably due to the same disorder of motility. Also an irregularity sometimes reported as the pre-diverticular stage can merely be due to abnormal motility. The erroneous label of diverticulitis must be avoided as it increases the anxiety of patients.

The fear of missing organic disease which previously led to unnecessary operations now results in a battery of futile investigations. Indeed one patient had had three ERCPs to exclude pancreatitis—apart from other tests—before someone talked to the patient and discovered the typical history of irritable colon.

Treatment. Simple psychotherapy—explanation and reassurance is the mainstay of treatment—the 'talking cure.' Reassurance is essential as many fear cancer or are frightened by mucus. Explanation is most important for many have been confused by numerous investigations and by being given different diagnoses. The pain can be described as 'spasm due to a sensitive bowel'. Extra residue, either in the form of a high fibre diet or by bran, produces changes in motility with improvement of symptoms but this may have to be continued for at least 3 months before benefit is felt. Some have been prescribed low residue diets in the past and it may be difficult to get them to accept the opposite idea. The importance of bran on colonic function can be discussed and the idea put forward that bran soothes the colon and reduces the pain.

Drugs are seldom necessary and the effect of drugs is difficult to assess because any new drug, whether placebo or otherwise, may have an effect, at any rate temporarily. Antispasmodics are often prescribed, either the anticholinergics which act through the autonomic nervous system or the musculotropics that have a direct effect on the colon. The former which includes propantheline bromide and dicyclomine amongst many others show a variable clinical response and may cause undesirable side effects. Mebeverine and peppermint oil belong to the latter group which act directly upon the smooth muscle of the colon. Sedatives or antidepressants are often prescribed if an underlying psychoneurosis is thought to be significant. A psychiatrist may be needed especially if a depressive state is present. The patient will have to be protected from unnecessary operations and a convincing diagnosis may save him travelling from one physician to another.

Prognosis. The outlook may depend upon the type of diagnosis. If a confident diagnosis is made soon after the start, the outlook is probably good, especially compared with patients who have gone from doctor to doctor with no definite diagnosis over many years. Many continue to have symptoms but no longer worry about them, and are able to lead a normal life. A few, perhaps 10%, become hypochondriacs.

Proctalgia fugax

This name is given to recurring attacks of distressing rectal pain without organic disease. Attacks, which often awake the patient at night, may be severe, and last for 10–15 min. A fruitless desire to empty the rectum is followed by the passage of flatus and an increased erotic feeling. The pain can be agonizing and cause syncope. The cause may be rectal spasm as is sometimes seen with irritable colon, or vascular as in migraine. Relief of pain is sometimes brought about by direct or firm pressure on the anus, by assumption of the genu-pectoral position, or by nitroglycerine tablets.

Self-induced diarrhoea

Deliberate disability is easily missed unless the index of suspicion is acute. It usually occurs in otherwise responsible paramedicals like nurses and can mimic various organic diseases. It is usually impossible to persuade the patient to admit having taken any purgatives and the locker may have to be searched to find the tablets, or a marked thermometer used to detect the faking of a temperature—Crohn's disease is then easily suspected. Often patients have been painstakingly investigated with negative findings and this diagnosis is only considered as a last resort. One woman was intensively investigated for malabsorption but it was noticed during a routine faecal fat estimation that the addition of alkali to the faecal aliquot turned it pink; this was due to phenolphthalein. In another, two bottles of cascara were found when a young woman's locker was searched in hospital; although cascara was present in the urine, she denied taking purgatives—but this revelation cured the diarrhoea. Tests for cascara or phenolphthalein can easily be done on the urine or faeces.

Diverticular disease of the colon

The incidence of diverticulosis increases directly with age. The average age of patients when first seen is 55 years, so diverticulitis will become an increasing problem in an ageing population. There is no obvious sex difference, and any connection between obesity and diverticulosis is a tradition and not a fact.

Aetiology

The geographical distribution of diverticulosis suggests that it is due to lack of fibre in the refined Westernized diet; for diverticular disease is hardly ever seen in underdeveloped countries where plenty of vegetables and fruit are eaten instead of refined carbohydrate, sugar, white flour and confectionery. Unknown in rural African communities, it is appearing in Africans living in towns. Moreover, the black races who eat the same food as other inhabitants of the USA develop diverticulosis like others. When the contents of the colon lack bulk, the muscle contracts on an empty lumen so that segmental rings of contraction cause areas of high pressure, producing balloon-like bulges at weak sites—usually where blood vessels penetrate—as in a damaged bicycle tyre.

Motility studies show an increased intraluminal pressure, and the thickening of smooth muscle seen especially in the sigmoid colon is due to work hypertrophy.

This disordered motility explains why some patients suffer from colonic pain like irritable colon long before diverticulosis presents.

Symptoms. Diverticulosis is usually symptomless. Diverticulitis follows inflammatory changes which start in the diverticula when their outlets are blocked by a faecal bolus or by spasm. Then there may be signs like localized pain or tenderness, with fever, leucocytosis, a raised ESR and X-ray changes.

Pain is the main symptom, usually in the left iliac fossa or lower abdomen. It may be aggravated by constipation and relieved by defaecation. With peritoneal involvement, it becomes continuous and more severe; a tender mass like carcinoma may be present. Bowel action is altered, constipation being more common than diarrhoea.

Other symptoms are due to complications (Fig. 18.6). Perforation of a diverticulum may be gradual so that a protective wall of inflammatory or fibrous tissue develops with abscess formation, or it may be sudden and followed by fatal peritonitis. A diverticular abscess may penetrate into the bladder and cause a vesico-colic fistula, with pneumaturia; or more commonly, symptoms of cystitis if the inflamed colon lies adjacent to the bladder. Similarly, a vagina-colic fistula may develop. Haemorrhage occurs intermittently, fresh blood being passed, but consistently positive occult blood in the stools is unlikely, in contrast to the positive results in carcinoma of the colon. Massive bleeding, severe enough to need operation, occasionally occurs; the blood usually comes from the inflamed mucosa or sometimes from a vessel passing over the neck of the diverticulum. Intestinal obstruction may be due to spasm or oedema rather than fibrosis and often responds to conservative measures. Bowel symptoms in diverticulitis may be minimal or absent, and the condition may then present as pyrexia of unknown origin.

Diagnosis. Diverticula may be present in up to 50% of patients over the age of 60 years when barium studies are done. It may be impossible to distinguish diverticulitis from diverticulosis by barium enema but pointers towards it are fixation of the bowel, distortion of the diverticula and persistent narrowing. The openings of diverticula can rarely be seen at sigmoidoscopy, and colonoscopy has to be practised with caution because of the risk of entering a diverticulum and perforating it.

Treatment. When diverticulitis is discovered as an incidental finding in a patient where the diagnosis is probably irritable colon, reassurance is given and a high residue diet prescribed. Attacks of diverticulitis are treated by bed rest and antibiotics. A low roughage diet is traditionally prescribed but there is no evidence that it helps and it may worsen symptoms by causing constipation. In fact, trials suggest that a high residue diet benefits diverticular disease as well as preventing it. Antispasmodic drugs can be used to relieve pain. Many lose their symptoms when a regular bowel action is obtained by diet or, if necessary, by hydrophilic colloids like Isogel or liquid paraffin.

Diverticulitis is treated medically unless complications make surgery necessary. The diagnosis must be established beyond doubt and where there is a narrow tubular segment, colonoscopy or resection may be required to exclude cancer. There is also a real danger of cancer of the colon being overlooked because of the incidental presence of diverticulosis. Other indications for operation are:

1 Complications like perforation, abscess formation, haemorrhage or fistula.
2 Persistent trouble localized to a segment of the colon, or when stenosis is developing.

Prognosis. Diverticulosis starts in the pelvic colon. As years go by, a progressive involvement of the colon affects about one-third of the patients, but in the others the extent of diverticulosis may not change. Generally, the course is benign and occasional attacks of diverticulitis interfere little with the patient's life. Complications occur in about 5%. The prognosis is related to the number of diverticula—the more diverticula the greater the opportunity for complications to arise—and it may be improved by change to a high residue diet.

Megacolon and Hirschsprung's disease

Children, or occasionally adults, with these disorders have severe constipation, sometimes without a bowel action for two months or longer. The colon may be enormously distended with faeces, and easily felt and seen through a prominent abdomen (Fig. 18.7). Barium enema may require 5 litres or more of fluid to fill the colon. Correct diagnosis is essential as the treatment of megacolon and Hirschsprung's disease differs.

Megacolon

This is the commoner and starts in infancy or childhood after a period of normal bowel action. It is a form of constipation (p. 16) due to faulty bowel habits so that the rectum becomes insensitive to the presence of faeces. The accumulating faecal mass gradually spreads backwards from the rectum into the colon (Fig. 18.7a). Constipation may begin when the child ignores the call to stool during the summer holiday or when starting school, or because of a painful anal fissure. Sometimes the child is erroneously diagnosed as suffering from diarrhoea or scolded for soiling the bed at night; this spurious diarrhoea is due to faecal fluid leaking past impacted faeces. Emotional factors are sometimes important.

Diagnosis. A glance at the anus may sometimes be sufficient for faeces may be seen to be dilating and even extruding from it and the faecal mass may easily be felt by rectal examination. Hypothyroidism and neurological lesions must be excluded.

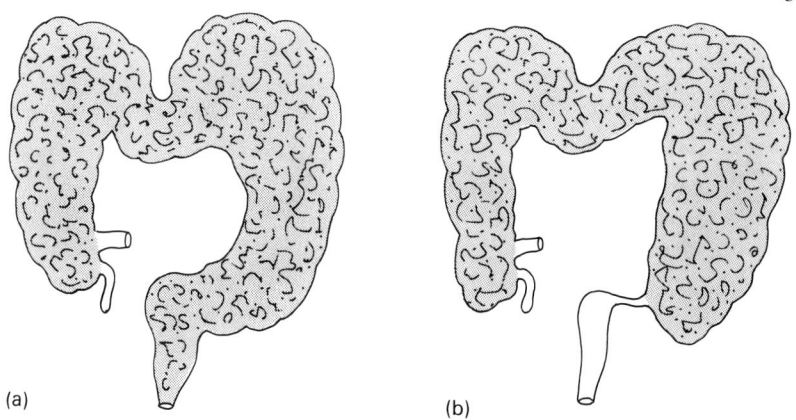

Fig. 18.7. (a) Megacolon (faeces reach anus); (b) Hirschsprung's disease (rectum empty and aperistaltic segment in sigmoid colon)

Treatment. The treatment is as for ordinary constipation but must be *persistent*. Neostigmine may be helpful as it increases smooth muscle contraction. Manual removal of stools and saline washouts are often necessary. Large enemas of tap water carry the danger of water intoxication. It is important to avoid overlooking painful lesions of the anus and psychological factors.

Hirschsprung's disease (aganglionic megacolon)
Hirschsprung's disease (Fig. 18.7b) is due to an aganglionic segment of bowel due to lack of development of the ganglion cells of Auerbach's and Meissner's plexus. This segment, which is of variable length and usually in the upper rectum and pelvic colon, is persistently contracted and fails to relax before the oncoming peristaltic wave, so obstruction results. It is similar to achalasia of the cardia and some suffer from this as well or from involvement of the ureter and bladder. A similar condition is seen as a late complication of Chagas' disease (South American trypanosomiasis) due to destruction of ganglia caused by a tissue reaction to the parasite.

Symptoms. These may start at birth. The passage of meconium may be delayed for several days or episodes of obstruction may occur. Later, the life of these unfortunates is chequered with chronic constipation and crises of subacute obstruction. Peritonitis and death may follow from perforation of the stercoral ulcer and iron deficiency anaemia may be due to bleeding. If the child survives and reaches the later teens, growth may be severely retarded and sexual development delayed. The abdomen progressively enlarges and the costal margins are flared. Colonic peristalsis may be visible.

Diagnosis. Rectal examination shows the rectum to be empty, in contrast to the faecal impaction of megacolon. A plain film of the abdomen should confirm that the distension is due to faeces. The narrow segment can be outlined by barium enema using a thin suspension of barium. Pressure studies when available confirm the aperistaltic segment. Biopsy of the wall of the narrow segment deep enough for ganglia through the anus and perhaps under general anaesthesia will demonstrate the absence of ganglia. Treatment is by resection of the affected segment of bowel.

Chapter 19
Tumours and Other Conditions of the Colon, Rectum and Anus

Cancer of the colon

More cancer deaths arise from the alimentary tract than from any other system. Those affecting the large bowel are common; they are next in frequency to cancer of the lung and so are the second commonest cause of death from malignant disease in Britain.

Tumours may occur at any age and can easily be overlooked in the young. There is little difference in the sexes: women are slightly more commonly affected than men though the incidence is about equal with rectal cancer. The sigmoid colon is a common site but the rectum accounts for one-third of all large bowel cancers. Five per cent of these are multiple. It is especially important to avoid missing cancer of the colon as the outlook after surgery is better than from malignant growths elsewhere in the alimentary tract, except for the visible lesions in the mouth or anus which can be diagnosed early.

Causative factors

Known causes are adenomas (though it is impossible to estimate how often cancer may arise in these), the rare familial polyposis coli and inflammatory bowel disease, especially in total ulcerative colitis after 10 years and rarely in Crohn's disease.

There is also increasing evidence that its prevalence is related to diet. It occurs more in industrialized countries where the food is high in protein and refined carbohydrates, but low in bulk, whereas it is rare in developing countries where bulky and mainly vegetarian food is eaten. The latter causes a short transit time; this avoids faecal stasis and may diminish the effect of carcinogens in the diet or which form in the lumen of the colon—for organisms, especially anaerobic Gram-negative ones of the bacteroides group, flourish in the colon of those on low residue diet and can alter bile salts to substances known to be carcinogenic in animals. A high residue diet results in large odourless stools which pass swiftly through the colon. Other correlations with food are being studied and an observation suggests that a low blood cholesterol, though protecting against heart disease, may make cancer of the colon more likely.

Types of tumour

Most are adenocarcinomas, usually of low or average grade of malignancy, about 15% being malignant, but a few are so slow growing as to show mucoid degeneration.

331

Dukes' classification is shown in Fig. 19.1. The cancer may spread as follows:

1   By direct infiltration to adjacent structures such as stomach, bladder, or pelvic wall.

2   By lymphatics to the pericolic and mesocolic lymph nodes.

3   By the bloodstream usually to the liver.

Clinical features

Suspicion of cancer must always arise when patients complain of a change in bowel habit, either constipation or diarrhoea, if the explanation is not apparent. Symptoms (Table 19.1) vary according to the site of the growth (Fig. 19.2). In the distal colon, where faeces are solid and the constrictive annular cancer more apt to occur, intestinal obstruction is to be expected, preceded by vague colicky pains and constipation. In the caecum and ascending colon where contents are fluid and the proliferative growth is more likely, the bowel upset may be slight with alternating

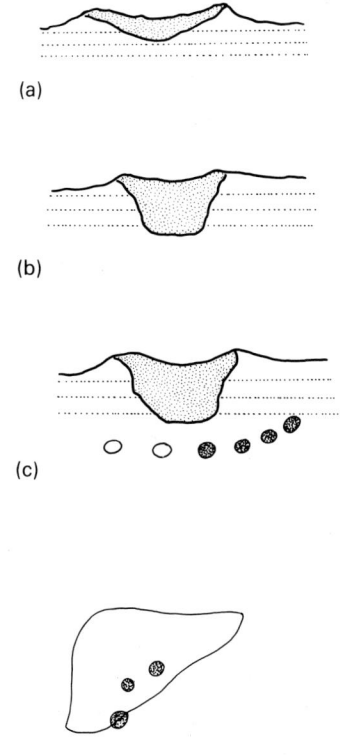

(a)

(b)

(c)

(d)

Fig. 19.1. Dukes' classification. (a) Tumour involves mucosa and submucosa only, good prognosis. (b) Tumour has completely penetrated the muscularis propria, moderate prognosis. (c) Metastatic tumour in lymph nodes: poor prognosis. (d) Distant metastases.

Table 19.1. Symptoms of carcinoma of colon.

1   Change in bowel habit.
2   Iron-deficient anaemia.
3   An emergency (usually intestinal obstruction sometimes perforation).
4   Abdominal mass.
5   Pyrexia of unknown origin.

constipation and diarrhoea, or absent altogether. It then may become large and easily palpable before causing pain, its surface ulcerating and bleeding so that anaemia may be the first sign, or infection-provoked fever and tenderness on palpation. Obvious blood and mucus in the stool is only seen when growths occur in the rectum or distal colon.

Some patients first present with ascites, jaundice, or hepatomegaly due to secondary deposits.

Diagnosis
Diagnosis of rectal or sigmoid cancer is made by sigmoidoscopy and barium enema (Fig. 19.3), but a barium enema can be negative, so a further X-ray—especially

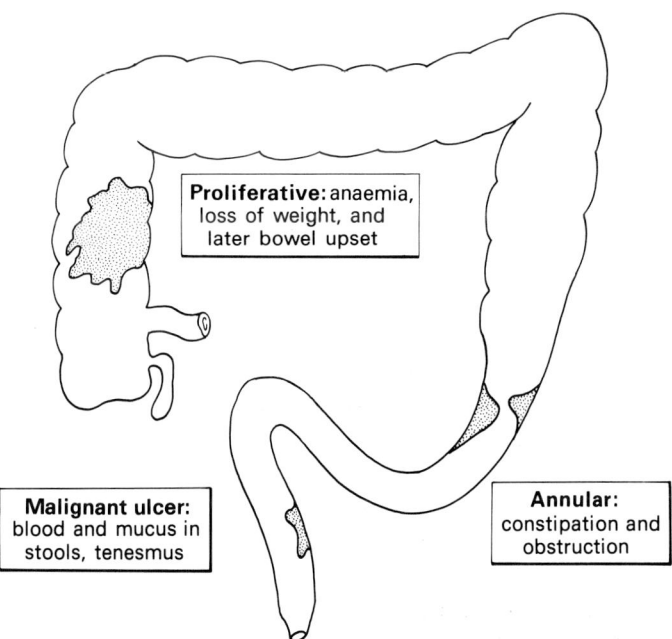

Proliferative: anaemia, loss of weight, and later bowel upset

Malignant ulcer: blood and mucus in stools, tenesmus

Annular: constipation and obstruction

Fig. 19.2. Types of carcinoma and likely symptoms.

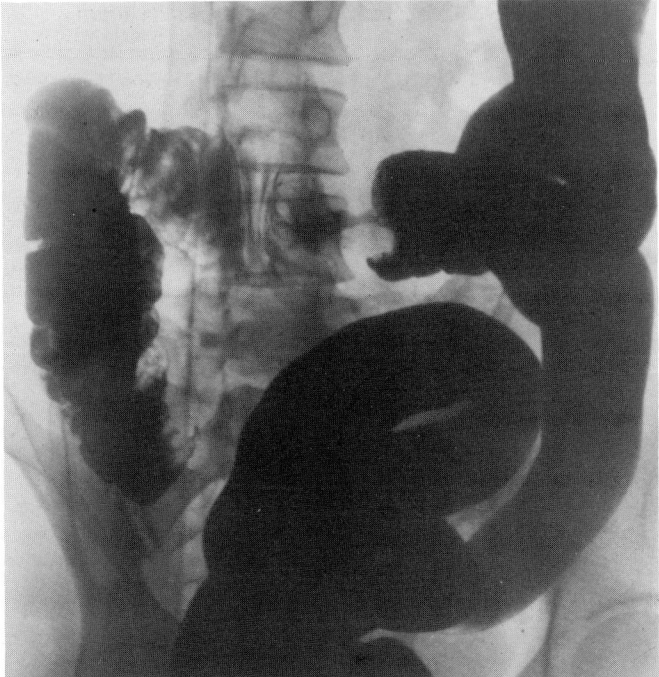

Fig. 19.3. Barium enema showing typical carcinoma of transverse colon.

double-contrast—or colonoscopy may be necessary. Rectal growths should be discovered early if rectal examination and sigmoidoscopy are done on everyone under suspicion. Occult blood is usually present in the stool but a negative result does not exclude an early growth. The carcino-embryonic antigen (CEA) estimation has no place in diagnosis but may help in detecting secondary carcinoma after resection of the primary growth. Computerized tomography is the best way for detecting metastases in the liver and usually better than ultrasound or isotope liver scan.

Differential diagnosis
Other causes of diarrhoea and constipation have to be considered. Diverticulitis may result in a carcinoma of the sigmoid colon being missed or it can, like Crohn's disease, cause a hard mass which mimics a growth. Sometimes the tumour may be due to secondary invasion from an adjacent carcinoma: stomach, bladder, uterus or ovary.

Treatment
Wide resection of the involved segment of the colon and an end-to-end anastomosis is usually done and it is seldom necessary to leave the patients with a colostomy

unless the rectum is involved. The operability rate for wide resection is about 70% and the overall 5 years survival rate for colonic and rectal cancer 20%. When a radical colonic resection can be done 40% of patients survive at 5 years. The operative mortality is around 5% but this depends upon the extent of the growth, the degree of sepsis, and condition of the patient, and can be much higher. Obviously it depends upon how early the growth is diagnosed. A permanent cure is possible in more than 90% if the tumour is detected at the stage of Dukes' classification A. The presence of liver metastases does not necessarily imply a hopeless prognosis; sometimes the patient lives surprisingly long when the primary tumour is removed or the metastases may be solitary and potentially resectable. Irradiation and cytotoxic drugs may have to be considered in the incurable patient, enthusiasm for treatment being tempered by the quality of life which is likely to result.

Prophylaxis
Studies are taking place as to the value of screening the healthy population by occult blood tests. Screening those especially at risk by barium enema or colonoscopy is not practicable but the fibreoptic sigmoidoscope would make it possible to check the following groups every 6 or 12 months:
1 Those who have already developed one or more polyps or a carcinoma of the colon.
2 Patients with long-standing ulcerative colitis.
3 Those with a strong family history of cancer of the colon.

Polyps in the colon and rectum
A *polyp* is defined as any mass of tissue that bulges or projects outwards from the normal surface level. These usually simple tumours may bleed or cause colicky pains. The commonest form is the *adenoma* where tumour cells form glands or gland-like structures in the stroma. A *papilloma* is an epithelial tumour consisting of villous outgrowths with a fibrovascular stroma. Rarely, there are *tumours of connective tissue origin*—lipomas, fibromas, haemangiomas, and neurofibromata; these, especially in the ileum, may cause intussusception into the colon.

Adenomas
These tend to become pedunculated by traction due to peristalsis. A solitary one may occur at any age, especially in the young, and be a cause of rectal bleeding. Adenomas in adults, usually benign, are probably an important cause of carcinoma of the colon. Their premalignant role is suggested by the following:
1 They occur in the same areas as carcinoma.
2 They are often in close relation to a carcinoma.
3 Satellite adenomas occur in up to 30% of carcinoma of the colon.
4 Microscopically a focal cancer may be found. This depends upon the size; only

about 1% of adenomas under 1 cm undergo malignant change but this rises to 50% in those over 2 cm.

5   Familial polyposis is a proven premalignant condition.

Rectal bleeding is usually caused by haemorrhoids but sigmoidoscopy should be done to exclude a polyp. Fibreoptic colonoscopy makes it possible to snare a pedunculated adenoma without open operation. If histology shows malignancy, formal resection is then indicated. A single adenoma does warn of an unstable colonic epithelium and is a sign to search for other adenomas elsewhere in the colon.

Familial polyposis of the colon

This rare condition is transmitted in Mendelian fashion by a dominant gene. In an afflicted family 50% of the offspring, both male and female, are likely to develop polyposis but only those who have it can transmit it. The polypi develop from puberty upwards and diarrhoea is the usual symptom. If untreated, cancer develops at about 35 years with death at 40 years.

Diagnosis is made at sigmoidoscopy and by barium enema. The presence of haustra separates it from the acquired polyposis of ulcerative colitis (Fig. 19.4). The term Gardner's syndrome is used when other congenital anomalies are present: subcutaneous lumps (either lipomas or fibromas) or bony tumours like osteomas.

Management is as follows:

1   A family tree is composed to keep a check on affected members.

2   Routine examination is started at 10 years of age and repeated every 2 years; most who have inherited the gene will have polypi before 20 years.

3   The best time for prophylactic operation is between leaving school and taking up work as no case of cancer has been recorded before 20 years. Surgery may be: (a) total colectomy plus excision of rectum with permanent ileostomy; total colectomy with preservation of rectum and ileorectal anastomosis; this has to be followed by a routine check of the rectum every 3 or 6 months to treat polyps by diathermy.

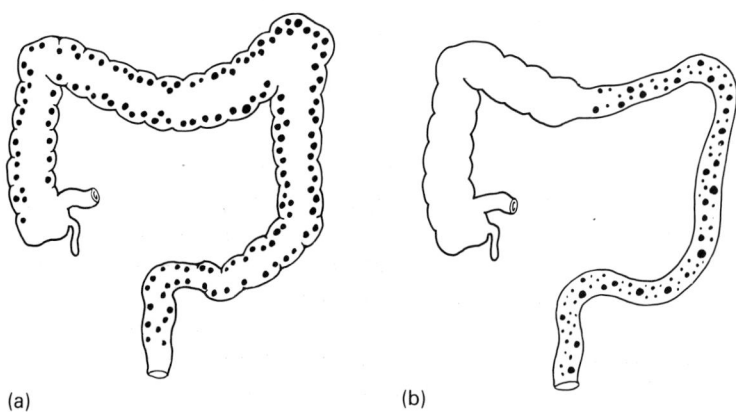

(a)   (b)

Fig. 19.4. Polyposis of the colon. (a) Familial polyposis with normal haustra. (b) Pseudopolyposis of ulcerative colitis with absent haustra.

Villous papilloma

This, rarer than adenomas, is seen in the rectum as a soft tumour with frond-like processes which may occupy much of the lumen. It is usually benign but there is a risk of malignant change in long-standing cases. Typically it produces a profuse watery diarrhoea with up to 2 litres of fluid lost daily; this may lead to dehydration, electrolyte depletion and especially hypokalaemia. If not too large it can be removed per anum.

Other rare conditions

Polyps occur throughout the alimentary tract, more in the upper part, in the *Peutz-Jeghers syndrome*. This is familial and usually recognized by looking at the face, especially the mouth where there is typical mucocutaneous pigmentation. It is usually benign but may cause pain from intussusception in children and anaemia from blood loss.

Pneumatosis intestinalis is a curious condition of gas-filled cysts in the bowel walls. These, seen at sigmoidoscopy or laparotomy, resemble a cluster of grapes and collapse when biopsied. The source of the gas (mainly nitrogen) is air originating either from a lesion of the alimentary tract where the continuity of the mucosa is broken or from rupture of lung alveoli as in asthma or emphysema. Treatment is directed towards the primary disease, for the cysts themselves are symptomless and resection of the bowel is not indicated. Hyperbaric oxygen can be used.

Peri-anal and anal canal disorders

Symptoms which indicate anorectal disease are soreness, discomfort or pain, pruritus, a swelling, prolapse, discharge, but most important of all is bleeding; but there are other important causes of rectal bleeding as well as local lesions (Table 19.2). Fortunately, most patients will have minor problems of the anal canal such as haemorrhoids or fissure, but a few will have potentially dangerous disease such as cancer or ulcerative colitis. So that every case must be carefully examined and investigated if necessary.

Haemorrhoids (Piles)

Piles are normal vascular cushions and we all have them. The word piles comes from the Latin for a pill or a ball and implies the complaint of a lump whereas haemorrhoids comes from the Greek meaning the flowing of blood. These normal structures containing veins become symptomatic because of the laxity of fixation of the vascular mucosa to the wall of the rectum and upper anal canal, and tightness of the anal sphincter. Fixation is normally very lax and the cushions may even have muscular fibres within them that pull them back to the safety of the upper anal canal after defaecation. When the veins become congested, hypertrophy with engorgement occurs and an increased tone of the anal sphincter hinders retraction.

Table 19.2. Causes of lower intestinal bleeding.

Common
    Haemorrhoids
    Anal fissure
    Carcinoma
    Ulcerative colitis
    Polyps
Occasional
    Crohn's disease
    Diverticulitis
Rare
    Meckel's diverticulum
    Small intestinal tumours
    Vascular abnormalities (e.g. angiodysplasia of the colon)
    Solitary rectal ulcer
    Ischaemic colitis

(Upper gastrointestinal bleeding usually causes *melaena* but occasionally patients with rapid bleeding may pass red blood.)

Symptoms. These are due to complications:
1 Congestion may cause discomfort and easy bleeding.
2 Failure to return to the anal canal after defaecation leaves exposed mucous membranes with consequent discharge and skin maceration—bacterial or fungal invasion may then cause pruritus; prolapse or thrombosis causes the lump from which the name is derived.

Treatment. This is as follows:
1 Regulation of bowel habits to avoid constipation and straining at defaecation. This is achieved by a high residue diet together with bran or other bulk laxative or hydrophilic substances. To avoid straining, glycerine suppositories may be needed to break the habit.
2 Local applications are of doubtful value; antibiotics, steroids, and antiseptics have been tried and though topical anaesthetic ointment gives temporary relief of symptoms, it can cause a hypersensitivity reaction with further pruritus.
3 Injection sclerotherapy is used for early piles (first degree).
4 Large second degree piles may be treated with elastic band ligation; ligation is an ancient treatment first used by Hippocrates.
5 For third degree piles, haemorrhoidectomy is the only curative treatment.
6 Other methods used are cryosurgery, manual dilatation of the anus, and lateral partial internal sphincterotomy, but their value is not yet established.

Peri-anal haematoma

This is an acutely painful condition due to rupture of one of the vessels in the external haemorrhoidal venous plexus. Its edge is well demarcated and it is entirely covered by peri-anal skin. It can be evacuated under local anaesthesia at the start but bleeding may be a problem afterwards. Without treatment, it usually resolves during the following 4–6 weeks.

Skin tags

There are usually symptomless and of no significance. If they become swollen and sore because of being scratched, they can usually be excised under local anaesthetic. Sometimes they occur in Crohn's disease and have a bluish-crimson tinge. Also venereal disease may be accompanied by anal 'warts' in the homosexual.

Fissure

This is the commonest form of anal ulceration and can usually be seen by parting the anal margin and asking the patient to bear down. Passing a proctoscope is painful without local anaesthetic ointment and usually unnecessary. Fissure is usually accompanied by a skin tag—the sentinal pile—or by a hypertrophied anal papilla or fibrous polyp.

Treatment is by relaxing the internal sphincter either by an anal dilator lubricated with a local anaesthetic which the patient can do at home or by dilatation under an anaesthetic, or by sphincterotomy.

Crohn's disease

Appearances (Table 19.3) are characteristic with a blue discoloration of the peri-anal skin, oedematous skin tag, fissures, ulceration and fistula formation. The rectum may be involved.

Other causes of ulceration

A syphilitic ulcer causes laxity of the anal sphincter in contrast to the spasm associated with a fissure. It occurs in the first stage (more likely in homosexuals) and motile spirochaetes may be found by dark-ground microscopy. Tuberculosis is

Table 19.3. Anal appearances in Crohn's disease.

1 Inflamed oedematous tags.
2 Chronic fissure.
3 External opening of a fistula.
4 Anal ulceration or bluish discolouration with or without oedematous peri-anal skin.
5 Peri-anal or ischio-rectal abscess.
6 Sometimes scars of previous operations.

unlikely to be seen except with obvious tuberculosis in the lungs or elsewhere. Malignant conditions (e.g. epithelioma) may also involve the anus.

Peri-anal abscess and fistula

An abscess may resolve completely as abscesses do elsewhere in the body, but sometimes it produces a chronic fistula, usually associated with Crohn's disease or ulcerative colitis.

Warts

These are usually due to a virus. They take different forms and some are called condylomata; they may complicate inflammatory bowel disease or be a later stage of syphilis.

Prolapse

Anorectal prolapse may be caused by polyps, intra-anal condylomata, redundant mucosa, or tumours of the rectum and sigmoid colon such as adenomas or occasionally carcinomas. Complete rectal prolapse resembles an intussusception. Treatment is by re-education of bowel habit or operation either by ligature and excision, or abdominal rectopexy.

Pruritus ani

Itching is a symptom of many conditions. Anorectal disease such as fissures or fistulae have to be excluded. The following should also be considered: skin diseases such as psoriasis, contact dermatitis including allergic reactions to agents used to treat the pruritus, infection and parasites like threadworm, and systemic diseases especially diabetes mellitus (causing a fungal infection) and chronic liver disease. Some are thought to have pruritus because of irritant stools; normal faeces are weakly acid and a change to alkaline as in diarrhoea is thought to cause an irritation, though other substances in loose stools could do this. No cause is found in many patients and there is sometimes an element of neurosis.

Some improve with 1% hydrocortisone, especially at night when itching is worse; otherwise careful hygiene after defaecation together with regulation of bowel action with a high residue diet usually suffices.

Faecal incontinence

This distressing symptom can occur in children, being due to megacolon where the rectum is full of faeces (spurious diarrhoea) and rarely to other conditions affecting the spinal cord. Damage to the anal sphincter may result from local lesions or be the consequence of past obstetric injury or anal surgery.

Incontinence may, however, be a symptom of any severe diarrhoea. It is most common in the elderly, particularly after strokes or brain failure. Faulty bowel habits may occur in any geriatric institution and rectal examination is necessary to exclude impacted faeces. Proctoscopy is usually indicated and, if facilities are available, anal canal manometry may help in unexplained cases.

Treatment is often unsatisfactory. Regulation of bowel function perhaps by a high residue diet or bulk laxative and sometimes by codeine phosphate may help. A routine of taking the patient to the toilet may be necessary in the elderly. Operation may be needed to reconstruct the anorectal area. Patients can be taught pelvic floor exercises and electrical stimulus to the external sphincter has been used.

Chapter 20
Miscellaneous Problems

Endocrinology and the gut

The gut has many associations with endocrinology. The idea that physiological functions are regulated by blood-borne substances was first suggested by the classical experiments of Bayliss and Starling in 1902. They observed that instillation of acid into the duodenum or intravenous injection of small bowel extracts induced a flow of bicarbonate-rich juice from a denervated pancreas. They called the blood-borne messenger secretin and coined the term hormone.

Gastrointestinal hormones

By now a large number of gastrointestinal hormones have been described and each year sees additions (Table 20.1). Most exist in many tissues including the brain and gut. They may act as hormones, neurotransmitters or local regulators by intercellular diffusion.

The active agents are derived from amino acids and are either amines (e.g. 5-hydroxytryptamine) or peptides. Each is produced by characteristic cells which may be scattered and isolated within the gastrointestinal mucosa or clustered as in the islets of Langerhans. Included within the islets of Langerhans are beta cells which produce insulin, A cells which produce glucagon, G cells which produce gastrin and D cells which produce somatostatin.

Hormonal actions. After attaching to specific plasma membrane receptors, gut hormones act in one of the following ways to produce stimulus-response coupling (e.g. secretion) by the target cell.

1 Increase of cytosolic Ca^{++} from stores is mediated by cyclic adenosine monophosphate (cAMP), prostaglandins or products of phosphatidyl inositol metabolism.

2 Activation of adenyl cyclase. This enzyme stimulates formation of cyclic AMP (cAMP) from ATP. cAMP stimulates phosphorylation of enzymatic proteins which catalyse the response to the hormone.

Most cells appear to be responsive to many stimuli. For instance, acid secretion by the gastric parietal cell occurs in response to histamine, gastrin and vagal release of acetyl choline. Combination of a hormone which acts via Ca^{++} release and a hormone which acts by stimulating adenyl cyclase has a potentiating effect, i.e. the combined response exceeds the sum of their individual responses.

Rarely tumours occur which produce an excess of one or more gastrointestinal

Table 20.1. Gastrointestinal hormones.

Peptide	Main target organ response
Gastrin	Gastric acid secretion
CCK/PZ (cholecystokinin–pancreozymin)	Pancreatic enzyme secretion and gallbladder contraction
Secretin	Pancreatic bicarbonate secretion
Glucagon	Hepatic glycogenolysis
Somatostatin	Inhibition of gastric and pancreatic secretion. Inhibits release of many gut hormones
VIP (vasoactive intestinal peptide)	Ileal secretion
Motilin	Stimulates gut motility
GIP (gastric inhibitory polypeptide)	Augments glucose-induced insulin release
PP (pancreatic polypeptide)	Inhibits pancreatic bicarbonate and enzyme secretion
Enteroglucagon	Stimulates intestinal villus growth
Neurotensin	
Bombesin	
Enkephalin	
Substance P	

hormones (Table 20.2). The carcinoid syndrome results from tumour production of amines, not peptides, and is therefore excluded from Table 20.2.

Endocrine causes of diarrhoea

Rarely a *gastrinoma* causes diarrhoea without features of the Zollinger–Ellison syndrome. There are two pathogenetic mechanisms. Watery diarrhoea results from the sheer volume of gastric acid secretion and the pancreatic secretory response to duodenal acidification. Gastric aspiration abolishes this watery diarrhoea.

Secondly excessive acidity of duodenal and jejunal contents inhibits normal digestion by destroying pancreatic lipase activity, producing diarrhoea due to fat malabsorption.

Vasoactive intestinal peptide (VIP) secreted by a tumour (vipoma) produces severe watery diarrhoea. The commonest cause of this rare syndrome is a pancreatic tumour (hence the old term pancreatic cholera), but in children ganglion neuromas are often responsible. VIP is a powerful stimulant of adenyl cyclase within the ileum, resulting in secretion of large amounts of sodium bicarbonate and water into the intestinal lumen. Diarrhoea is watery and may amount to several litres per day when its major differential diagnosis is purgative abuse or, in appropriate countries,

Table 20.2. Tumour production of gastrointestinal peptide hormones.

Tumour type	Hormone	Clinical features
Insulinoma	Insulin	Hypoglycaemia
Gastrinoma	Gastrin	Zollinger–Ellison syndrome
Vipoma	VIP	Watery diarrhoea, hypokalaemia
Glucagonoma	Glucagon	Necrotizing migratory erythema weight loss
		Impaired glucose tolerance
Somatostatinoma	Somatostatin	Abdominal discomfort
		Weight loss
		Mild diabetes

cholera. This produces hypokalaemia, often with an acidosis, and reduced gastric acid production.

In the *carcinoid syndrome* secretion of 5-hydroxytryptamine may cause troublesome diarrhoea. The tumour probably releases other active substances including kinins, e.g. bradykinin, to account for the flushing and wheezing that some patients experience. Although carcinoid tumours are not infrequently removed as incidental findings during abdominal surgery, they never produce symptoms until the liver has been massively involved by metastatic tumour. Heart murmurs may arise from fibrosis of the pulmonary and tricuspid valves. The typical patient has bluish telangiectasis of the malar areas and a large firm liver without jaundice or other signs of liver failure.

In *thyrotoxicosis* diarrhoea is usually associated with weight loss despite an excellent appetite. Other symptoms and signs of thyrotoxicosis (goitre with a bruit, fine tremor, sweating, tachycardia, lid lag, proptosis etc.) may or may not be present.

Diabetes mellitus is sometimes associated with troublesome diarrhoea which is often worse at night. Several possible mechanisms are involved including a motility disorder with bacterial overgrowth due to an autonomic neuropathy; pancreatic exocrine insufficiency; ischaemic enteropathy and a side-effect of therapeutic agents, most notably metformin.

Adrenal insufficiency (Addison's disease) occasionally presents with diarrhoea. Vomiting is often severe with primary adrenal failure. Patients usually have marked pigmentation involving the palmar skin creases and buccal mucosa, but this is not seen when pituitary function is impaired, e.g. after prolonged steroid therapy. Remember that vomiting in a patient receiving long-term corticosteroid therapy may rapidly produce an adrenal crisis if steroids are not available systemically.

There is usually hypovolaemia with postural hypotension and hyponatraemia may also be apparent.

Phaeochromocytoma may cause weight loss and diarrhoea. Diagnosis is by measurement of 24-h urinary metadrenaline excretion.

Medullary carcinoma of the thyroid when advanced also causes a secretory diarrhoea. Though the mechanism is not understood, prostaglandins appear to be involved in stimulation of intestinal secretion, and diarrhoea may be relieved by prostaglandin synthetase inhibitors, e.g. indomethacin. Nutmeg also has a favourable effect.

Immunology

Normal immunological defence mechanisms

The intestine and liver have important immune functions affecting both cellular and humoral immunity.

Cellular

Gut. Antigens from the intestinal lumen traverse specialized 'M' cells to the underlying Peyer's patches (Fig. 20.1). There they stimulate immunocytes (lymphocytes and plasma cells) which then travel via the lymphatics to the bloodstream before returning to populate the lamina propria of the gut.

Liver. Kupffer cells are phagocytic cells of the reticuloendothelial (RE) system which stride hepatic sinusoids, removing debris including antigen–antibody complexes. They constitute 15% of all liver cells. Experiments show that they react differently from RE cells in other organs, e.g. spleen, since antigenic haptens fed orally induce a state of immunological tolerance which does not occur after porto-caval anastomosis. This may be a mechanism whereby the body normally avoids a state of hypersensitivity to a large number of dietary antigens. Impairment of Kupffer cell function, e.g. in cirrhosis, is often associated with hypergammaglobulinaemia, including high levels of antibodies to many types of *E. coli* present within the intestinal lumen.

Humoral

Immunoglobulin A (IgA). IgA is the major secretory immunoglobulin of intestinal secretions and bile. It is normally secreted as a dimer bound to secretory component derived from the mucosal cell (Fig. 20.2). There is also evidence that dimeric IgA derived from intestinal plasma cells is removed from the portal bloodstream and secreted in bile. This may be a biological method which produces a high level of antibody in the proximal intestine to antigens encountered more distally.

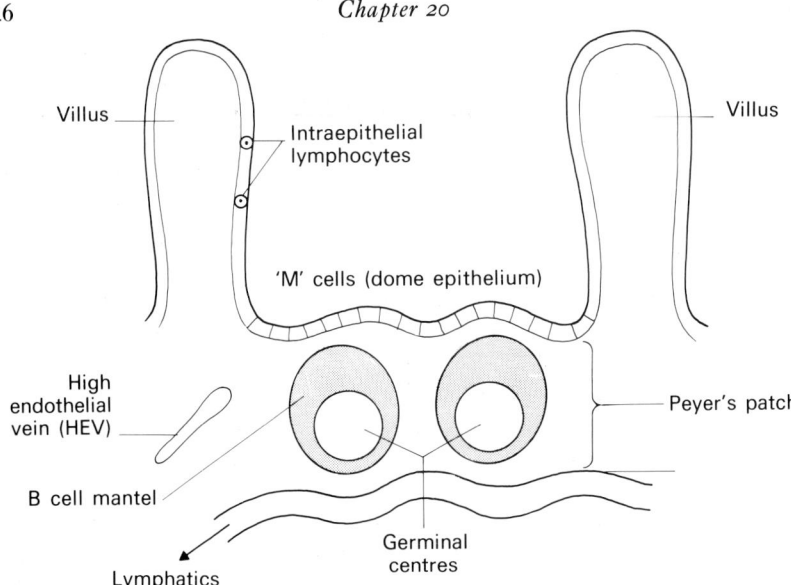

Fig. 20.1. The gut mucosa overlying Peyer's patches consists of specialized cuboidal microfold 'M' cells. 'M' cells are permeable to many antigens which challenge lymphoblasts within Peyer's patches. After antigen challenge, lymphoblasts circulate through the thoracic duct and blood circulation before returning to the gut via high endothelial veins to populate the lamina propria as mature IgA-secreting plasma cells.

Disturbed immunity and the gut

In selective IgA deficiency serum levels of IgA are low or absent, but levels of IgG and IgM are usually normal. Selective IgA deficiency is sometimes associated with adult coeliac disease, bronchiectasis and sinusitis, nodular lymphoid hyperplasia of the intestine and giardiasis.

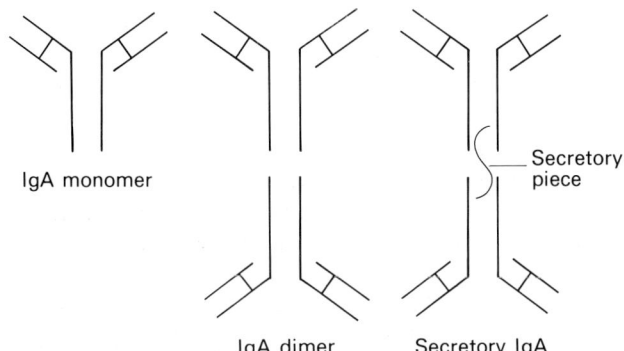

Fig. 20.2. Circulating IgA is normally in monomeric or dimeric form. IgA secreted into the lumen of the gut, bile or bronchi is bound to secretory piece to form secretory IgA.

Hypogammaglobulinaemia. Levels of serum IgA, IgG and IgM are all reduced. Patients may present with malabsorption and diarrhoea due to bacterial overgrowth. Rarely hypogammaglobulinaemia may be associated with pernicious anaemia, or pancreatic insufficiency when cyclical neutropenia may also be a feature. In AIDS (acquired immune deficiency syndrome) hypogammaglobulinaemia and helper T cell deficiency is associated with diarrhoea due to rare opportunistic infections, e.g. cryptosporidiosis.

Alpha-chain disease is an apparently neoplastic disease affecting intestinal plasma cells which produce the heavy chain of IgA devoid of either κ or λ (kappa or lambda) light chains. It is a rare disease which is almost entirely confined to areas of the world where intestinal infestation with parasites is common, e.g. Mediterranean countries. Patients may present with features of malabsorption, systemic illness or local symptoms due to the tumour, e.g. perforation, obstruction or intussusception.

Lymphoproliferative disorders affecting the gastrointestinal tract may present with features of malabsorption with weight loss and diarrhoea, with systemic symptoms, e.g. fever and malaise, or with local symptoms due to the tumour tissue such as an intestinal obstruction, perforation or intussusception. Lymphoma of the small intestine is a well-recognized complication of adult coeliac disease and should be suspected in a coeliac who has an apparent relapse of clinical symptoms despite adherence to a gluten-free diet.

Immunological aspects of adult coeliac disease

The following factors suggest involvement of the immune system in causation or response to adult coeliac disease:

1 Serum antibodies to reticulin and to various dietary antigens.
2 Association in a few patients with selective IgA deficiency.
3 Increased incidence of tissue type HLA-B8.
4 Splenic and reticular atrophy.
5 Complicating lymphoma.
6 Dermatitis herpetiformis with skin deposition of IgA, C_3 and fibrin.
7 Circulating immune complexes.
8 An apparent Arthus reaction in the intestine following gluten challenge.

Gastrointestinal food allergy

Cow's milk intolerance is well documented in some young children who develop diarrhoea, abdominal pain and distension following its ingestion. Symptoms and signs disappear following withdrawal of all milk products. The condition is largely confined to children.

There is often a family history of atopy with asthma, eczema and hay fever. Skin challenge may give a positive response and antibodies to lactoglobulin are detectable in the serum by appropriate tests. The intolerance may follow infective gastroenteritis and be transient with complete spontaneous remission. Oral disodium cromoglycate may be useful in relieving symptoms. The condition must not be confused with hypolactasia which may produce similar abdominal symptoms following milk ingestion.

Follicular (or nodular) lymphoid hyperplasia (NLH)
This group of conditions is characterized by proliferation of the lymphoid follicles of the intestine which is sufficient to produce impressions on the lumen on X-ray, or polyps visible macroscopically at endoscopy or on direct inspection. Though some cases are not easily classified they appear to be divisible into three groups:
1   Lymphoid hyperplasia of the rectum, colon and terminal ileum in children. This is a benign reversible (probably reactive) lesion.
2   NLH of the entire small bowel sometimes with involvement of the colon and rectum in common variable hypogammaglobulinaemia. Selective IgA deficiency is frequently present, giardiasis common, and lymphomatous transformation very rare.
3   NLH of the small bowel in the absence of a detectable abnormality in humoral immunity. This is the rarest of the three forms, is frequently complicated with intestinal lymphoma, and has been described in peoples of the same geographical origin as alpha chain disease.

Detection of auto-antibodies as a diagnostic aid
Several conditions are associated with serum auto-antibodies and there is an increased incidence in the patient or close relatives of other autoimmune disease, e.g. Hashimoto's thyroiditis, Addison's disease and vitiligo. Detection of these auto-antibodies is often helpful in confirming the diagnosis (Table 20.3) although

Table 20.3. Diagnostic value of serum auto-antibody detection.

Disease	Auto-antibody	Incidence
Pernicious anaemia	Parietal cell	75–90%
	Intrinsic factor	50–70%
'Lupoid' chronic active hepatitis	Smooth muscle	70%
	Anti-nuclear factor	80%
Primary biliary cirrhosis	Mitochondrial	95%
Coeliac disease (gluten-sensitive		70–100% in children
enteropathy)	Reticulin	50–70% in adults

the use of reticulin antibodies in this context is usually confined to small children and any others in whom it is not possible to perform a jejunal biopsy.

The skin and the gut
Many gastrointestinal conditions occur in association with skin disorders which may give the clue that first suggests the correct diagnosis. The following are examples:

Diarrhoea

Erythema nodosum. Painful, raised red areas on shins. Associations: Crohn's, ulcerative colitis, tuberculosis, sulphasalazine toxicity.

Pyoderma gangrenosum. Acute blood blisters breaking down to give large areas of skin necrosis. Associations: ulcerative colitis.

Rose-red spots. Around the umbilicus on the seventh to tenth day of fever are characteristic of infection with *Salmonella typhi*.

Neurofibromatosis. Lumps in or under the skin and café au lait spots. Associations: medullary carcinoma of the thyroid, phaeochromocytoma.

Creeping necrolysis of the skin. Initial erythema gives way to spreading necrosis of the skin with bullous formation. Association: glucagonoma.

Acrodermatitis enteropathica. Rash of extremities, oral and peri-anal regions in infants. Associations: zinc deficiency.

Malabsorption

Dermatitis herpetiformis. Intensely itchy vesicular rash on the extensor aspects (elbows, shoulders, buttocks, knees). Responds to dapsone. Associations: adult coeliac disease, partial or subtotal villous atrophy of jejunum.

Systemic sclerosis. Scleroderma with tense skin, small mouth.

Crest syndrome. Calcinosis cuti (calcification in soft tissues visible on X-ray of the hand, Raynaud's, oesophageal disorder, sclerodactyly and telangectasia). Reflux oesophagitis may lead to peptic stricture formation. Barium swallow in the Trendelenberg (head down) position shows free gastro-oesophageal reflux and a shortened aperistaltic oesophagus. Smooth muscle atrophy with impaired contractibility and progressive dilatation of the intestine involves the small bowel (malabsorption due to bacterial overgrowth) and colon (constipation). There is also an association between systemic sclerosis and primary biliary cirrhosis.

Abdominal pain

Peutz–Jeghers syndrome. Freckle-like spots on the lips. Association: small bowel polyps usually presenting with intussusception.

Hereditary angio-oedema. Large swellings resembling allergic angio-oedema associated with hereditary Cı esterase inhibitor deficiency. Association: abdominal pain with features depending on the site of swelling/obstruction.

Generalized pigmentation

Liver disease. Haemochromatosis, primary biliary cirrhosis.

Malabsorption. Adult coeliac disease, Whipple's disease.

Gastrointestinal bleeding

Hereditary telangiectasia (Rendu–Osler–Weber syndrome). Red spots on lips, tongue and elsewhere. Association: chronic slow bleeding with Fe deficiency.

Pseudoxanthoma elasticum. Highly extensible skin variously likened to crepe-bandage or plucked chicken skin in the antecubital fossae and on the neck. Association: upper gastrointestinal bleeding with poor response to surgery and generally poor prognosis.

Henoch-Schönlein purpura. Purpuric spots occur on the legs in association with nephritis. Association: bleeding into the intestine may give abdominal pain and/or bleeding per rectum.

Malignancy

Dermatomyositis. Heliotrope (violaceous) discolouration of the eye lids, forehead and knuckles with myositis. Association: in patients over 50 years old this frequently (60%) occurs with malignancy (pancreas, stomach and other primary sites).

Acanthosis nigricans. Blackish discoloration especially of the axillae and nape of neck. Association: malignancy of the gastrointestinal tract may be present.

Liver disease

Xanthelasma and palmar xanthomas. Cholesterol deposits. Association: biliary cirrhosis (primary or secondary).

Haemochromatosis. The bronze colour of bronze diabetes.

Porphyria cutanea tarda. Fragile blisters on exposed areas with scar formation on healing. Association: liver disease of alcoholism and iron overload.

Vitiligo. Areas of depigmentation due to loss of melanin. Association: autoimmune disorders, especially pernicious anaemia and primary biliary cirrhosis (also thyroid, adrenal auto-antibodies).

Pruritus

This may be a presenting complaint with any of the following:
1 Cholestasis.
2 Dermatitis herpetiformis.
3 Creeping eruption: hookworm or similar helminthic infestation.
4 Lymphoproliferative disorder.

Drugs and the liver

There are many important interrelationships between the liver and pharmacological agents which need to be borne in mind when prescribing. Many drugs exert an important influence on normal liver metabolism. Conversely, liver dysfunction has a profound effect on the bioavailability of many therapeutic agents.

Influence of drugs on the healthy liver

Enzyme induction

Exposure of the liver to enzyme-inducing drugs (e.g. phenobarbitone, phenytoin, rifampicin, alcohol) considerably alters the pharmacology of many other therapeutic agents, e.g. addition of rifampicin may (a) make oral contraception ineffective by reducing the half-life of oestrogens, (b) increase the hepatotoxicity of isoniazid by increasing its metabolism to toxic hydrazine derivatives, (c) reduce the anticoagulant effect of warfarin by increasing the rate at which it is degraded by the liver, (d) reduce the effectiveness of tranquillizers or night sedation.

Hepatic blood flow

This may be altered, e.g. vasopressin, β-adrenergic blockers.

Competitive inhibition

Bilirubin competes for uptake by the hepatocyte with rifampicin and flavaspidic acid (extract of male fern).

Influence of liver disease on drug metabolism (Table 20.4)

Generally speaking, drugs normally inactivated by the liver and excreted in bile will have their *effect prolonged* by liver disease or cholestasis. Thus impaired hepatic metabolism of chloramphenicol may produce high blood levels which correlate with the drug's direct toxic effect upon the bone marrow, though not with the idiosyncratic reaction which produces agranulocytosis or aplastic anaemia.

The concept of first-pass extraction is important to the understanding of many drug actions. If a drug has a high first-pass extraction a vastly greater dose will need to be given orally (even allowing for complete absorption) to obtain the same systemic concentrations that result from its parenteral administration. Porto-systemic shunting and decreased hepatocellular function both tend to diminish first-pass extraction of absorbed drugs and thus increase their pharmacologic availability and potency.

Table 20.4. Effects of liver disease on drug metabolism.

---

1   An increased volume of distribution (with fluid retention).
2   Decreased protein binding (with hypoproteinaemia).
3   Displacement from binding sites (e.g. bilirubin competes with numerous drugs for binding sites on serum albumin).
4   Partitioning.
5   Decreased metabolism.
6   Decreased biliary excretion.
7   Decreased first pass extraction.

Drug-induced liver disease
The following examples (Table 20.5) demonstrate the wide spectrum of liver injury that may be produced in this way. Hence the importance of a careful drug history in all patients presenting with a liver complaint.

Sex hormones and the liver
Sex hormones may affect the liver in several ways.

Cholestasis
This is produced by oestrogens and certain androgens, e.g. methyltestosterone. Oral contraceptive-induced jaundice has the clinical picture of a pure intrahepatic cholestasis, i.e. bile secretory failure in the absence of obstruction or inflammation. Its onset usually occurs within the first 2 or 3 monthly cycles and jaundice is usually preceded by pruritus. Liver function returns to normal by stopping the pill. Patients who have suffered from pill-jaundice are also liable to develop cholestasis of pregnancy and it is therefore likely that oestrogenic steroids are the cause.

Adenoma
Hepatic *adenoma* formation occurs in association with oral contraception. Tumours may present as a mass, but are also subject to bleeding either internally (causing pain) and a fall in the haematocrit, or intraperitoneally (causing collapse). They may be multiple. Regression often follows withdrawal of hormonal therapy.

Carcinoma
Hepatocellular *carcinoma* complicates androgenic steroid usage, e.g. oxymetholone treatment of aplastic anaemia. There may also be a weak link between this tumour and oral contraception but the association has not been proven.

Table 20.5. Hepatoxic drug reactions.

Type of injury	Examples
Acute hepatitis	Paracetamol (overdose)
	Halothane
	Isoniazid
	Monoamine oxidase inhibitor
	Dantrolene
Chronic hepatitis	Alpha methyl dopa
	Isoniazid
	Nitrofurantoin
	Oxyphenisatin
Cholestasis	Chlorpromazine
	Oestrogenic and androgenic steroids
	Erythromycin estolate
Hyperbilirubinaemia	Rifampicin
	Novobiocin
	Flavaspidic acid
Large droplet fatty liver (e.g. ethanol)	Perhexilene maleate
Small droplet fatty liver (e.g. Reye's syndrome. Acute fatty liver of pregnancy)	Tetracycline (i.v.)
	Valproic acid
Portal fibrosis	Methotrexate
Granulomatous hepatitis	Phenylbutazone
	Allopurinol
Hepatic vein thrombosis (Budd–Chiari syndrome)	Oestrogenic steroids
Hepatic adenoma	Oestrogenic steroids
Hepatocellular carcinoma	Androgenic steroids, e.g. oxymetholone
Gallstones	Oestrogenic steroids
	Clofibrate

Peliosis hepatitis
In which hepatic sinusoids dilate to give abnormal endothelial lined blood lakes within the parenchyma; it occurs in patients exposed to androgenic steroids.

Hepatic vein thrombosis
This occurs in some patients receiving oral contraceptives: the Budd–Chiari syndrome. There is widespread involvement of small hepatic venules in association with a hypercoagulability state.

Gallstones

These occur more commonly when oestrogen levels are high, i.e. women generally more than men, and especially in association with pregnancy or oestrogen therapy.

Chronic intestinal ischaemia

This now is rare but may become more common as the number of middle-aged and elderly increases. It is usually due to atheroma but may occur in patients with arteritis, from an embolus (Fig. 17.8) or in women on the contraceptive pill.

Arterial insufficiency of the small intestine may be a cause of unexplained pain, usually postprandial, perhaps radiating to the back and causing anorexia and loss of weight. It should only be considered when carcinoma, peptic ulcer, nervous dyspepsia, irritable colon, and biliary or pancreatic disorders have been excluded. It has been called 'intestinal angina'. The only abnormal sign may be a systolic bruit over the upper abdomen but this can occur in the healthy. Aortography may confirm it but the superior mesenteric artery can be completely obliterated without causing symptoms. In the rare proved case, endarterectomy or bypass has been performed.

Ischaemia of the colon can mimic other types of colitis but especially affects the left transverse and splenic flexure. It can be transient, result in a segmental colitis like Crohn's disease, cause a stricture, or as elsewhere in the gut result in gangrene. It causes pain in the left abdomen, loose motions with dark blood and clots. A plain X-ray may show thumb printing of the gas shadows and mucosal irregularities which may be confirmed by barium enema. The rectum is normal. Angiograms may not be helpful. Treatment is 'expectant'.

Aneurysms of the abdominal aorta

These are usually incidental and dual pathology is common in older age groups. An aneurysm is, however, worth detecting as elective operation may be indicated. Aneurysms may cause the following:
1   The patient notices a pulsatile swelling.
2   There is an alteration of bowel habit, perhaps from ischaemia of the colon.
3   Abdominal and back pain are caused.
4   Pain may radiate to the groin, testicles, perineum or legs.
5   Distension, vomiting or weight loss may occur from stretching of the third part of the duodenum over the aneurysm.
6   Haematemesis, not necessarily disastrous, may be a symptom.
7   Erosion of one or more lumbar vertebra may be noticed on an X-ray.

Many aneurysms do not pulsate because of clot formation. Careful judgement is needed to decide whether symptoms are relevant or not.

Intestinal parasites

The gut with its warmth and supply of food provides a peaceful haven for parasites. These are especially common in deprived areas of the world where education and sanitation is inadequate. They are symptomless in about 90% of cases and should not be blamed unfairly for causing vague abdominal symptoms. It is also easy to attribute malabsorption to their presence, but 'the tropical intestine' is virtually a normal variation in hot areas of the world; the villi are shorter, broader and show leaf forms and ridges together with an increased number of chronic inflammatory cells in the lamina propria. Indeed, any definition of a normal intestinal mucosa must take geographical variations into account.

The screening of immigrant children in the UK has shown that nearly half may be carriers of parasites: helminths such as ascaris (roundworm) and trichuris (whipworm), ancylostomiasis (hookworm), enterobius (pinworms) and hymenolepis (dwarf tapeworms). Occasionally symptoms occur and vary from pruritus ani to serious disease. The following are the more important ones to consider.

Ascariasis (roundworm)

This is the largest of intestinal nematodes and adults may measure up to 45 cm in length. There may be one or two or hundreds in the intestine and their life span is about 18 months. The female produces about 200,000 ova daily; these are passed by the host in the stool and may last in soil for some years. A large part of the world's population is infected, especially in warm climates, children being especially affected. Ascaris is a marker of rural poverty.

Clinical picture. After ingestion, the eggs hatch in the duodenum and the larvae penetrate the intestinal wall where they enter the venous circulation and are carried to the lungs. Then a patchy pneumonia may occur—an eosinophilic pneumonitis called Loffler's syndrome; this may cause cough, fever and other pulmonary symptoms with eosinophils in the sputum.

The larvae then migrate across the alveolar capillary walls, travel up the respiratory tree to the epiglottis; then they are swallowed and returned to the small intestine where they mature (Fig. 20.3). Vague symptoms such as diarrhoea and anorexia may occur and malabsorption in children has been described.

A bolus of worms in the bowel is the commonest cause of intestinal obstruction in the tropics, far commoner than malignant disease. Other serious problems are intussusception, volvulus, and appendicitis. The worms may migrate into the bile or pancreatic duct, causing cholangitis or pancreatitis.

Diagnosis. The ova are usually found on microscopic examination of the stool. Sometimes a patient will have seen a worm passed in the stool or vomit one. The presence of eosinophilia is unreliable, as are serological tests.

Treatment. Piperazine salts have been used for over a quarter of a century and are

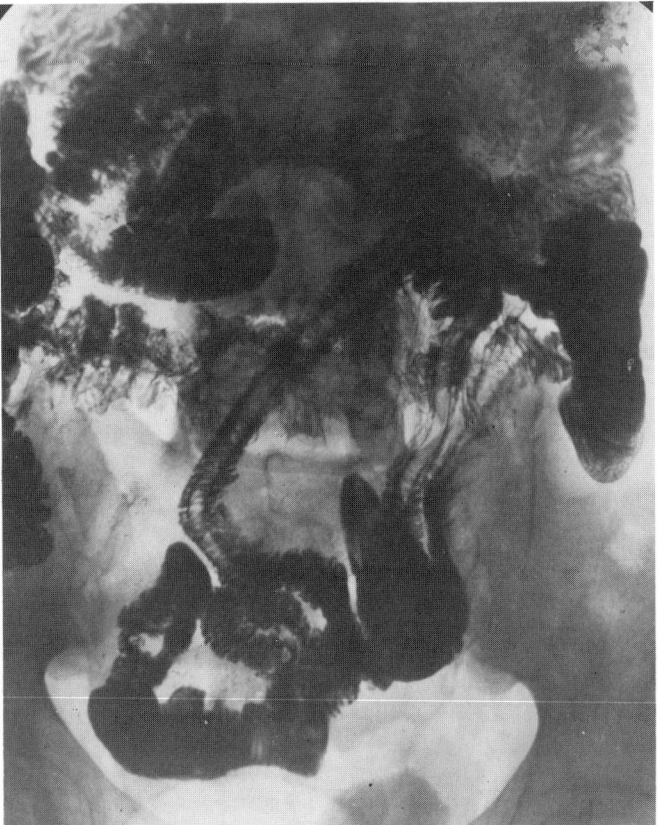

Fig. 20.3. Roundworm in ileum mimicking Crohn's disease.

highly effective in a single dose, equivalent to 4 g of piperazine hydrate. Bephenium is also effective: 2.5 g may be given as a single dose or divided into two doses separated by 2–3 days. Side-effects from either of these are unlikely.

Ancylostomiasis (hookworm disease)
This is endemic in the tropics and subtropics, although epidemics have occurred amongst miners in Cornwall, Germany and Switzerland. Adult worms are thread-like (Fig. 20.4) and about 10 mm long. They live in the small intestine with their mouths fixed to villi from which they feed on blood; ova are passed in the faeces and the larvae hatch in a warm moist soil. Man is usually infected through the skin of the feet when in contact with mud; vegetables may also be infected so that infection can occur orally. After penetrating the skin, the filariform larvae pass into the bloodstream to the lung, up the trachea and down the oesophagus to develop into adult worms in the upper small gut.

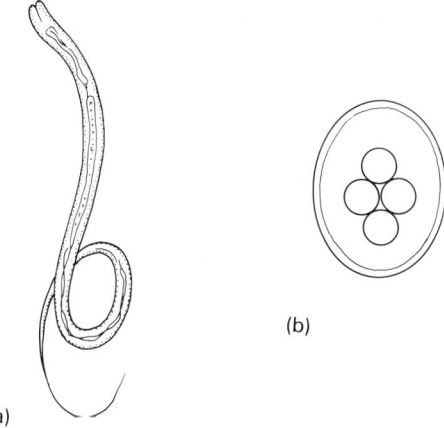

(b)

(a)

Fig. 20.4. Ancylostoma duodenale (hookworm). (a) Larva; (b) ova.

Symptoms. Local dermatitis or 'ground itch' may occur where the larvae penetrate the skin. This may be followed by pulmonary symptoms as in roundworm infection, and urticaria.

Chronic ancylostome infection is commonly symptomless. The important complication is hypochromic anaemia due to blood loss; there may also be abdominal discomfort and poor nutrition in children.

Diagnosis. The ova can usually be detected in the faeces and the severity of the infestation may be gauged by counting the number of eggs per gram of stool.

Treatment. Tetrachloroethylene is still the most widely used drug and is best given in a suspension rather than in capsules so the effective action of the drug on the worms in the duodenum can be assured. Alcohol and fatty food have to be avoided as they increase the absorption and hepatotoxicity of the drug. Other drugs are bephenium and bitoscanate. The anaemia responds to iron such as ferrous sulphate.

Strongyloidiasis
This is a tiny worm about 2 mm long and its life cycle is similar to that of the hookworm and infection is acquired in the same way. However, the adult female does not live within the lumen of the bowel but burrows into the jejunal mucosa where she lays her eggs. The ova hatch within the mucosa, liberating larvae which are passed in the stool.

Pulmonary symptoms with eosinophilia may occur during the early stages of infestation. Chronic infections are often symptomless but may cause colic. Also a segment of the lower duodenum and upper jejunum can become grossly oedematous with enlarged lymph nodes draining the segments. Filariform larvae can be seen in all these tissues and a barium meal may show the affected gut as a rigid tube; steatorrhoea, hypoalbuminaemia, and electrolyte imbalance may be caused but without eosinophilia. The condition can be fatal. Other symptoms may be urticaria and pruritus ani.

Diagnosis depends upon finding the larvae either in the stools, sometimes in the sputum, in duodenal aspirate and by histological section of the mesenteric lymph nodes as when an occasional patient needs laparotomy. A positive complement fixation reaction is given in 75% of infected patients.

Treatment may be difficult because the rhabdidiform larvae may transform into infective filariform within the bowel so that a cycle of autoinfection is set up. Thiabendazole is the drug of choice.

Trichuriasis

This infection, which is particularly common amongst children and adults in institutions, is caused by a whipworm—so called because of its shape: the posterior end is stout and the anterior hair-like, resembling the lash of a whip. It is 3–5 cm long. The adults inhabit the colon, particularly the caecum. Infection of man usually takes place from the pollution of water or vegetables. The ova hatch in the intestine and the larvae mature into adults which fix themselves to the bowel wall by means of the fine anterior end which is inserted into the mucosa. They can sometimes be seen on the bowel wall at endoscopy; the visible white worms on the oedematous mucosa have given the condition the name 'coconut cake' appearance.

The average infection is symptomless but there may be vague pain and diarrhoea. In undernourished children heavy infections may cause anaemia, volvulus and prolapse of the rectum. Worms have also been reported to obstruct the appendix and cause acute appendicitis.

Diagnosis is by finding the egg in the stool or by seeing the worms at sigmoidoscopy. Eosinophilia is common.

The drug of choice is merbendazole; side effects are very uncommon, but it has to be avoided in children under 2 years and pregnant women.

Giardiasis

Giardia lamblia has been found in the intestinal contents in people with diarrhoea for many years but its pathogenic significance has been uncertain. Recent outbreaks of diarrhoeal disease have, however, given definite epidemiological evidence of the association between giardia and disease.

Now giardiasis is the commonest protozoal disease reported in Britain. It affects people of all ages and may cause a clinical picture in children resembling coeliac disease with changes in the jejunal villi. It also accounts for some patients suffering from traveller's diarrhoea, especially if the infection does not clear up in a few days. The main source of infection is untreated drinking water, which need not be demonstrably contaminated by human excreta. Infection has been acquired from the water of remote mountain streams. Transmission may also occur by the faecal–oral route within families or institutions.

The illness starts 1 or 2 weeks after exposure as an explosive watery diarrhoea without blood or mucus but often accompanied by fatty stools and abdominal pain. It may clear up in 3 or 4 days.

The protozoa (Fig. 20.5) flourish in their thousands in the duodenum and upper jejunum and are perhaps attracted to this locality by its hydrogen ion concentration. They attach themselves by their peristomes to the mucosa, and their bodies and flagella are in constant motion. Diagnosis can be made by duodenal aspiration and

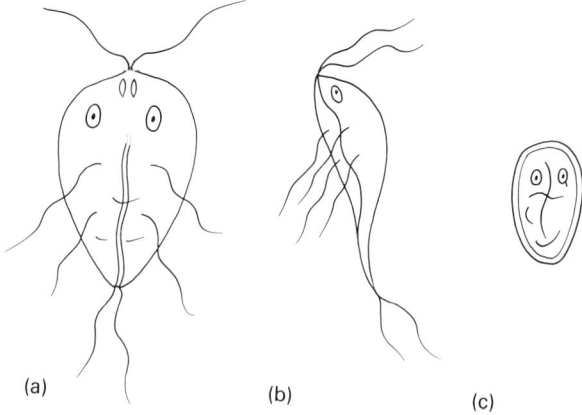

(a) (b) (c)

Fig. 20.5. *Giardia lamblia.* (a) and (b) frontal and lateral view of trophozoite; (c) cyst.

the trophozoites may sometimes be seen in a jejunal biopsy specimen (Fig. 20.6), when the cysts are not obvious in the stool. Metronidazole 2 g orally for 3 days is the best treatment.

Traveller's diarrhoea

Traveller's diarrhoea is no respecter of persons, or race. Mexicans call it Montezuma's revenge (Montezuma was the last of the Aztec emperors and succumbed to Spanish invaders, who presumably were attacked in turn by traveller's diarrhoea); elsewhere colourful synonyms include Delhi belly, Rangoon runs, and Tokyo trots. If contracted in one's own country, change of water or strength of the seaside air is wrongly blamed. When caught abroad it is attributed, often correctly, to bad hygiene. Perhaps because of its rarity in Britain, no-one has coined terms like Glasgow gripes or Gloucester gallops. Perhaps some of the visitors do suffer but politely do not mention it. Factors responsible are poor personal cleanliness in food handlers (the importance of washing hands after visiting the WC should be taught in schools everywhere), bad sanitation, and hot weather.

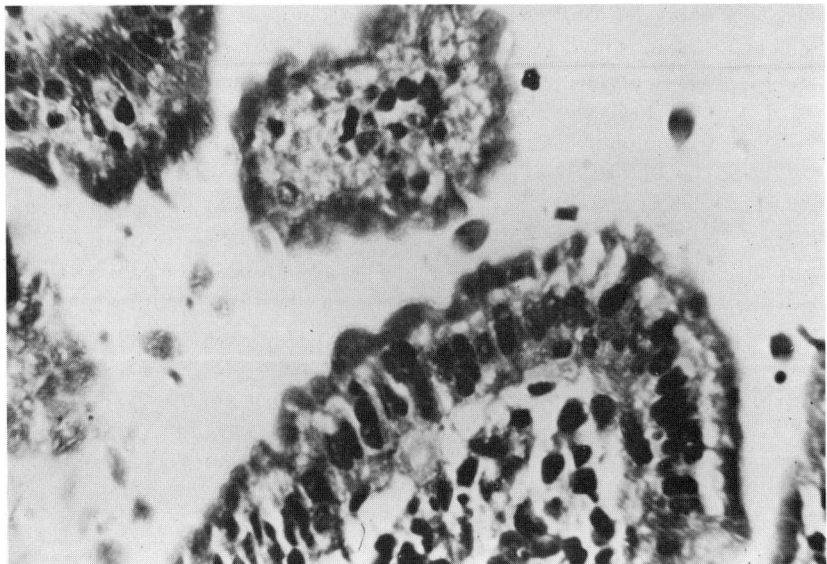

Fig. 20.6. Jejunal biopsy with *Giardia lamblia*.

No single organism is responsible and stools are often negative for pathogenic organisms, perhaps being examined too late. Salmonellas and campylobacter species are the usual causes in travellers from Mediterranean countries, while those returning from the tropics may also suffer from giardiasis or, rarely, amoebiasis. Enterotoxin-producing *E. coli* of different, non-'enteropathogenic' serotypes are thought to be a common cause though it is difficult to prove the case against a strain of a mundane organism like *E. coli* to which the host is unaccustomed.

The affliction lasts about 5 days; one-fifth of the sufferers are confined to bed and about one-third have to change their activities. Assessing therapy in a short self-limiting disorder is fraught with difficulties. All that is usually needed is plenty of fluid and additional salt if in a hot country. Some believe in taking an opiate or other drugs commonly used for diarrhoea (p. 21).

A drug which will shield the traveller completely is not available. Most remedies such as enterovioform are just placebos. Antibiotics should give some protection. So far, controlled trials have given varying results, probably because of the different pathogens. Streptotriad started before the visit showed some promise in one trial; however, sulfonamide can produce side-effects as unpleasant as the diarrhoea itself, and could cause crystal deposition in the kidney in a hot climate with a poor fluid intake, although the risk is remote in a small dose such as 0.5 g twice daily.

Some are fortunate and travel throughout the world without heeding what they eat or drink, for they never get diarrhoea. Little is known about protective mechanisms. The change in pH of the stomach and duodenum accounts for the relative sterility of the small intestine, and this is maintained partly by IgA-producing cells in the mucosa and the peristaltic sweeps. Many travellers ask advice about the precautions, but the need for these depends on the risk in the country visited, and tourist agents do not include this information in their glossy brochures. Those who are staying in a high-risk area should avoid dishes known to transmit the usual forms of food poisoning: raw foods, salad, ice cream of uncertain origin, ice itself, prepared meat dishes, and meat pies that have been inadequately reheated. Safer foods are those whose handling is minimal or whose germs have been destroyed by adequate cooking—tinned foods or fish or meat well-cooked just before serving. If cleanliness of water is suspect, bottled drinks or water chlorinated with a suitable tablet can be taken instead. Water from the hot tap should be safe if fairly hot and so disinfected. Obviously such deprivations are unnecessary in areas where the risk is low. Then travellers will abandon themselves to the pleasures of the table, relying only on an aperitif or wine to stimulate a flow of hydrochloric acid sufficient to destroy organisms before they can disturb the tranquility of the gut.

List of Abbreviations

Alk Phos (or SAP)	Serum alkaline phosphatase
AST (or SGOT)	Aspartate aminotransferase ⎱ transaminases
ALT (or SGPT)	Alanine aminotransferase ⎰
BAO	Basal acid output
BSP	Bromsulphthalein
CBD	Common bile duct
CCK/PZ	Cholecystokinin/pancreozymin
CEA	Carcinoembryonic antigen
CMV	Cytomegalovirus
CT	Computerized tomography
DNA	Deoxyribonucleic acid
DU	Duodenal ulcer
ECF	Extracellular fluid
ERCP	Endoscopic retrograde cholangiopancreatography
ESR	Erythrocyte sedimentation rate
FHVP	Free hepatic venous pressure
γGT	Gamma glutamyl transpeptidase
HCl	Haemoglobin
HC$_I$	Hydrochloric acid
HCO$_3$	Bicarbonate
HIDA	Iminodiacetic acid derivative
HMGCoA	Hydroxymethylglutaryl coenzyme A
ICF	Intracellular fluid
ITU	Intensive Therapy Unit
IVC	Inferior vena cava
K$^+$	Potassium
LOS	Lower oesophageal sphincter
LDH	Lactate dehydrogenase
MAO	Maximal acid output
MCH	Mean corpuscular haemoglobin
MCHC	Mean corpuscular haemoglobin concentration
MCV	Mean corpuscular volume
Na$^+$	Sodium
PGV	Proximal gastric vagotomy
PSE	Porto-systemic encephalopathy
PT	Prothrombin time

PTC	Percutaneous transhepatic cholangiography
PTT	Partial thromboplastin time
S	Secretin
TIBC	Total iron binding capacity
UDPGT	Uridine diphosphate glucuronyl transferase
VIP	Vasoactive intestinal peptide
WHVP	Wedged hepatic venous pressure

Bibliography

References

Beaumont W. (1833) *Experiments and Observations on the Gastric Juice and Physiology of Digestion.* F.P. Allen, Plattsburgh.

Cleave T.L. (1974) *The Saccharine Disease.* J. Wright & Sons, Bristol.

Crohn B.B., Ginzburg L. & Oppenhemer G.D. (1932) Regional ileitis: a pathologic and clinical entity. *JAMA* **99**, 1323–9.

Fry J. (1979) *Common Diseases: the Nature, Incidence and Care.* 2nd ed. MTP Press, Lancaster.

Gerber A., Apt M.K. & Craig P.H. (1983) The Kock continent ileostomy. *Surg. Gyn. Obst.* **156**, 345–350.

Holdsworth C.D. (1981) Sulphasalazine desensitization. *Brit. Med. J.* **i**, 110.

Salter R.H., Cole T.P., Scott-Harden W.G., Girdwood T.G. & Reid M.A. (1975) Patient-orientated gastroenterology. *Brit. Med. J.* **1**, 130–2.

Szasz T.A. (1968) The psychology of persistent pain. In *Proc. Internat. Symp. Pain.* Organized by the Laboratory of Psychophysiology, Faculty of Science, Paris (ed. by A. Soulairac, J. Cahn & J. Charpentier). Academic Press, London.

Wolf S. & Wolff H.G. (1947) *Human Gastric Function.* Oxford University Press, London.

Suggestions for further reading

Allan R.N., Keighley M.R.B., Alexander-Williams J. & Hawkins C. (1983) *Inflammatory Bowel Disease.* Churchill Livingstone, Edinburgh.

Cotton P.B. & Williams C.B. (1982) *Practical Gastrointestinal Endoscopy*, 2nd ed. Blackwell Scientific Publications, Oxford.

Dykes D.P. & Keighley M.R.B. (1981) *Gastrointestinal Haemorrhage.* J. Wright & Sons, London.

Sherlock S. (1981) *Diseases of the Liver and Biliary System*, 6th ed. Blackwell Scientific Publications, Oxford.

Sileu W. (1983) *Cope's Early Diagnosis of the Acute Abdomen*, 16th ed. Oxford University Press, New York.

Index